FWRC
R
899
.H472
2020
c.2

TRI-STATE UNIVERSITY

P9-ASK-241

WITHDRAWN

LEARNING RADIOLOGY

LEARNING RADIOLOGY

Recognizing the Basics

4th Edition

William Herring, MD, FACR

Vice Chairman and Residency Program Director (retired)
Einstein Healthcare Network
Philadelphia, Pennsylvania

Trine University
Health Education Center - FWRC
1819 Carew Street
Fort Wayne, IN 46805

ELSEVIER

LEARNING RADIOLOGY, FOURTH EDITION   ISBN: 978-0-323-56729-9

Copyright © 2020 by Elsevier, Inc. All rights reserved.

No part of this publication may be reproduced or transmitted in any form or by any means, electronic or mechanical, including photocopying, recording, or any information storage and retrieval system, without permission in writing from the publisher. Details on how to seek permission, further information about the Publisher's permissions policies and our arrangements with organizations such as the Copyright Clearance Center and the Copyright Licensing Agency, can be found at our website: www.elsevier.com/permissions.

This book and the individual contributions contained in it are protected under copyright by the Publisher (other than as may be noted herein).

Notices

Knowledge and best practice in this field are constantly changing. As new research and experience broaden our understanding, changes in research methods, professional practices, or medical treatment may become necessary.

Practitioners and researchers must always rely on their own experience and knowledge in evaluating and using any information, methods, compounds, or experiments described herein. In using such information or methods they should be mindful of their own safety and the safety of others, including parties for whom they have a professional responsibility.

With respect to any drug or pharmaceutical products identified, readers are advised to check the most current information provided (i) on procedures featured or (ii) by the manufacturer of each product to be administered, to verify the recommended dose or formula, the method and duration of administration, and contraindications. It is the responsibility of practitioners, relying on their own experience and knowledge of their patients, to make diagnoses, to determine dosages and the best treatment for each individual patient, and to take all appropriate safety precautions.

To the fullest extent of the law, neither the Publisher nor the authors, contributors, or editors, assume any liability for any injury and/or damage to persons or property as a matter of products liability, negligence or otherwise, or from any use or operation of any methods, products, instructions, or ideas contained in the material herein.

Previous editions copyrighted 2016, 2012, and 2007.

International Standard Book Number: 978-0-323-56729-9

Content Strategist: Marybeth Thiel
Senior Content Development Specialist: Ann Ruzycka Anderson
Publishing Services Manager: Catherine Albright Jackson
Senior Project Manager: Claire Kramer
Design Direction: Bridget Hoette

Printed in Canada

Last digit is the print number: 9   8   7   6   5   4   3   2

1600 John F. Kennedy Blvd.
Ste 1600
Philadelphia, PA 19103-2899

 Working together
to grow libraries in
developing countries

www.elsevier.com • www.bookaid.org

To my wife Patricia,

and our family

CONTRIBUTORS

Debra Copit, MD
Former Director of Women's Imaging
Einstein Healthcare Network
Philadelphia, Pennsylvania

Daniel J. Kowal, MD
Chief and Medical Director of Ultrasound
Baystate Health
Assistant Professor
University of Massachusetts Medical
School–Baystate
Springfield, Massachusetts

Trevor Lewis, MD
Resident in Diagnostic and Interventional
    Radiology
Beth Israel Deaconess Medical Center/
    Harvard Medical School
Boston, Massachusetts

Peter Wang, MD
Section Head of Body CT and MRI
Assistant Residency Program Director
Einstein Healthcare Network
Philadelphia, Pennsylvania

Jeffrey L. Weinstein, MD
Section of Interventional Radiology
Beth Israel Deaconess Medical Center
Program Director, Vascular and
    Interventional Radiology Fellowship and
    Residency Programs
Instructor in Radiology
Harvard Medical School
Boston, Massachusetts

This fourth edition of *Learning Radiology: Recognizing the Basics* features numerous changes and additions while adhering to its core design of presenting key, fundamental material in a concise, uncomplicated format.

Three completely new chapters have been added to this edition. Almost all the photos in the text have been fine tuned to highlight the findings. Key sections have been reorganized to strengthen teaching in the vital, cross-sectional modalities of computed tomography, magnetic resonance imaging, and ultrasound.

The three new chapters will expand your understanding of the growing use of ultrasound, enable you to appreciate the role of image-guided interventions in clinical care, and introduce you to mammographic imaging.

Scattered throughout relevant chapters in the text are mini "clinical-scenarios" that invite you to examine how image-guided interventions might be helpful in solving everyday clinical problems. The solutions to these clinical challenges are revisited in the new chapter on interventional radiology.

Trauma has been reorganized into three consecutive chapters, bringing together related material to cover this critical topic in a cohesive manner.

Please pay particular attention to the wealth of additional and complementary material available online to registered users of the textbook starting, of course, with full-access to the entire text and all of its photos.

Online, you will also find two dozen interactive quizzes that reinforce essential elements found throughout the text; an interactive anatomy section that helps you learn key, normal, radiographic structures; and another two dozen clinical cases to challenge and sharpen your imaging skills.

There is also an online-only chapter on Nuclear Medicine and an in-depth algorithm for diagnosing adult heart disease using conventional radiography that should be very helpful.

There are online glossaries and an appendix that links to lists of the most appropriate imaging study to order for each of a myriad of clinical situations. This information should prove indispensable on clinical rounds.

We have always believed that this text and its online extras allow you to rapidly begin recognizing abnormalities and making diagnoses that will impress your mentors and peers and astonish your friends and relatives. With this new edition, you hold the potential to be even more astounding.

Prepare to amaze.

ACKNOWLEDGMENTS

I am again grateful to the many thousands of you whom I have never met but who first found a website called LearningRadiology helpful and made it so popular that it played a role leading from the first edition of this text to what is now its fourth edition.

For his help and suggestions, I would like to thank Stacy White, MD, one of my former radiology residents, who made invaluable suggestions about how this edition could be improved and then helped in improving it. Peter Wang, MD, contributed two chapters on ultrasound, augmenting and expanding the material from the last edition. Daniel Kowal, MD, again did a wonderful job in simplifying the complexities of MRI for the chapter he wrote. Debra Copit, MD, FACR, contributed a terrific, new chapter on mammography. Jeffrey Weinstein, MD, an attending physician at Beth Israel Deaconess Medical Center along with resident Trevor Lewis, MD, also at Beth Israel Deaconess, added an important new chapter on image-guided interventions in medicine.

I want to thank Brooke Devenney Cakir, MD, Mindy Horrow, MD, FACR, and Huyen Tran, MD, for their assistance in this edition.

I certainly want to recognize and again thank Jim Merritt from Elsevier for his long-term support and Ann Anderson, Claire Kramer, and Marybeth Thiel from Elsevier for their assistance.

I also wanted to acknowledge the hundreds of radiology residents and medical students who, over the years, provided me with an audience of motivated learners without whom a teacher would have no one to teach.

Finally, I want to thank my wonderful wife, Pat, who has encouraged me throughout the project, and my family.

CONTENTS

VIDEO CONTENTS

Recognizing Anything
An Introduction to Imaging Modalities

This chapter provides a brief introduction to the major imaging modalities. Accompanying most of the modalities is a **Case Quiz** that uses that modality. A number 2 pencil is not necessary for the quiz. The answers to the quizzes are at the very end of this book. If you do not know the answers to any of the quizzes, that is perfectly fine because you are about to learn about each of these imaging modalities, how to approach imaging studies, and much more as you complete this text.

MANY SHADES OF GRAY

- In 1895, Wilhelm Röntgen (or Roentgen), working in a darkened laboratory in Würzburg, Germany, noticed that a screen painted with a fluorescent material and located a few feet away in the same room as a cathode ray tube he had energized and made lightproof, started to glow (fluoresce). After repeating the experiment, he recognized that the screen was responding to the nearby production of a form of energy transmitted invisibly through the room. He named the new rays **"x-rays"** using the mathematical symbol "x" for something unknown. It did not take long before almost everyone was taking x-rays of almost everything imaginable (Fig. 1.1).
- Like today, **conventional radiographic images** (usually shortened to **x-rays**) were produced by a combination of **ionizing radiation** and **light** striking a **photosensitive surface** which, in turn, produces a **latent image** that is subsequently **processed** to become visible. For about a hundred years after the discovery of x-rays, radiographic images survived their birth as a burst of ionizing radiation by resting comfortably on a piece of **film.**
- At first, the processing of film was carried out in a darkroom containing trays with various chemicals, and the films were then, literally, hung up to dry.
    - When an immediate reading was requested, the films were interpreted while still dripping with chemicals and the term *wet reading* for a "stat" interpretation was born.
- Films were then viewed on **lighted view boxes** (almost always backward or upside down if the film placement was being done as part of a movie or television show). In a few places, film is the medium still used, but it is much less common because it has some **major drawbacks.**
    - It required a great deal of **physical storage space** for the ever-growing number of films. Even though each film was

very thin, many films in thousands of patients' folders took up a great deal of space (eFig. 1.1)
- The other drawback was that the radiographic films could physically be in only **one place at a time**, which was not necessarily where they might be needed to help in the care of the patient.
- Eventually **digital radiography** came into being, in which the photographic film was replaced by a **photosensitive cassette or plate** that could be processed by an **electronic reader,** and that image could be stored in a **digital format.** This electronic processing no longer required a darkroom to develop the film or a large room to store the films. Countless images could be stored in the space of one, spinning, hard disk on a computer server. Even more importantly, the images could be viewed by anyone with the right to do so, anywhere in the world, at any time.
- The studies were maintained on computer servers on which the images could be **archived** for posterity, from which they could be **communicated** to others and in which they could be **stored.** This system is called a *PACS* system, for **picture archiving, communications and storage** system.
- With PACS systems, images from all modalities can be stored and retrieved, including conventional radiographs (CR), CT

Fig. 1.1 Wilhelm Roentgen Discovers X-Rays. Wilhelm Roentgen in his laboratory in Germany is shown in this photograph from 1895, the year in which (on November 8), he discovered a new, invisible source of electromagnetic radiation he called *x-rays*. For his discovery, he was awarded the very first Nobel Prize for Physics in 1901.

scans, ultrasound images, MRI studies, fluoroscopy studies, and nuclear medicine studies.

* We will look briefly at each of these modalities.

CONVENTIONAL RADIOGRAPHY (PLAIN FILMS)

* Images produced through the use of ionizing radiation (i.e., the production of x-rays, but without added **contrast material** like barium or iodine) are called *conventional radiographs* or, more often, **plain films.**
* The major advantage of conventional radiographs is that the images are relatively **inexpensive** to produce, can be obtained almost **anywhere** with portable or mobile machines, and are still the most widely obtained imaging studies.
* Radiographs require a **source** to produce the x-rays (the "x-ray machine"), a method to **record** the image (a film, cassette, or photosensitive plate), and a way to **process** the recorded image (either with chemicals or a digital reader).
* Common uses for conventional radiography include the ubiquitous chest x-ray, plain films of the abdomen, and virtually every initial image of the skeletal system to evaluate for fractures or arthritis. Fig. 1.2 contains our **first Case Quiz,** this one related to conventional radiography (Fig. 1.2).
* The major disadvantages of conventional radiography are the **limited range of densities** it can demonstrate and its reliance on **ionizing radiation.**

THE FIVE BASIC DENSITIES

* Conventional radiography is limited to demonstrating five basic densities, arranged here from least to most dense (Table 1.1):
  * **Air,** which appears the blackest on a radiograph
  * **Fat,** which is a lighter shade of gray than air

* **Soft tissue or fluid** (because both soft tissue and fluid appear the same on conventional radiographs, it is impossible to differentiate the heart muscle from the blood inside of the heart on a chest radiograph)
* **Calcium** (usually contained within bones)
* **Metal,** which appears the whitest on a radiograph
* Metallic densities are not normally present in the body. Radiologic **contrast media** and **prosthetic knees or hips** are examples of **metallic densities** artificially placed in the body (Fig. 1.3 **Case Quiz 2**).

TABLE 1.1	Five Basic Densities Seen on Conventional Radiography	
Density	**Appearance**
Air	Absorbs the least x-rays and appears "blackest" on conventional radiographs
Fat	Gray, somewhat darker (blacker) than soft tissue
Fluid or soft tissue	Both fluid (e.g., blood) and soft tissue (e.g., muscle) have the same density on conventional radiographs
Calcium	The most dense, naturally occurring material (e.g., bones); absorbs most x-rays
Metal	Usually absorbs all x-rays and appears the "whitest" (e.g., bullets, barium)

Fig. 1.2 CASE QUIZ 1. This patient is a 24-year-old male who came to the emergency department after experiencing sharp, left-sided chest pain and shortness of breath. This conventional chest radiograph (x-ray) was obtained. A major abnormality that requires immediate attention is shown. Are you able to recognize it? See the answer at the end of this book.

Fig. 1.3 CASE QUIZ 2: THE "CASE OF THE DISAPPEARING HEART." This is an obviously abnormal chest radiograph of a 43-year-old female who had undergone surgery about 2 years previously for a bronchogenic carcinoma. Why are we unable to see the heart? (**Spoiler alert:** The heart was not removed at the time of surgery!) The answer can be found at the end of this book.

- Although conventional radiographs are produced by ionizing radiation in relatively low doses, radiation has the **potential** to produce cell mutations that could lead to many forms of cancer or anomalies. Public health data on lower levels of radiation vary as to their assessment of risk, but in general, only medically necessary diagnostic examinations should be performed, and studies with x-rays should be avoided during potentially teratogenic times, such as pregnancy. (**Registered users can learn more about radiation dose and safety in a bonus online module.**)

COMPUTED TOMOGRAPHY

- CT or CAT scanners, first introduced in the 1970s, brought a quantum leap to medical imaging.
- With the use of a **gantry** with a rotating x-ray beam and multiple detectors in various arrays (which themselves are rotating continuously around the patient), along with sophisticated computer algorithms to process the data, a large number of two-dimensional (2D), slice-like images (each millimeters in size) could be formatted in multiple imaging planes (eVideo 1.1).
- **The CT scanner** is connected to a **computer,** which processes the data though various **algorithms** to produce **images** of diagnostic quality.
- A **CT** image is composed of a matrix of thousands of tiny squares called *pixels*, each of which is computer-assigned a *CT number* from –1000 to +1000 measured in something called *Hounsfield units (HU)*, after Sir Godfrey Hounsfield, the man credited with developing the first CT scanner (for which he won the Nobel prize in Medicine in 1979, along with Allan Cormack).
  - The CT number will **vary according to the density of the tissue** scanned and is a **measure of how much of the x-ray beam is absorbed** by the tissues at each point in the scan.

By convention, **air is assigned a Hounsfield number of –1000 HU,** and **bone is about 400 to 600 HU** (fat is –40 to –100; water is 0; and **soft tissue, 20 to 100**).

- CT images are displayed or viewed with a range of Hounsfield numbers pre-selected to best demonstrate the tissues being studied (e.g., from –100 to +300) and anything within that range of CT numbers is displayed over the levels of density in the available gray scale. This range of displayed densities is called the *window.*
- **Denser substances** that absorb more x-rays have **high CT numbers.** They are said to demonstrate *increased attenuation* and are displayed as **whiter densities** on CT scan images.
  - On conventional radiographs, these substances (like **metal** and **calcium**) would also appear whiter and be said to have *increased density* or be *more opaque.*
- **Less-dense substances** that absorb fewer x-rays have **low CT numbers.** They are said to demonstrate *decreased attenuation* and are displayed as **blacker densities** on CT scan images.
  - On conventional radiographs, these substances (like **air** and **fat**) would also appear blacker and be said to have *decreased density* (or *increased lucency*).
- CT scans can also be windowed in a way that optimizes the visibility of different types of pathology **after** they are obtained, a benefit called *post-processing* that digital imaging, in general, markedly advanced. Post-processing allows for additional manipulation of the raw data to best demonstrate the abnormality **without repeating a study** and without re-exposing the patient (Fig. 1.4).
- Traditionally, CT images were viewed mostly in the axial plane. Now, because of volumetric acquisition of data, CT images can be shown in any plane: **axial, sagittal,** or **coronal.** Volumetric data consist of a series of thin sections that can be **reassembled** for a 3D reconstruction. Surface and volume

Fig. 1.4 Windowing the Thorax. Chest CT scans are usually "windowed" and displayed in several formats in order to optimize anatomic details. (A) **Lung windows** are chosen to maximize our ability to image abnormalities of the lung parenchyma and to identify normal and abnormal bronchial anatomy (*black circle*).(B) **Mediastinal windows** are chosen to display the mediastinal, hilar, and pleural structures to best advantage (*white circle*). (C) **Bone windows** are used as a third way of displaying the data, visualizing the bony structures to their best advantage (*white arrow* and *oval*). It is important to recognize that the displays of these different windows are manipulations of the data obtained during the **original scan** and **do not** require re-scanning the patient.

rendering in 3D can produce CT images of amazing realistic quality (Fig. 1.5).

- One of the major benefits of CT scanning over conventional radiography is its ability to **expand the gray scale,** which enables us to differentiate many more than the five basic densities available on conventional radiographs (Fig. 1.6 **Case Quiz 3**).

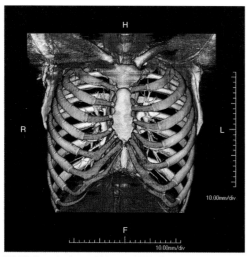

Fig. 1.5 CT 3D Rendering of Normal Rib Cage. This is a color version of a 3D surface rendering of the rib cage made possible by the acquisition of multiple thin CT sections through the body that can then be digitally reconstructed to demonstrate surface anatomy, as in this illustration. The same data set could have been manipulated to show the heart or lungs (which are digitally removed here) and not the rib cage. Such renderings are especially helpful in demonstrating the exact anatomic relationships of structures, especially for surgical planning. *F,* Foot; *H,* head; *L,* left; *R,* right.

Fig. 1.6 CASE QUIZ 3. This patient is a 67-year-old male who developed sudden loss of motor function involving his left arm along with difficulty speaking. This is a single axial image of a CT scan of the brain. The brain, never directly visible with plain films, is now seen because of the wide latitude of densities visible by CT. The white densities in the brain are physiologic calcifications, unrelated to the patient's condition. What has caused his symptoms? See the answer at the end of this book.

- Because of increasingly sophisticated arrays of detectors and acquisition of hundreds of slices simultaneously, **multislice CT scanners permit very fast imaging** (head to toe in less than 10 seconds) that has allowed for the development of new applications for CT, such as *virtual colonoscopy* and *virtual bronchoscopy*, *cardiac calcium scoring,* and *CT coronary angiography* (eVideo 1.2).

- These examinations can contain a thousand or more images so that the older method of filming each image for study on a viewbox became impractical and such examinations are almost always viewed on computer workstations where it is possible to study many images by scrolling.

- **CT scans are the cornerstone of cross-sectional imaging** and are **widely available,** although not as yet truly portable. To produce CT images requires an expensive scanner, a space dedicated to its installation, and sophisticated computer processing power. As with conventional radiography, CT scanners **also use ionizing radiation** (x-rays) to produce their images.

ULTRASOUND

- Ultrasound probes use **acoustic energy** above the audible frequency of humans to produce images, instead of using ionizing radiation as both conventional radiography and CT scans do (**see Chapter 19**).

- An ultrasound **probe** or **transducer** both produces the ultrasonic signal and records it. The signal is processed for its characteristics by an on-board computer. Ultrasound images are recorded digitally and are easily stored in a PACS system. Images are displayed either as static images or in the form of a movie (cine) (eVideo 1.3).

- Ultrasound scanners are relatively **inexpensive** compared with CT and MRI scanners. They are **widely available** and can be made **portable** to the point of being handheld.

- Because ultrasound uses no ionizing radiation, it is particularly useful in imaging women of **childbearing age** and **during pregnancy** and imaging **children.**

- **Ultrasound is widely used in medical imaging.** It is usually **the study of first choice** in imaging the female pelvis and pediatric patients, in differentiating cystic versus solid lesions in patients of all ages, in non-invasive vascular imaging, in imaging of the fetus and placenta during pregnancy, and for performing real-time, image-guided fluid aspiration and biopsies (Fig. 1.7 **Case Quiz 4**).

- Other common uses are in the evaluation of cystic versus solid breast masses, thyroid nodules, tendons and in the assessment of the brain, hips, and spine in newborns. Ultrasound is used everywhere from intraoperative scanning in the hospital surgical suite to the medical tent in the battlefield and in locations as remote as Antarctica.

- Ultrasound is generally considered to be **a very safe imaging modality** without any known major side effects when used at medically diagnostic levels.

MAGNETIC RESONANCE IMAGING

- MRI utilizes the potential energy stored in the body's **hydrogen atoms.** The atoms are manipulated by very strong magnetic

Fig. 1.7 CASE QUIZ 4. This patient is a 43-year-old female who developed right upper quadrant pain and tenderness. You are looking at a single image from an ultrasound examination of the right upper quadrant in the sagittal (longitudinal) plane. This is the patient's right upper quadrant. What has most likely caused her symptoms? See the answer at the end of this book. *F*, Foot; *H*, head.

fields and radio-frequency pulses to produce enough localizing and tissue-specific energy to allow highly sophisticated computer programs to generate 2D or 3D images (**see Chapter 21**).

- MRI scanners are **not as widely available** as CT scanners. They are **expensive** to acquire and require careful site construction to operate properly. In general, they also have a relatively **high, on-going operating cost**.
- However, they utilize **no ionizing radiation** and produce much higher contrast between different types of soft tissues than even CT can.
- MRI is widely used in **neurologic imaging** and is particularly sensitive in imaging **soft tissues** such as muscles, tendons, and ligaments (Fig. 1.8 **Case Quiz 5**).
- There are **safety issues** associated with the extremely strong magnetic fields of an MRI scanner, both for objects within the body (e.g., cardiac pacemakers) and for ferromagnetic projectiles in the MRI scanner environment (e.g., metal oxygen tanks in the room which, owing to the strength of the magnet, can become airborne "missiles"). There are also known side effects from the radiofrequency waves such scanners produce, and possible adverse effects from some MRI contrast agents.

FLUOROSCOPY

- Fluoroscopy (or "fluoro") is a modality that uses **ionizing radiation** (x-rays) in performing **real-time visualization** of the body in a way that allows for evaluation of the motion of body parts, real-time positioning changes of bones and joints, and the location and path of externally administered barium or iodine contrast agents through the gastrointestinal (GI) and genitourinary tracts and blood vessels. Images can be viewed as they are acquired on video screens and captured as either a series of static images or motion (video) images (eVideo 1.4).
- Fluoroscopy requires an x-ray unit specially fitted to allow for controlled motion of not only the x-ray tube, but also

Fig. 1.8 CASE QUIZ 5. This is an image from an MRI scan of the lower lumbar spine viewed in the sagittal plane. The 42-year-old patient had experienced sudden onset of low back pain radiating to the legs. The lumbar vertebral bodies are numbered. What has most likely caused his symptoms? The answer is at the end of this book.

Fig. 1.9 A Standard Radiology Room Equipped to Perform Both Conventional Radiographs and Fluoroscopy. The patient lies on the tabletop (*black arrow*), which has the capacity to tilt up or down. Images can be obtained with the sensor on the fluoroscopic carriage (*black oval*) that can be manipulated more-or-less freely by the operator to follow the barium column. Static images can be obtained with the overhead x-ray tube (*white circle*) that can be moved into place over an x-ray cassette that would be located under the patient (*white arrow*).

the imaging sensor **and the patient** to find the best projection to demonstrate the body part being studied. For this to be done, fluoroscopic tables are made to tilt, and the fluoroscopic tube is able to move freely back and forth to image the patient (Fig. 1.9).

- Instantaneous "snapshots" during the procedure are called *spot films* (usually obtained by the radiologist), and they are combined with other images obtained by an overhead x-ray machine in multiple projections (usually obtained by a radiologic technologist) during the performance of barium studies for whatever part of the GI tract is being studied, depending on the nature of the abnormality and the mobility of the patient (Fig. 1.10 **Case Quiz 6**).
- In **interventional radiology**, iodinated contrast is selectively injected into blood vessels, tubes, or other ducts that can be fluoroscopically imaged to demonstrate normal anatomy, pathology, or the position of catheters or other devices (eVideo 1.5).
- Fluoroscopy units can be made **mobile**, although they are still relatively large and heavy. They carry the same warnings of exposure to radiation as any modality with **ionizing radiation**.
- Radiation doses in fluoroscopy can be **substantially higher** than in conventional radiography because the equivalent of many static images is acquired for every minute of fluoroscopy time. Therefore the dose is reduced by the **shortest possible fluoroscopy time** being used to obtain diagnostic images.

NUCLEAR MEDICINE

- A **radioactive isotope (radioisotope)** is an unstable form of an element that emits radiation from its nucleus as it decays. Eventually, the end product is a stable, nonradioactive isotope of another element.

Fig. 1.10 CASE QUIZ 6: THE "CASE OF THE UPSIDE-DOWN STOMACH." The patient is a 71-year-old female who complained of recurrent episodes of vomiting over the course of several years. This is an image at the level of the diaphragm obtained during the course of an upper gastrointestinal examination in which the barium the patient drank is shown as black. The image is oriented correctly. What has most likely caused her symptoms? See the answer at the end of this book.

- Radioisotopes can be produced **artificially** (most frequently by neutron enrichment in a nuclear reactor or in a cyclotron) or may occur **naturally**. Naturally occurring radioisotopes include **uranium** and **thorium. Most radioisotopes** used in medicine are produced **artificially.**
- **Radiopharmaceuticals** are combinations of **radioisotopes** attached to a **pharmaceutical** that has binding properties that allow it to concentrate in certain body tissues (e.g., the lungs, thyroid, or bones). Radioisotopes used in clinical nuclear medicine are also referred to as *radionuclides, radiotracers,* or sometimes simply *tracers.*
- Various body organs have a specific affinity for, or absorption of, different biologically active chemicals. For example, the thyroid takes up **iodine**, the brain utilizes **glucose**, bones utilize **phosphates**, and **particles** of a **certain size** can be trapped in the lung capillaries (Fig. 1.11).
- After the radiopharmaceutical is carried to a tissue or organ in the body, usually via the bloodstream, its radioactive

Anterior   **Posterior**

Fig. 1.11 Bone Scan. Anterior and posterior views are frequently obtained for bone scans because each view brings different structures closer to the gamma camera for optimum imaging (e.g., the sternum on the anterior view [*solid white arrow*] and the spine on the posterior view [*dotted white arrow*]). Notice that the kidneys are normally visible on the posterior view (*white oval*). Unlike the convention used in viewing other studies in radiology, the patient's right side is not always on your left in nuclear medicine scans. On posterior views, the patient's right side is on your right. This can be confusing, so make sure you look for the labels on the scan. In many cases a white marker dot will be placed on the patient's right side (*white circles*).

emissions allow it to be measured and imaged with a detection device called a *gamma camera.*

- **Single photon emission computed tomography (SPECT)** imaging is a nuclear medicine study that is performed with a gamma camera to acquire many 2D images from **multiple angles,** which are then reconstructed by computer into a **3D data set** that can be manipulated to demonstrate thin slices in any projection. To acquire SPECT scans, the **gamma camera rotates around the patient.**

- **Positron emission tomography (PET)** scans operate on a molecular level to produce 3D images that depict the body's biochemical and metabolic processes. They are performed with a **positron (positive electron)** producing radioisotope attached to a targeting **pharmaceutical.** The most commonly used target molecule in PET scanning is an analog of glucose called *fluorodeoxyglucose* **(FDG).**

- PET scanning is most often used in the **diagnosis and treatment follow-up of cancer.** It is frequently used **to locate hidden metastases** from a known tumor or to **detect recurrence.** Oncologic PET scans make up about 90% of the clinical use of PET. Some tumors take up more of the radiotracer than others and are referred to as *FDG avid* tumors (eVideo 1.6).

- Since the radiopharmaceutical resides within the patient in these types of studies, the patient can briefly be the **source** of radiation exposure to others (e.g., technologists) with nuclear medicine studies. To limit exposure to others, the principles of **decreasing the time** in proximity to the patient, **increasing the distance** from the source (the patient), and appropriate shielding are used (**see online section on radiation dose and safety).**

- Compared with CT and fluoroscopy examinations, nuclear medicine studies, in general, produce **less patient exposure to radiation.** The types of scans that deliver the highest dose relative to other nuclear scans are cardiac studies and PET examinations. (**An additional online chapter on nuclear medicine is available to registered users online.**)

CONVENTIONS USED IN THIS BOOK

- And now, a word from our sponsor. **Bold type** is used liberally throughout this text to **highlight important points,** and because this is a book filled with numerous extraordinarily important points, **there is much bold type.**

- **Diagnostic pitfalls,** potential false–positive or false–negative traps on the sometimes-perilous journey to the correct interpretation of an image, are signaled by this icon: [!]

- **Important points** that are so important not even **boldface** type does them justice are signaled by this icon: [»]

- This symbol means there is additional or complementary instructional material available online for registered users (see inside front cover for instructions). Web-only extras include quizzes, imaging anatomy modules, expanded text and additional chapters, color photos, and videos.

- **"Take-home" points** at the end of chapters are signaled by this icon: [🏠]
  - You may take these points anywhere, not only your home.

🏠 TAKE HOME POINTS

Today, almost all images are stored electronically on a picture archiving and communications system called *PACS.*

Conventional radiographs (plain films) are produced with ionizing radiation generated by x-ray machines and viewed most commonly on a monitor.

Such x-ray machines are relatively **inexpensive,** are **widely available,** and can be made **portable.** The images are **limited as to the range** of densities and, therefore, the scope of findings they are capable of displaying.

There are **five basic radiographic densities,** arranged in order from that which is displayed the whitest to that which is displayed as the blackest: metal, calcium (bone), fluid (soft tissue), fat, and air.

CT uses rapidly spinning arrays of x-ray sources and detectors and sophisticated computer processing to increase the range of densities visible and display them in any geometric plane.

CT scanners have **become the foundation of cross-sectional imaging.** They are **moderately expensive** and also use **ionizing radiation** to produce their images.

Ultrasound produces its images using the acoustic properties of tissue and **does not use ionizing radiation.** It is thus safe for use in pregnant women, children, and women of childbearing age. It is particularly useful in analyzing soft tissues and blood flow.

Ultrasound units are **less expensive,** are in **widespread use,** and have been produced as small as **handheld devices.**

MRI produces its images based on the energy derived from hydrogen atoms placed in a very strong magnetic field and subjected to radio-frequency pulsing. The data are analyzed by powerful computer algorithms to produce its images in any plane.

MRI units are **relatively expensive,** require site construction for their placement, and are usually **higher in cost to operate.** They have become the **cornerstone of neuroimaging** and are of particular use in studying muscles, ligaments, and tendons.

Fluoroscopy uses **ionizing radiation** to produce real-time visualization of the body that allows for evaluation of motion, positioning, and the visualization of barium or iodine contrast agents moving through the GI and genitourinary tracts and blood vessels.

Nuclear medicine uses radioisotopes that have been given the property to "target" different organs of the body to evaluate the physiology and anatomy of those organs. Unlike other modalities that use ionizing radiation, the patient can briefly be the source of radiation exposure in nuclear medicine studies.

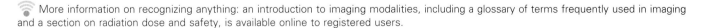

More information on recognizing anything: an introduction to imaging modalities, including a glossary of terms frequently used in imaging and a section on radiation dose and safety, is available online to registered users.

2

Recognizing a Technically Adequate Chest Radiograph

- This chapter will enable you to evaluate the technical adequacy of a chest x-ray by helping you become more familiar with the diagnostic pitfalls certain technical artifacts can introduce. This is important so that you don't mistake technical deficiencies for abnormalities.

EVALUATING THE CHEST RADIOGRAPH FOR TECHNICAL ADEQUACY

- Evaluating **five technical factors** will help you to determine if a chest radiograph is adequate for interpretation or whether certain artifacts may have been introduced which can lead you astray (Table 2.1):
  - **Penetration**
  - **Inspiration**
  - **Rotation**
  - **Magnification**
  - **Angulation**

PENETRATION

- Unless x-rays adequately pass through the body part being studied, you may not visualize everything necessary on the image produced.
  - To determine if a frontal chest radiograph is adequately penetrated, **you should be able to see the thoracic spine through the heart shadow** (Fig. 2.1).

! DIGNOSTIC PITFALLS

Pitfalls of Underpenetration (Inadequate Penetration)
- You can tell **if a frontal chest radiograph is underpenetrated** (too light) if you **cannot see the thoracic spine through the heart.**
- Underpenetration can introduce at least **two errors** into your interpretation:
  - First, the left hemidiaphragm may not be visible on the frontal image because the left lung base may appear opaque. This technical artifact could either mimic or hide true disease in the left lower lung field (e.g., left lower lobe pneumonia or left pleural effusion) (Fig. 2.3). To avoid such a problem, look at the **lateral chest radiograph** to confirm the presence of disease at the left base **(see "The Lateral Chest" in Chapter 3)**.
  - Second, the pulmonary markings, which are mostly the blood vessels in the lung, may appear more prominent than they really are. You may mistakenly think the patient is in congestive heart failure or has pulmonary fibrosis. To recognize this pitfall, look for **other radiologic signs of congestive heart failure (see Chapter 12)**.

Pitfall of Overpenetration
- If the study is overpenetrated (too dark), the lung markings may seem decreased or absent (Fig. 2.4). You could mistakenly think the patient has emphysema or

a pneumothorax or, if the degree of overpenetration is marked, it could render a pulmonary nodule almost invisible. To prevent this complication, look for other radiographic signs of emphysema **(see Chapter 11)** or pneumothorax **(see Chapter 25)**. Ask the radiologist if the film should be repeated.

INSPIRATION

- A full inspiration ensures a reproducible radiographic image for comparison from one study to the next and eliminates artifacts that may be confused for, or obscure, disease.
  - The **degree of inspiration** can be assessed by counting the number of **posterior ribs visible above the diaphragm** on the frontal chest radiograph.
    - To help in differentiating the anterior from the posterior ribs, see Box 2.1.

▶▶ IMPORTANT POINTS

- **If 10 posterior ribs are visible, it is an excellent inspiration** (Fig. 2.2).
  - In many **hospitalized patients, visualization of eight to nine posterior ribs** is a degree of inspiration usually **adequate** for accurate interpretation of the image.

Fig. 2.1 Technically Adequate Normal Frontal Chest. As explained in this chapter, the degree of **penetration** is adequate since we can see the spine (*solid white arrows*) through the heart. There is a good **inspiration** with almost ten (10) posterior ribs visible. The patient is **not rotated** because the spinous process of a thoracic vertebral body (*solid black arrow*) is projected midway between the heads of the clavicles (*dotted white arrows*). There is **little magnification** because this is a PA chest x-ray. The medial end of the clavicle (C) superimposes on the anterior first rib (1) so there is no **angulation**. Note that the left hemidiaphragm is visible (*dotted black arrow*) as it should be.

TABLE 2.1   What Defines a Technically Adequate Chest Radiograph?

Factor	What You Should See
Penetration	The spine through the heart
Inspiration	At least eight to nine **posterior** ribs
Rotation	Spinous process should fall equidistant between the medial ends of the clavicles
Magnification	Anteroposterior (AP) films (mostly portable chest x-rays) will magnify the heart slightly
Angulation	The clavicle normally has an "S" shape and the medial end superimposes on the 3rd or 4th rib

BOX 2.1   Differentiating Between Anterior and Posterior Ribs

Posterior ribs are immediately more apparent to the eye on frontal chest radiographs.

The posterior ribs are oriented more or less horizontally.

Each pair of posterior ribs attaches to a thoracic vertebral body.

Anterior ribs are visible, but are more difficult to see on the frontal chest radiograph.

Anterior ribs are oriented downward toward the feet.

Anterior ribs attach to the sternum or each other with cartilage, which is usually not visible on radiographs until later in life when the cartilage may calcify.

Fig. 2.3 Underpenetrated Frontal Chest Radiograph. The spine (*solid black arrow*) is not visible through the cardiac shadow. The left hemidiaphragm is also not visible (*dotted black arrows*), but the degree of underpenetration makes it impossible to differentiate between actual disease at the left lung base versus non-visualization of the left hemidiaphragm from underpenetration. A lateral radiograph of the chest would help to differentiate between artifact of technique and true disease.

Fig. 2.2 Adequate Inspiration. The posterior ribs are numbered in this photograph. Ten posterior ribs are visible above the right hemidiaphragm, an excellent inspiration. In most hospitalized patients, eight to nine visible posterior ribs seen in the frontal projection is an inspiration that is adequate for accurate interpretation of the image. When counting ribs, make sure you do not miss counting the second posterior rib, which frequently overlaps the first rib.

Fig. 2.4 Overpenetrated Frontal Chest Radiograph. The overpenetration makes lung markings difficult to see, mimicking some of the findings in emphysema or possibly suggesting a pneumothorax. How lucent (dark) the lungs appear on a radiograph is a poor way of evaluating for the presence of emphysema, in part because of artifacts introduced by technique. In emphysema, the lungs are frequently hyperinflated and the diaphragm flattened **(see Chapter 11)**. To diagnose a pneumothorax, you should see a **pleural white line (see Chapter 25)**.

! DIAGNOSTIC PITFALLS

Pitfall: Poor Inspiration
- A **poor inspiratory effort will compress and crowd the lung markings,** especially at the bases of the lungs near the diaphragm (Fig. 2.5). This may lead you to mistakenly think the study shows lower lobe pneumonia. To avoid this error, look at the lateral chest radiograph to confirm the presence of pneumonia **(see "The Lateral Chest Radiograph" in Chapter 3)**.

Fig. 2.5 Suboptimal Inspiration. Only eight posterior ribs are visible on this frontal chest radiograph. A poor inspiration may "crowd" and therefore accentuate the lung markings at the bases (*black arrows*) and may make the heart seem larger than it actually is. The crowded lung markings may mimic the appearance of aspiration or pneumonia. A lateral chest radiograph should help in eliminating the possibility, or confirming the presence, of basilar airspace disease, which is suggested in the frontal radiograph.

ROTATION

- The easiest way to assess whether the patient is rotated toward their left or right is by studying the relationship between the clavicles and the thoracic spine (Fig. 2.6).
- Fig. 2.7 demonstrates the position of the medial ends of each clavicle relative to the spinous process of the thoracic vertebral body between the clavicles on three chest radiographs. These relationships hold true regardless of whether the patient was facing the x-ray tube or facing the cassette at the time of exposure.

! DIAGNOSTIC PITFALLS

- **Significant rotation** (the patient turns the body to one side or the other) **may alter the expected contours of the heart and great vessels, the hila, and the hemidiaphragms. A pitfall of excessive rotation** is shown in (Fig. 2.8).

MAGNIFICATION

- Magnification usually is not an issue in assessing normal pulmonary anatomy but, depending on the position of the patient relative to the imaging cassette, magnification can play a role in assessing the size of the heart.

▶ IMPORTANT POINTS

- **The closer any object is to the surface on which it is being imaged, the more true to its actual size the resultant object will be.** As a corollary, **the farther any object is from the surface on which it is being imaged, the more magnified that object will appear.**

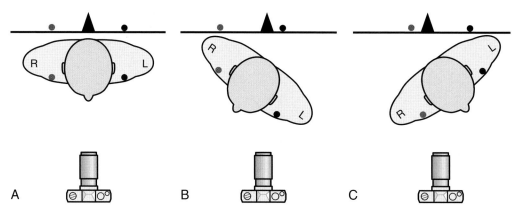

A   B   C

Fig. 2.6 How to Determine if the Patient Is Rotated. (A) The patient is not rotated and the medial ends of the right (*orange dot*) and left (*black dot*) clavicles are projected on the radiograph (*black line*) equidistant from the spinous process (*black triangle*). (B) The patient is rotated toward his **own right.** Notice how the medial end of the left clavicle (*black dot*) is projected closer to the spinous process than is the medial end of the right clavicle (*orange dot*). (C) This patient is rotated toward his **own left.** The medial end of the right clavicle (*orange dot*) is projected closer to the spinous process than is the medial end of the left clavicle (*black dot*). The camera icon (x-ray source) depicts this as an AP projection, but the same relationships would be true for a PA projection as well. Fig. 2.7 shows how this applies to radiographs.

Fig. 2.7 How to Evaluate for Rotation. (A) Close-up view of the heads of the clavicles demonstrates that each (solid white arrow for right and dotted white arrow for left) is about equidistant from the spinous process of the vertebral body between them (*black arrow*). This indicates the patient is not rotated. (B) Close-up view of the heads of the clavicles in a patient rotated toward his own right (remember that you are viewing the study as if the patient were facing you). The spinous process (*black arrow*) projects much closer to the left clavicular head (*dotted white arrow*) than to the right clavicular head (*solid white arrow*). (C) Close-up view of the heads of the clavicles in a patient rotated toward his own left. The spinous process (*black arrow*) is much closer to the right clavicular head (*solid white arrow*) than it is to the left (*dotted white arrow*).

Fig. 2.8 Distorted Appearance Due to Severe Rotation. This is a frontal chest radiograph of a patient markedly rotated toward her own right. Rotation can distort the appearance of the normal contours of the heart and hila. Notice how the left hemidiaphragm, being farther from the cassette than the right hemidiaphragm because of the rotation, appears higher than it normally would (*white arrow*). The hilum could also appear larger than its actual size because of rotation. The heart and the trachea (*black arrow*) appear displaced into the right hemithorax because of the rotation.

- In the standard **PA** chest radiograph (i.e., one obtained in the **posteroanterior projection**) **the heart,** being an anterior structure, **is closer** to the imaging surface and thus **truer to its actual size.** In a PA study, the x-ray beam enters at "P" (posterior) and exits at "A" (anterior). The standard frontal chest radiograph is usually a PA exposure (Fig. 2.9).
- On an AP image (i.e., one obtained in the anteroposterior projection) the heart is farther from the imaging cassette and is therefore slightly magnified. In an AP study, the x-ray beam enters at "A" (anterior) and exits at "P" (posterior). Portable, bedside chest radiographs are almost always AP.
- **To learn how to determine if the heart is really enlarged on an AP chest radiograph, see Chapter 4.**

ANGULATION

- Normally, the x-ray beam passes **horizontally (parallel to the floor) for an upright chest** study and, in that position, the **plane of the thorax** is **perpendicular** to the x-ray beam.
- If the patient is sitting or standing upright and the x-ray beam is angled upward, the image so obtained is called an **apical lordotic** view of the chest. If, on the other hand, the x-ray beam is horizontal but the patient is tilted backward, this produces the same apical lordotic effect.
- **Hospitalized patients**, in particular, may not be able to sit completely upright in bed so that **the x-ray beam may enter the thorax with the patient's head and thorax tilted backward.**
- On AP apical lordotic views, anterior structures in the chest (like the clavicles) are projected higher on the resultant radiographic image than posterior structures in the chest, which are projected lower (Fig. 2.10).

> **❗ DIAGNOSTIC PITFALLS**
>
> - **Pitfall of excessive angulation.** You can recognize an apical lordotic chest study when you see the **clavicles project at or above the first ribs on the frontal image.** An apical lordotic view distorts the appearance of the clavicles, straightening their normal "S" shape appearance (Fig. 2.11). To avoid this pitfall, know how to recognize technical artifacts and understand how they can distort normal anatomy. Consult with a radiologist about confusing images.

Fig. 2.9 Effect of Positioning on Magnification of the Heart. (A) Frontal chest radiograph done in the AP projection shows the heart to be slightly larger than in B, which is the same patient's chest exposed minutes later in the PA projection. In actual practice, there is very little difference in the heart size between an AP and PA exposure so long as the patient has taken an equal inspiration on both. Another reason the heart looks larger on a portable AP chest image than a standard PA chest radiograph is that the **distance between the x-ray tube and the patient is shorter when a portable AP image is obtained** (≈40 inches) **than** when a **standard PA chest radiograph** is exposed (taken by convention at 72 inches). The greater the distance the x-ray source is from the patient, the less the amount of magnification.

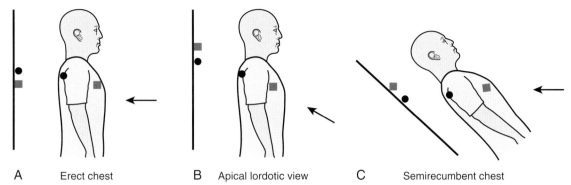

A   Erect chest   B   Apical lordotic view   C   Semirecumbent chest

Fig. 2.10 Diagram of Apical Lordotic Effect. (A) The x-ray beam (*black arrow*) is correctly oriented perpendicular to the plane of the cassette (*black line*). The *orange square* symbolizes an anterior structure (like the clavicles) and the *black circle* a posterior structure (like the spine). (B) The x-ray beam is angled upward, which is the manner in which an apical lordotic view of the chest is obtained. The x-ray beam is no longer perpendicular to the cassette, which has the effect of **projecting anterior structures higher on the radiograph than posterior structures.** (C) In this case, the x-ray beam is horizontal but the patient is tilted backward. This leads to the exact same result as B and is how semirecumbent, bedside AP studies are frequently obtained on patients who are not able to sit or stand upright. Anterior structures in C are projected higher than posterior structures

Fig. 2.11 Apical Lordotic Chest Radiograph. An apical lordotic view of the chest is most frequently obtained inadvertently using the portable technique in patients who are semirecumbent because they are bedridden and cannot stand. Notice how the clavicles are projected above the first ribs and their usual "S" shape is now straight (*white arrows*). The lordotic view also distorts the shape of the heart and produces spurious obscuration of the left hemidiaphragm (*black arrow*). Unless the artifacts of technique are understood, these findings could be mistaken for disease that does not exist.

🏠 TAKE HOME POINTS

Five parameters define an adequate chest examination and recognition of them is important to accurately differentiate abnormalities from technically produced artifacts. They are penetration, inspiration, rotation, magnification, and angulation.

- If the chest is adequately penetrated, you should be able to see spine through the heart; **underpenetrated** (too light) studies obscure the left lung base and tend to spuriously accentuate the lung markings; **overpenetrated** studies (too dark) may mimic emphysema or pneumothorax.
- If the patient has taken an **adequate inspiration**, you should see at least eight to nine posterior ribs above the diaphragm; poor inspiratory efforts may mimic basilar lung disease and may make the heart appear larger.

- The spinous process should fall equidistant between the medial ends of the clavicles to indicate the patient is **not rotated**; rotation can introduce numerous artifactual anomalies affecting the contour of the heart and the appearance of the hila and diaphragm.
- **Anteroposterior (AP)** films (mostly portable chest x-rays) will **magnify** the heart slightly compared with the standard **posteroanterior (PA)** chest radiograph (usually done in the radiology department).
- Frontal views of the chest obtained with the patient semiupright in bed (tilted backward) may produce **apical lordotic** images that distort normal anatomy.

 More information on recognizing normal chest anatomy and a technically adequate chest radiograph is available to registered users online.

3

Recognizing Normal Pulmonary Anatomy

In this chapter, you will learn the normal anatomy of the lungs as depicted by conventional radiographs and chest CT. To become more comfortable interpreting images of the chest, you should first be able to recognize fundamental, normal anatomy to differentiate it from what is abnormal (Box 3.1).

THE NORMAL FRONTAL CHEST RADIOGRAPH

- Fig. 3.1 displays some of the normal anatomic features visible on the frontal chest radiograph.

BOX 3.1 Which "System" Works Best

What is the best system to look at an imaging study, such as a chest x-ray? I'm glad you asked.

Some individuals systematically look at imaging studies, such as chest radiographs, from the outside of the image to the inside of the image; others look at them from the inside out or from top to bottom. Some systems for reminding you to examine every part of an image have catchy acronyms and mnemonics.

The fact is **it does not matter what system you use as long as you look at everything** on the image. So, **use whatever system works** for you, but be sure to look at everything. "Looking at everything," by the way, includes looking at **all of the views available in a given study**, not just everything on *one* view (do not forget the lateral chest radiograph in a two-view study of the chest).

Experienced radiologists usually have no system at all. "Burned-in" images are bad for computer monitors, but they are great for radiologists. "Burned" into the neurons of a radiologist's brain are mental images of what a normal frontal chest radiograph looks like, what thoracic sarcoidosis looks like, and so on. Radiologists frequently use a **"gestalt"** impression of a study that they see in their mind's eye within seconds of looking at an image. If the image does or does not correspond to the mental image that resides in their brains, **then** they systematically study the images. This is not magic; this ability comes only with experience so, at least for now, you are probably not quite ready to use the "gestalt" approach.

The most important part of the "system" you use in interpreting images is a **system in which you routinely increase your knowledge.** If you do not know what you are looking for, you can stare at an image for hours or days or, in the case of the lateral chest radiograph, you can ignore an image entirely, and the result will be the same: you will not see the findings. There is an axiom in radiology: **You only see what you look for and you only look for what you know.** So, if you do not know what to look for, you will never recognize the finding no matter what system you use or how long you stare at the image.

By reading this book, you will gain the knowledge that will allow you to recognize what it is you are looking at—the best system of all.

- Fig. 3.2 shows **vessels and bronchi—normal lung markings.**
  - **Virtually all of the "white lines"** you see in the lungs on a chest radiograph **are blood vessels.** Blood vessels characteristically branch and taper gradually from the hila centrally to the periphery of the lung. You cannot accurately differentiate between pulmonary arteries and pulmonary veins on a conventional radiograph.
  - **Bronchi are mostly invisible** on a normal chest radiograph because they are normally very **thin-walled,** they **contain air,** and they are **surrounded by air.**

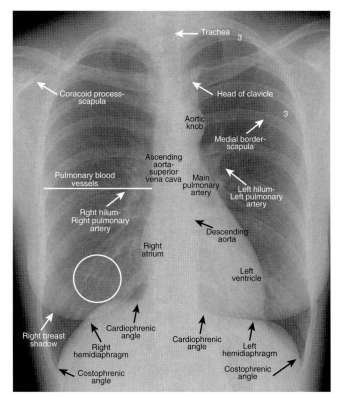

Fig. 3.1 Well-Exposed Frontal View of a Normal Chest. Notice how the spine is just visible through the heart shadow. Both the right and left lateral costophrenic angles are sharply and acutely angled. The white line demarcates the approximate level of the minor or horizontal fissure, which is usually visible on the frontal view. There is no minor fissure on the left side. The white circle contains lung markings that are blood vessels. Note that the left hilum is normally slightly higher than the right. The white numeral 3 lies on the posterior third rib, whereas the black numeral 3 lies on the anterior 3rd rib.

- **Pleura: normal anatomy**
  - The **pleura is composed of two layers, the outer parietal and inner visceral layers with the pleural space between them.** The visceral pleura is adherent to the lung and enfolds to form the **major (oblique)** and **minor (horizontal) fissures.**
  - Normally there are **several milliliters of fluid, but no air, in the pleural space.**
  - **Neither the parietal pleura nor the visceral pleura is normally visible** on a conventional chest radiograph, except where the two layers of visceral pleura enfold to form the fissures. Even then, they are **usually no thicker than a line you could draw with the point of a sharpened pencil.**

Normal Pulmonary Vasculature

> ### IMPORTANT POINTS
>
> - In the **upright position,** the blood flow to the **bases** is normally **greater** than the flow to the apices because of the effect of gravity. Therefore the vessels at the **base are normally larger in size** than the vessels at the apex of the lung.

- Normally, blood vessels branch and taper gradually from central (the hila) to peripheral (near the chest wall) (Fig. 3.2).
- Changes in pressure or flow can alter the normal dynamics of the pulmonary vasculature, some of which are described in **Chapter 12.**
- **For more on recognizing normal pulmonary vasculature and an imaging approach to diagnosing heart disease in adults, registered users can view "The ABCs of Heart Disease" online.**

THE NORMAL LATERAL CHEST RADIOGRAPH

- As part of the standard two-view chest examination, patients usually have an **upright, frontal** chest radiograph and an upright, **left lateral** view of the chest. A **left lateral chest x-ray** (the patient's left side is against the detector) is of **great diagnostic value** but is **sometimes ignored by beginners** because of their lack of familiarity with the findings visible in that projection.
- **Why look at the lateral chest?**
  - It can help you **determine the location** of disease you already identified as being present on the frontal image.
  - It can **confirm the presence of disease** you may be unsure of on the basis of the frontal image alone, such as a mass or pneumonia.
  - It can **demonstrate disease not visible on the frontal image** (Fig. 3.3).

Fig. 3.2 Normal Pulmonary Vasculature. The right lung is shown. In the upright position, the lower lobe vessels (*black circle*) are larger in size than the upper lobe vessels (*white circle*) and all vessels taper gradually from central to peripheral (*white arrow*). Alterations in pulmonary flow or pressure may change these relationships.

Fig. 3.3 The Spine Sign. Frontal (A) and lateral (B) views of the chest demonstrate air space disease on the lateral image (B) in the left lower lobe that may not be immediately apparent on the frontal image (look closely at A and you may see the pneumonia in the left lower lobe behind the heart). Normally, the thoracic spine appears to get **"blacker"** as you view it from the neck to the diaphragm because there is less dense tissue for the x-ray beam to traverse just above the diaphragm than in the region of the shoulder girdle (see Fig. 3.4). In this case, a **left lower lobe pneumonia** superimposed on the lower spine in the lateral view (*white arrow*) makes the spine appear **"whiter"** (more dense) just above the diaphragm. This is called the **spine sign.** Note that on a well-positioned lateral projection, the right and left posterior ribs almost superimpose on each other (*black arrow*), a sign of a true lateral.

- Figs. 3.4 and 3.5 display some of the normal anatomic features visible on the lateral chest radiograph.

Five Key Areas on the Lateral Chest X-Ray (See Fig. 3.4 and Table 3.1)

- **The retrosternal clear space**
- **The hilar region**
- **The fissures**
- **The thoracic spine**
- **The diaphragm and posterior costophrenic sulci**

The Retrosternal Clear Space

- Normally, there is a relatively lucent crescent just behind the sternum and anterior to the shadow of the ascending aorta. **Look for this clear space to "fill-in"** with soft-tissue density when there is an **anterior mediastinal mass** present (Fig. 3.6).

TABLE 3.1 **The Lateral Chest: A Quick Guide of What to Look for**	
Region	**What You Should See**
Retrosternal clear space	Lucent crescent between sternum and ascending aorta
Hilar region	No discrete mass present
Fissures	Major and minor fissures should be pencil point thin, if visible at all.
Thoracic spine	Rectangular vertebral bodies with parallel end plates; disk spaces maintain height from top to bottom of thoracic spine
Diaphragm and posterior costophrenic sulci	Right hemidiaphragm slightly higher than left; sharp posterior costophrenic sulci

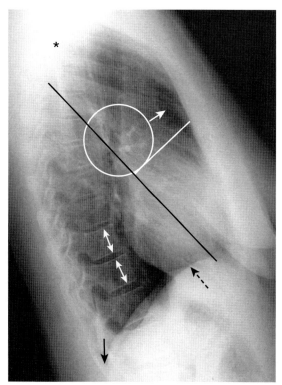

Fig. 3.4 Normal Left Lateral Chest Radiograph. There is a clear space behind the sternum (*solid white arrow*). The hila produce no discrete shadow (*white circle*). The vertebral bodies are approximately of equal height and their end plates are parallel to each other (*double white arrows*). The posterior costophrenic angles (*solid black arrow*) are sharp. Notice how the thoracic spine appears to become blacker (darker) from the shoulder girdle (*black star*) to the diaphragm because there is less dense tissue for the x-ray beam to traverse at the level of the diaphragm. The superior surface of the right hemidiaphragm is frequently seen continuously from back to front (*dotted black arrow*) because it is not obscured by the heart, whereas the heart normally touches the anterior aspect of the left hemidiaphragm and obscures **(silhouettes)** it. Notice the normal space posterior to the heart and anterior to the spine; this will be important in assessing cardiomegaly (see Chapter 12). The black line represents the approximate location of the major fissure; the white line is the approximate location of the minor fissure. Both are frequently visible on the lateral view.

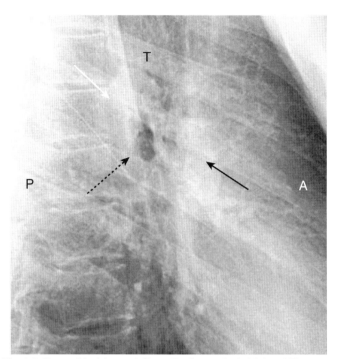

Fig. 3.5 Normal Left Lateral Chest Radiograph, Additional Findings. The left main pulmonary artery *(white solid arrow)* arches over the air-filled left main bronchus *(dotted black arrow)*, superior and posterior to the right main pulmonary artery *(solid black arrow)*. Normally, the right main pulmonary artery produces an opacity anterior to the distal trachea *(T)*, but there should be only aerated lung posterior and inferior to the distal trachea. *A,* Anterior; *P,* posterior.

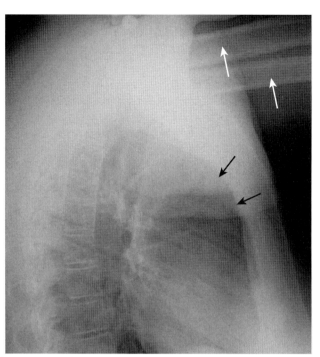

Fig. 3.7 Arms Obscure Retrosternal Clear Space. In this example, the patient was not able to hold her arms over her head for the lateral chest examination, as patients are instructed to do in order to eliminate the shadows of the arms from overlapping the lateral chest. The humeri are clearly visible *(white arrows)* so even though the soft tissue of the patient's arms appears to fill in the retrosternal clear space *(black arrows)*, this should not be mistaken for an abnormality such as anterior mediastinal adenopathy

> **❗ DIAGNOSTIC PITFALL**
>
> • Be careful not to mistake the soft tissue of the patient's superimposed arms for "filling-in" of the clear space. Although patients are asked to hold their arms over their head for a lateral chest exposure, many are too weak to raise their arms. To avoid this pitfall, you should be able to identify the patient's arm by identifying the humerus (Fig. 3.7).

Fig. 3.6 Anterior Mediastinal Adenopathy. (A) A normal lateral view shows a clear space behind the sternum *(white arrow)*. (B) Left lateral view of the chest demonstrates a soft-tissue density which is filling in the normal clear space behind the sternum *(black arrow)*. This represents anterior mediastinal lymphadenopathy in a patient with lymphoma. Adenopathy is probably the most frequent reason the **retrosternal clear space** is obscured. Thymoma, teratoma, and substernal thyroid enlargement also can produce anterior mediastinal masses, but do not usually produce exactly this appearance.

The Hilar Region

- The hila may be difficult to assess on the frontal view, especially if both hila are slightly enlarged because comparison with the opposite normal side is impossible. The lateral view may help. Most of the hilar densities are made up of the pulmonary arteries. Normally, no discrete mass is visible in the hilar region on the lateral view (see Fig. 3.5).
- When there is a hilar mass, such as might occur with enlargement of hilar lymph nodes, the hilum (or hila) will cast a distinct, lobulated, mass-like shadow on the lateral radiograph (Fig. 3.8).

The Fissures

- On the **lateral** projection, both the **major and minor fissures may be visible** as smooth, fine, white lines. The fissures demarcate the upper and lower lobes on the left and the upper, middle, and lower lobes on the right.
- The **major fissures** course obliquely, roughly **from the level of the fifth thoracic vertebra to** a point on the diaphragmatic surface of the pleura **a few centimeters behind the sternum.**

- The **minor fissure lies at the level of the fourth anterior rib** (on the right side only) and is **horizontally** oriented (see Fig. 3.4).
- **Both** the major and minor fissures may be visible on the **lateral view,** but because of the oblique plane of the major fissure, **only the minor fissure** is usually visible on the **frontal view.**
- **When a fissure contains fluid or develops fibrosis from a chronic process, it will become thickened** (Fig. 3.9). **Thickening of the fissure by fluid is almost always associated with other signs of fluid in the chest,** such as Kerley B lines and pleural effusions (**see Chapter 12). Thickening of the fissure by fibrosis** is the more likely cause if there are **no other signs of fluid in the chest.**

The Thoracic Spine

- Normally, the **thoracic vertebral bodies are** roughly **rectangular in shape, and each** vertebral body's endplate **parallels the endplate of the vertebral body above and below it. Each intervertebral disk space becomes slightly taller than or**

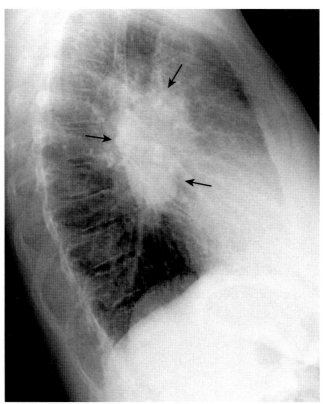

Fig. 3.8 Hilar Mass on Lateral Radiograph. Left lateral view of the chest shows a discrete, lobulated mass in the region of the hila *(black arrows)*. Compare this with the normal hilum in Fig. 3.5. This patient had bilateral hilar adenopathy from sarcoidosis, but any cause of hilar adenopathy or a primary tumor in the hilum would have a similar appearance.

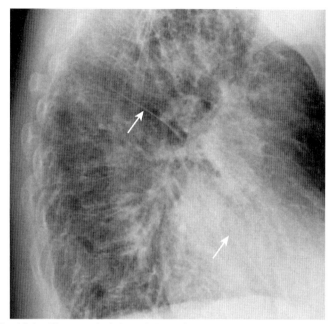

Fig. 3.9 Fluid in the Major Fissures. Left lateral view of the chest shows thickening of both the right and left major fissures *(white arrows)*. This patient was in congestive heart failure and this thickening represents **fluid** in the fissures. Normally, the fissures are either invisible or, if visible, they are fine, white lines of uniform thickness no larger than a line made with the point of a sharpened pencil. The course of the major fissure is usually from the level of the fifth thoracic vertebral body to a point on the anterior diaphragm about 2 cm behind the sternum. Notice the increased interstitial markings that are visible throughout the lungs, which are due to fluid in the interstitium of the lung.

remains the same as the one above it throughout the thoracic spine.

- **Degeneration** of the disk can lead to narrowing of the disk space and the development of small, bony spurs *(osteophytes)* at the margins of the vertebral bodies.
- When there is a **compression fracture,** most often from osteoporosis, the vertebral body loses height. Compression fractures very commonly first involve depression of the superior endplate of the vertebral body (Fig. 3.10).
- **Do not forget to look at the thoracic spine when studying the lateral chest radiograph** for valuable clues about systemic disorders (**see Chapter 22**).

The Diaphragm and Posterior Costophrenic Sulci

- Because the **diaphragm** is composed of soft tissue (muscle) and the abdomen below it contains soft-tissue structures such as the liver and spleen, only the **upper border** of the diaphragm, abutting an air-filled lung, is usually visible on conventional radiographs.
- Even though we have one diaphragm that separates the thorax from the abdomen, we do not usually see the entire diaphragm from side-to-side on conventional radiographs because of the position of the heart in the center of the chest. Therefore radiographically we refer to the **right-half** of the diaphragm as the *right hemidiaphragm* and the **left-half** of the diaphragm as the *left hemidiaphragm.*
- **How to tell the right from the left hemidiaphragm on the lateral radiograph:**

Fig. 3.10 Osteoporotic Compression Fracture and Degenerative Disk Disease. Do not forget to look at the thoracic spine when studying the lateral chest radiograph for valuable information about a host of systemic diseases. In this study, there is loss of stature of the eighth thoracic vertebral body owing to osteoporosis *(black arrow)*. Compression fractures frequently involve the superior endplate first. There are small osteophytes present at multiple levels from degenerative disk disease *(white arrows)*.

Fig. 3.11 Blunting of the Posterior Costophrenic Sulcus by a Small Pleural Effusion. Left lateral view of the chest shows fluid blunting the posterior costophrenic sulcus *(solid white arrow)*. The other posterior costophrenic angle *(solid black arrow)* is sharp. The pleural effusion is on the right side because the involved hemidiaphragm can be traced anteriorly farther forward *(dotted black arrow)* than the other hemidiaphragm (the left), which is normally silhouetted by the heart and not visible anteriorly.

- The **right hemidiaphragm is usually visible for its entire length from front to back.** Normally, the **right hemidiaphragm is slightly higher than the left,** a relationship that tends to hold true on the lateral radiograph as well as the frontal.
- The **left hemidiaphragm** is seen sharply posteriorly but **is silhouetted by the muscle of the heart anteriorly** (i.e., its edge disappears anteriorly) (Fig. 3.11).
- **Air in the stomach or splenic flexure of the colon appears immediately below the left hemidiaphragm.** The liver lies below the right hemidiaphragm and bowel gas is usually not seen between the liver and the right hemidiaphragm.

The Posterior Costophrenic Sulci (Posterior Costophrenic Angles)

- Each hemidiaphragm produces a rounded dome that indents the central portion of the base of each lung, like the bottom of a wine bottle. This produces a depression or *sulcus* that surrounds the base of each lung and represents the lowest point of the pleural space when the patient is upright.
- On a frontal chest radiograph, this sulcus is most easily viewed at the outer edge of the lung as the *lateral costophrenic sulcus* (also called the *lateral costophrenic angle*) and on the lateral radiograph as the *posterior costophrenic sulcus* (also known as the *posterior costophrenic angle*) (see Figs. 3.1 and 3.4).
- **Normally, the costophrenic sulci are sharply outlined and acutely angled.**

- **Pleural effusions** accumulate in the deep recesses of the costophrenic sulci with the patient upright, filling in their acute angles. This is called *blunting of the costophrenic angles* **(see Chapter 8).**
- It requires only about **75 mL** of fluid (or less) to **blunt the posterior costophrenic angle** on the lateral projection, whereas it takes about **250 to 300 mL** to **blunt the lateral costophrenic angles** on the frontal projection (see Fig. 3.11 and Table 3.1).

NORMAL CT ANATOMY OF THE CHEST

- By convention, **CT scans of the chest,** like most other radiologic studies, **are viewed** with the **patient's right on your left and the patient's left on your right.** If the patient is scanned in the supine position, as most usually are, the **top** of each image is **anterior** and the **bottom** of each image is **posterior.**

> **⊗ IMPORTANT POINTS**
>
> - Chest CT scans are usually "windowed" and **displayed in** at least **two formats** designed to be viewed as parts of the same study, in order to optimize anatomic definition.

- *Lung windows* are chosen to maximize our ability to image abnormalities of the **lung parenchyma** and to identify **normal and abnormal bronchial anatomy.** The mediastinal structures frequently appear as a homogenous white density on lung windows.
- *Mediastinal windows* are chosen to display the **mediastinal, hilar, and pleural structures** to best advantage. The lungs usually appear completely black when viewed with mediastinal windows.
- *Bone windows* are also used often as a third way of displaying the data, demonstrating the bony structures to their best advantage.
- It is important to know that the displays of these different windows are **manipulations of the data** obtained during the **original scan** and **do not require rescanning the patient** (see Fig. 1.4).

Normal CT Anatomy of the Lungs

- CT scans of the lungs reveal additional and more detailed anatomy than conventional radiographs. With computer reconstruction of thin-section CT images, the lungs can be visualized in any plane, although the three most common are the **axial (transverse), sagittal (lateral),** and **coronal (frontal)** (Fig. 3.12).
- Blood vessels are visible for almost their entire course from hilum to pleural surface. Pulmonary arteries can be differentiated from pulmonary veins (Fig. 3.13).
- Bronchi and bronchioles are also visible and, as a rule, **bronchi are normally smaller** than their **accompanying pulmonary artery** (Fig. 3.14).
- The **trachea** is usually oval in shape and about 2 cm in diameter.

Fig. 3.12 Axial (A), Coronal (B), and Sagittal Views (C) of the Thorax. The three standard planes for imaging the thorax are shown above. Remember that the data were all acquired at the time of the same scanning session, but thin-section acquisition allows digital reformatting in any plane. The left main bronchus (*black arrow*) and the right main bronchus (*white arrow*) are seen in A. *Ao,* Aorta; *LA,* left atrium; *LV,* left ventricle; *PA,* pulmonary artery; *RA,* right atrium; *S,* superior vena cava.

Fig. 3.13 MIP of Pulmonary Vasculature. MIP (or MIPs if pleural) stands for **maximum intensity projections**; it is a way to display certain structures of a given density preferentially making them stand out more easily. It is a computer post-processing manipulation of the same data acquired at the time of the original scan. It produces an image that looks like an angiogram and is used particularly for CT angiography (as here) and is also utilized for finding pulmonary nodules **(see also Video 3.1).**

Fig. 3.14 Bronchus-Artery Relationship. The normal relationship between the **bronchus** *(solid white arrow)* and its accompanying **pulmonary artery** *(dotted white arrow)* is that the artery is usually larger than the bronchus. In bronchiectasis, that relationship is reversed with the bronchus becoming larger than the artery **(*signet-ring sign*) (see Chapter 11).**

- In most people, there is a space visible just underneath the arch of the aorta but above the pulmonary artery, which is called the *aorto-pulmonary window.* The aortopulmonary window is an important landmark because it is a favorite location for **enlarged lymph nodes to appear.** At or slightly below this level, the trachea bifurcates at the **carina** into the **right and left main bronchi** (Fig. 3.15).
- Slightly more inferior are the **right and left main bronchi** and the **bronchus intermedius.** The **right main bronchus** will appear as a circular, air-containing structure which will then become tubular as the **right upper lobe** bronchus comes into view. There should be nothing but lung tissue posterior to the **bronchus intermedius.** The **left main bronchus** will appear as an air-containing circular structure on the left (Fig. 3.16).

The Fissures

- Depending on slice thickness, the **fissures** will be visible either as **thin white lines or** by an **avascular band** up to 2 cm thick as they travel obliquely through the lungs (Fig. 3.17).

- The **major fissure** demarcates the upper lobe from the lower lobe on the left and the lower and middle lobes on the right. On the right, the minor fissure demarcates the middle lobe. The middle lobe's analog on the left is the lingular segment of the left upper lobe. (Fig. 3.18).
- The **minor fissure** travels in the same horizontal plane as the plane of an axial CT image so the minor fissure is normally not visible except in the sagittal or coronal planes. Although as with the major fissures, the **location of the minor fissure can be inferred by an avascular zone** between the right upper and middle lobes (see Fig. 3.17A).

Fig. 3.15 Coronal and Axial CT at Carina. A. The trachea (T) bifurcates at the carina (C) into the right main bronchus (RMB) and left main bronchus (LMB). After the origin of the right upper lobe bronchus *(dotted white arrow)*, the bronchus intermedius (BI) gives rise to the right lower lobe bronchus *(dotted black arrow)* and middle lobe bronchus (not shown). The left upper lobe bronchus is shown *(solid black arrow)*. The **aortopulmonary "window"** *(solid white arrow)* lies between the aorta (Ao) and the pulmonary artery (PA). B. Just distal to the carina, the right main bronchus (RMB) gives rise to the upper lobe bronchus *(white arrow)*. The left main bronchus (LMB) is also seen at this level.

Fig. 3.16 Bronchus Intermedius. Distal to the origin of the right upper lobe bronchus is a short bronchial section called the **bronchus intermedius** *(solid black arrow)*. The bronchus intermedius divides into the middle and lower lobe bronchi more caudal to this image. There is normally nothing but lung tissue posterior to the bronchus intermedius; soft tissue in this location would suggest a tumor or adenopathy. The left main bronchus is shown by the dotted black arrow.

Fig. 3.17 Fissures Seen on Axial and Coronal Reformatted Views. (A) The major fissure is seen as a thin white line on the axial view of the right lung *(solid white arrow)* and the minor fissure can be seen anterior to the major fissure *(dotted white arrow)*. (B) The minor fissure is seen as a faint white line *(dotted white arrow)*, whereas the major fissure travels obliquely at this level and is represented by an avascular zone that surrounds the fissure *(solid white arrows)*. *RLL,* Right lower lobe; *RML,* right middle lobe; *RUL,* right upper lobe.

Fig. 3.18 Lobes and Fissures-Sagittal of Right (A) and Left (B) Lungs. (A) The major fissure *(solid white arrows)* demarcates the right lower lobe (RLL) from the upper (RUL) and middle lobes (RML). On the right, the minor fissure *(dotted white arrows)* demarcates the middle lobe, separating the upper and lower lobes anteriorly. (B) The major fissure is seen on the left *(solid white arrows)*. The analog of the middle lobe on the left is the lingula, part of the left upper lobe. A portion of the heart (H) is seen on the left. *LLL,* Left lower lobe; *LUL,* left upper lobe.

TAKE HOME POINTS

- The best **"system"** to use for carefully looking at any imaging study is one based on a solid knowledge base of the appearance of **normal anatomy** and the most common deviations from normal.
- Virtually all of the lung markings on chest radiographs are composed of **pulmonary blood vessels;** most **bronchi** are too thin-walled to be visible on conventional radiography.
- Normal pulmonary vasculature **tapers gradually** from central to peripheral and the vessels are normally larger at the base than at the apex on an **upright** chest radiograph.
- The **lateral chest radiograph** can provide invaluable information and should always be studied, when available.
- Five key areas to inspect on the lateral projection include the retrosternal clear space, hilar region, fissures, thoracic spine, and diaphragm/posterior costophrenic sulci.
- There is normally a **retrosternal "clear space"** on a lateral radiograph that can "fill-in" with a mediastinal mass or adenopathy, such as in lymphoma.
- Although the pulmonary arteries themselves can normally be seen in the hila on the lateral projection, a discrete mass in the hilum is abnormal and should alert to the possibility of tumor or adenopathy.
- The **minor fissure,** not the major fissure, will usually be visible on a frontal view. On the lateral view, both the major and minor fissures can be seen normally. When visible, they are very thin lines of uniform size about 1 to 2 mm in thickness.
- The thoracic spine should **appear to become blacker** from the upper to the lower portion of the spine, owing to greater overlying soft tissue more superiorly. Increased density at the base, such as a pneumonia, can produce the reverse of this normal pattern, which is called the *spine sign.*
- On the lateral view, the **left hemidiaphragm** will be obscured (silhouetted) anteriorly by the heart. The **right hemidiaphragm** is usually higher than the left and can be seen in its entirety from front to back.
- The **costophrenic angles** are normally acute and sharply outlined. Pleural effusions and scarring may cause blunting of the costophrenic angles.
- CT scans of the chest display much more detail than conventional radiographs and, owing to rapid acquisition of very thin slices, can be displayed in any plane using the original data set. The planes most commonly used are the **axial, sagittal, and coronal.**
- The normal anatomy of the trachea and main bronchi is outlined.
- Both the major and minor fissures are visible on CT either as **thin white lines** or **avascular bands** depending on the orientation of the fissure relative to the plane in which the scan is displayed.

More information on recognizing normal pulmonary anatomy is available to registered users online.

4

Recognizing Normal Cardiac Anatomy

Emphasizing conventional radiography first, we will begin with an assessment of heart size, then describe the normal and abnormal contours of the heart on the frontal radiograph and, finally, discuss the normal anatomy of the heart as seen on computed tomography (CT) and magnetic resonance imaging (MRI).

EVALUATING THE HEART ON CHEST RADIOGRAPHS

Recognizing a Normal-Sized Heart

> **» IMPORTANT POINTS**
>
> - You can estimate the size of the cardiac silhouette on the frontal chest radiograph using the ***cardiothoracic ratio,*** which is a measurement of the **widest transverse diameter of the heart** compared with the **widest internal diameter of the rib cage** (from inside of rib to inside of rib at the level of the diaphragm) (Fig. 4.1).

- In most normal adults at **full inspiration,** the cardiothoracic ratio is **less than 50%.** That is, the size of the heart is usually less than half of the internal diameter of the thoracic rib cage.

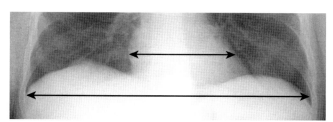

Fig. 4.1 The Cardiothoracic Ratio. To estimate the cardiothoracic ratio, the widest diameter of the heart (*upper double arrow*) is compared with the widest **internal** diameter of the thoracic cage from the inside of the right rib to the inside of the left rib (*lower double arrow*). The widest internal diameter of the thorax is usually at the level of the diaphragm. The cardiothoracic ratio should be **less than 50%** in most normal adults on a standard PA frontal radiograph taken with an adequate inspiration (about nine posterior ribs showing).

The Normal Cardiac Contours

- The **normal cardiac contours** comprise a series bumps and indentations visible on the frontal chest radiograph. They are demonstrated in Fig. 4.2.

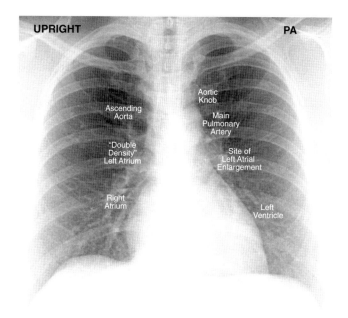

Fig. 4.2. Normal Cardiac Contours Seen in the Frontal Projection. On the right side of the heart, the first contour is the **ascending aorta**. Where the contour of the ascending aorta meets the contour of the right atrium, there is usually a **slight indentation** which is where the left atrium may appear when it enlarges (called the ***double-density sign***). The right heart border is formed by the **right atrium**. On the left, the first contour is the **aortic knob**, a radiographic structure formed by the foreshortened aortic arch superimposed on a portion of the proximal descending aorta. The next contour below the aortic knob is the **main pulmonary artery**, before it divides into a right and left pulmonary artery. Just below the main pulmonary artery segment there is normally a **slight indentation** where an enlarged left atrium/left atrial appendage may appear on the left side of the heart. The last contour of the heart on the left is formed by the **left ventricle.** The descending aorta almost disappears with the shadow of the spine.

▶▶ IMPORTANT POINTS

Key Points About the Cardiac Contours
- The **ascending aorta** should normally not project farther to the right than the right heart border (i.e., the right atrium).
- The **aortic knob** is normally less than 35 mm (measured from the edge of the air-filled trachea) and will normally push the trachea slightly to the right.
- The **main pulmonary artery** segment is usually concave or flat. In **younger, females** it may **normally be convex** outward.
- The **normal left atrium** does not contribute to the border of the heart on a nonrotated frontal chest radiograph.
- An **enlarged left atrium** and left atrial appendage "fills-in" and straightens the normal concavity just inferior to the main pulmonary artery segment and may sometimes be visible on the right side of the heart as well.
- The lower portion of the left side of the heart border is made up of the **left ventricle.** Remember that the left ventricle is really a **posterior** ventricle and the **right ventricle** is an **anterior** ventricle.
- Normally, the **descending aorta** parallels the spine and is barely visible on the frontal radiograph of the chest. When it becomes **tortuous** or **uncoiled**, it swings farther away from the thoracic spine toward the patient's left (Fig. 4.3).

Therefore the heart may **not** appear enlarged at first with lesions such as **aortic stenosis, coarctation of the aorta, pulmonic stenosis,** or **systemic hypertension.** When the ventricular wall becomes thicker, the lumen actually becomes smaller and it is only when the muscle begins to fail and the heart decompensates that the heart visibly enlarges on chest radiographs.

- **Cardiomegaly,** as recognized on chest radiographs, refers to enlargement of the cardiac silhouette produced by **ventricular enlargement,** not by isolated enlargement of the atria. For example, the cardiac silhouette usually appears normal in size when there is isolated atrial enlargement, such as left atrial enlargement in early mitral stenosis.
- In general, **the most marked chamber enlargement will occur from volume overload** rather than **pressure increases** so that the largest chambers are usually produced by **regurgitant valves** rather than **stenotic valves.** Therefore the heart will usually be larger as a result of aortic regurgitation than aortic stenosis and the left atrium will usually be larger in mitral regurgitation than mitral stenosis (Fig. 4.4).

GENERAL PRINCIPLES

- As you interpret cardiac abnormalities, no matter what imaging modality is being used, the following principles hold true:
  - The **ventricles respond to obstruction** to their outflow **by first undergoing hypertrophy** rather than dilatation.

EVALUATING THE HEART ON CARDIAC CT

- **CT scanning of the heart** is done using a fast, multislice CT scanner, usually with intravenous iodinated contrast and electrocardiographic (ECG)-gated acquisition to reduce motion artifacts.

Fig. 4.3 Appearances of the Aorta. (A) **Normal.** The ascending aorta is a low-density, almost straight edge (*solid white arrow*) and does not project beyond the right heart border (*dotted white arrow*). The aortic knob is not enlarged (*double arrow*) and the descending aorta (*solid black arrow*) almost disappears with the shadow of the thoracic spine. (B) **Aortic stenosis.** The ascending aorta is abnormal as it projects convex outward (*solid white arrow*) almost as far as the right heart border (*dotted white arrow*). This is secondary to *post-stenotic dilatation*. The aortic knob (*double arrow*) and descending aorta (*solid black arrow*) remain normal. (C) **Systemic hypertension.** Both the ascending (*solid white arrow*) and descending aorta (*solid black arrow*) project too far to the right and left, respectively. The aortic knob is enlarged (*double black arrow*).

Fig. 4.4 Heart Size with Stenotic Versus Regurgitant Valve. (A) There is **post-stenotic dilatation** of the ascending aorta (*white arrow*) from turbulent flow in this patient with **aortic stenosis**. Notice that the cardiac silhouette is not enlarged (*dotted black double arrows*) even though this lesion produces left ventricular hypertrophy. (B) This patient has **aortic regurgitation**. Note the enlarged cardiac silhouette (*solid black double arrows*) due to an extremely large left ventricle. Volume overload will cause a greater increase in chamber size than will increased pressure alone.

- Both cardiac CT and cardiac MRI use ECG-gating, which allows for a series of images to be obtained either prospectively or retrospectively over several cardiac cycles and parsed together with powerful computer algorithms.
- Cardiac CT can be used to evaluate the **coronary arteries, valves** and search for cardiac **masses.** By reconstructing multiple phases of the cardiac cycle, it is also possible to analyze **wall motion** and evaluate **ejection fraction** and **myocardial perfusion.**
- The three standard planes for viewing CT images of the heart are the **axial, sagittal,** and **coronal.** Figs. 4.5 to 4.10 demonstrate the major normal CT anatomy of the heart and great vessels.

Normal Cardiac CT Anatomy

- We cover only a few of the major anatomic landmarks demonstrable on chest CT, and all of the scans used will be *contrast-enhanced* (i.e., in the scans shown, the patient will have had an injection of intravenous contrast to opacify the heart chambers and blood vessels). It is best to read the text in conjunction with its associated photograph. Any references to "right" or "left" mean the patient's right or left side, not yours.
- We will start at the top of the chest and progress inferiorly, highlighting the major structures visible at **six key levels.** This is a good way to systematically study every CT study of the chest.

Five-Vessel Level (Fig. 4.5)

- At this level, you should be able to identify the **lungs, the trachea, and the esophagus.** The **trachea** is black because it contains air; it is usually oval in shape and about 2 cm in diameter. The **esophagus** lies posterior and either to the left or right of the trachea. The esophagus is usually collapsed, but may contain swallowed air.

Fig. 4.5 Five-Vessel Level. At this level, you should be able to identify the lungs, the **trachea (T)** and the **esophagus** (*white arrow*). Depending on the exact level of the image, several of the great vessels will be visible. The **right brachiocephalic vein (R)** is the vessel to the right of the **trachea (T).** The **left brachiocephalic vein (L)** lies just posterior to the sternum. From the patient's right to the patient's left, the arteries you see may include the **innominate artery (I), left common carotid (C), and left subclavian arteries (S).**

Fig. 4.6 Aortic Arch Level. (A) **Mediastinal window and** (B) **lung window.** (A) At this level, you should be able to identify the **aortic arch (AA), superior vena cava (S), and azygos vein** (A). The white arrow points to air in the esophagus. (B) The same image as (A), but windowed to better visualize lung anatomy. Lung windows are chosen to maximize our ability to image abnormalities of the lung parenchyma and to identify normal and abnormal bronchial anatomy. *T,* Trachea.

• Depending on the exact level of the image, several of the great vessels will be visible. The **venous structures** tend to be more **anterior than the arterial.** The **brachiocephalic (innominate) veins** lie just posterior to the sternum.

Aortic Arch Level (Fig. 4.6)

• At this level, you should be able to identify the **aortic arch, superior vena cava, and azygos vein.**
• The *aortic arch* forms an upside-down U-shaped tube. If the scan skims the very top of the arch, it will appear as a comma-shaped tubular structure with roughly the same diameter anteriorly as posteriorly. To the right of the trachea will be the *superior vena cava* into which the *azygos vein* drains.

Aortopulmonary Window Level (Fig. 4.7)

• At this level you should be able to identify the **ascending and descending aorta, superior vena cava,** and **uppermost aspect of the left pulmonary artery** (maybe).

⯈ IMPORTANT POINTS

• As we scan lower and through the opening of the upside-down U-shaped aortic arch, the **ascending aorta** will appear as a rounded density **anteriorly,** whereas the descending aorta will appear as a separate rounded density posterior and to the **left** of the spine. The **ascending aorta** usually measures **2.5 to 3.5 cm** in diameter and the **descending aorta** is slightly smaller at **2 to 3 cm.**

• In most people, a space is visible just underneath the arch of the aorta, but above the pulmonary artery called the *aortopulmonary window.* The aortopulmonary window is an important landmark because it is a favorite location for **enlarged lymph nodes** to appear.
• At or slightly below this level, the trachea bifurcates at the **carina** into the **right and left main bronchi.**

Main Pulmonary Artery Level (Fig. 4.8)

• At this level (it may require more than one image to see all of these structures), you should be able to identify the **main, right and left pulmonary arteries,** the **right and left main bronchi,** and the **bronchus intermedius.**
• The **left pulmonary artery** is higher than the right and appears as a direct continuation of the main pulmonary artery. The **right pulmonary artery** originates at a 90° angle to the main pulmonary artery and crosses to the right side.
• On the **right,** the **main bronchus** will appear as a circular, air-containing structure that will then become tubular as the **right upper lobe** bronchus comes into view. The **bronchus intermedius** then gives rise to the right middle and lower lobe bronchi. There should be nothing but lung tissue posterior to the bronchus intermedius. On the **left,** the **main bronchus** will appear as an air-containing circular structure.

Fig. 4.7 Aortopulmonary Window Level, Axial (A) and Coronal Views (B). (A) At this level you should be able to identify the **trachea (T)**, **ascending (AA)** and **descending aorta (DA)**, **superior vena cava (S)**, and possibly the uppermost aspect of the **left pulmonary artery (P)**. In most people, there is a space visible just under the arch of the aorta and above the pulmonary artery called the **aortopulmonary window** (*white arrow*). (B) Coronal reformatted CT enables us to also see the **right atrium (RA)**, **superior vena cava (S)**, **pulmonary artery (P)**, **left ventricle (LV)**, aortic valve (*black arrow*), **left atrial appendage** (*white arrow*), and origin of the great vessels (*white circle*).

Fig. 4.8 Main Pulmonary Artery Level (A) Mediastinal Window and (B) Lung Window. (A) At this level, you should be able to identify the **main (MPA)**, **right (RPA)**, and **left pulmonary arteries (LPA)**, the **right (RB)** and **left main bronchi (LB)**, and the **superior vena cava (S)**. The left pulmonary artery passes anterior to the **descending aorta (DA)**. The right pulmonary artery passes posterior to the **ascending aorta (AA)** and crosses to the right side. (B) Distal to the takeoff of the right upper lobe bronchus is the **bronchus intermedius (BI)**. The posterior wall of the right upper lobe bronchus is 2 to 3 mm in thickness with only aerated lung normally posterior to it (*white arrow*).

Fig. 4.9 High Cardiac Level. At this level, you should be able to identify the **left atrium (LA), right atrium (RA), aortic root (Ao)**, and **right ventricular outflow tract (RVOT)**. The **left atrium** occupies the posterior and central portion of the heart. One or more **pulmonary veins** may be seen to enter the left atrium (*white arrow*). The right atrium produces the right heart border and lies anteriorly and to the right of the left atrium. DA, Descending thoracic aorta; *LV*, Left ventricle.

Fig. 4.10. Low Cardiac Level. At this level, you should be able to identify the **right atrium (RA), right ventricle (RV), left ventricle (LV)**, and **interventricular septum (IVS)**. The right ventricle is more **heavily trabeculated** (*solid white arrow*) and has a **thinner wall** (*dotted white arrow*) than the wall of the left ventricle (*solid black arrows*). *DA*, Descending thoracic aorta.

High Cardiac Level (Fig. 4.9)

- At this level, you should be able to identify the **left atrium, right atrium, aortic root,** and **right ventricular outflow tract.**

> ### ⟩⟩ IMPORTANT POINTS
>
> - An important anatomic relationship is the relative locations of the right ventricular outflow tract (and pulmonic valve) and the aortic root, especially in congenital cardiac lesions. The **right ventricular outflow tract** lies **anterior, lateral,** and **superior** to the root of the aorta. The **P**ulmonic valve lies **A**nterior, **L**ateral and **S**uperior to the aortic valve (you can remember that relationship using the acronym "PALS").

Low Cardiac Level (Fig. 4.10)

- At this level, you should be able to identify the **right atrium, right ventricle, left ventricle,** and **interventricular septum.**
- The **right atrium** continues to form the right border of the heart. The **right ventricle** is anteriorly located, just behind the sternum, and demonstrates **more trabeculation** than the **smoother-walled left ventricle.** The left ventricle produces the left border of the heart and normally has a thicker wall than the right ventricle.
- With intravenous contrast filling the chambers, you should be able to see the **interventricular septum** between the right and left ventricles.

- When seen, the **normal pericardium** is about **2 mm thick** and is usually outlined by **mediastinal fat** outside the pericardium and **epicardial fat** on its inner surface.

USES OF CARDIAC CT

- Cardiac CT scanning is used for evaluation of the coronary arteries, the presence of **cardiac masses,** abnormalities of the aorta (including **aortic dissection**), and **pericardial diseases.**
- Cardiac CT also allows for the imaging and three-dimensional reconstruction of the **coronary arteries** and quantitative measurement of the amount of **coronary artery calcium.** The administration of intravenous contrast allows for evaluation of vessel patency with identification of thrombus in the lumen or plaque in the vessel wall.

Calcium Scoring

- **Calcium scoring** is based on the premise that the amount of calcium detectable in the coronary arteries is related to the degree of coronary atherosclerosis and that quantifying the amount of calcium may help **predict** future cardiac events related to coronary artery disease, such as **heart attack.** The scoring is usually done by calculations that combine the **amount** and **density** of calcium in the coronary arteries visualized on unenhanced CT of the heart. The **absence** of coronary artery calcification has a **high negative predictive**

Fig. 4.11 Coronary Artery Calcification and Scoring. (A) Dense calcification is seen, mostly in the left anterior descending coronary artery (*white circle*). (B) The **calcium scores** are shown superimposed on the areas of calcification. A score of zero means no calcium is detectable, which correlates with a low likelihood of a cardiac event in the near future. The higher the calcium score, the higher the risk of adverse cardiac events in the long term. Scores of 100 to 300 correlate with a mild to moderate risk of a heart attack or other cardiac events over the next 3 to 5 years. A score greater than 300 indicates the greater likelihood of severe disease and a heart attack risk, as is seen in this image.

value for significant luminal narrowing. The higher the calcium score, the greater the risk for a future cardiac event (Fig. 4.11).

- Although calcium scoring is primarily used for risk analysis of asymptomatic patients, **coronary CT angiography (CCTA)** is primarily used in patients with **acute or chronic chest pain.** Like calcium scoring, a **negative CCTA** has a **high negative predictive value** (i.e., a negative study effectively excludes obstructive coronary artery disease).
- One potential drawback to cardiac CT is the **radiation dose** delivered to the patient, which historically had been relatively high. Numerous methods are now being utilized to reduce that dose so that the procedure can now be performed at a dose well below the average annual background radiation dose.

Coronary CT Angiography: Normal Anatomy

- Coronary CT angiography (CCTA) compares favorably in accuracy with invasive (catheter) coronary angiography, long held as the reference standard in studying the coronary arteries (eVideo 4.1).
- Normal coronary artery anatomy has many variations. Only the most common branching is described here (Fig. 4.12).
- The two main coronary arteries are the **left** (also known as the left main) and the **right coronary artery.**

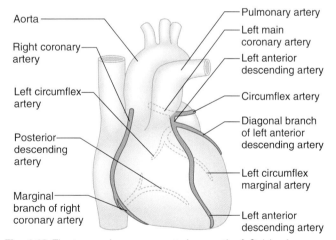

Fig. 4.12 The two main coronary arteries are the **left** (also known as the **left main**) and the **right coronary artery**. The left coronary artery divides almost at once into the **circumflex artery** and **left anterior descending artery (LAD)**. The LAD, in turn, gives rise to **diagonal branches** and **septal branches** (not shown). The circumflex artery has **marginal branches**. The **right coronary artery** courses between the right atrium and right ventricle to the inferior part of the septum. It gives rise to a large acute **marginal branch** and, in most people, the **posterior descending artery (PDA)**. The PDA supplies the inferior wall of the left ventricle and inferior part of the septum. (Revised from Bruce NH, Ray R. Cardiovascular disease. In: Kumar P, Clark M, eds. *Kumar and Clark's Clinical Medicine*, 8th ed. London: Elsevier; 2012, pg. 673.)

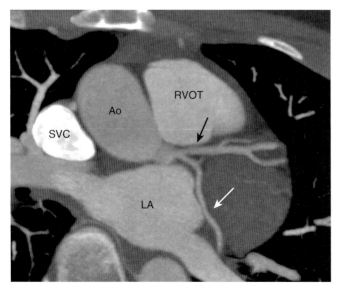

Fig. 4.13 CT Coronary Angiogram, Left Coronary Artery. The **left coronary artery (LCA)** arises from the left coronary cusp at the aortic valve. It divides almost at once into the **circumflex artery** (*white arrow*) and **left anterior descending artery (LAD)** (*black arrow*). *Ao,* Aorta; *LA,* left atrium; *RVOT,* right ventricular outflow tract; *SVC,* superior vena cava.

Fig. 4.14 CT Coronary Angiogram, Left Anterior Descending (LAD) Coronary Artery. The LAD (*white arrow*) travels in the **anterior interventricular groove** and continues to the apex of the heart. It supplies most of the left ventricle and also the AV-bundle. *Ao,* Aorta; *IVS,* interventricular septum; *LV lumen,* left ventricular lumen; *RV,* right ventricle.

- The **left coronary artery (LCA)** arises from the left coronary cusp at the aortic valve. It divides almost at once into the **circumflex artery** and **left anterior descending artery (LAD)** (Fig. 4.13). The LAD, in turn, gives rise to **diagonal branches** and **septal branches.** The **circumflex artery** has **marginal branches.**
- The LAD travels in the **anterior interventricular groove** and continues to the apex of the heart (Fig. 4.14). It supplies most of the left ventricle and also the atrioventricular (AV)-bundle, serving the anterior part of the septum with **septal branches** and the anterior wall of the left ventricle with **diagonal branches.**
- The **circumflex artery** (see Fig. 4.13) lies between the left atrium and left ventricle and supplies **obtuse marginal** vessels to the lateral wall of the left ventricle.
- The right aortic sinus gives rise to the **right coronary artery (RCA),** which courses between the right atrium and right ventricle to the inferior part of the septum (Fig. 4.15).
- In most people, the first branch of the RCA is the **conus branch** that supplies the right ventricular outflow tract. In most people, a **sinus node artery** arises as a second branch of the RCA. The next branches are **diagonals** that supply the anterior wall of the right ventricle.
- The large **acute marginal branch** supplies the lateral wall of the right ventricle and runs along the *margin* of the right ventricle above the diaphragm. The RCA continues in the AV groove posteriorly and gives off a branch to the AV node (see Fig. 4.12).
- In most people, the **posterior descending artery (PDA)** is a **branch of the RCA.** The PDA supplies the inferior wall of the left ventricle and inferior part of the septum (see Fig. 4.15).
- **Coronary artery dominance**
  - The artery that supplies the **posterior descending artery** determines **coronary artery dominance.**

- If the **posterior descending artery** is supplied by the **right coronary artery,** then the coronary circulation is said to be **right-dominant.**
- If the **posterior descending artery** is supplied by the **circumflex artery,** a branch of the left coronary artery, then the coronary circulation is called **left-dominant.**
- If the **posterior descending artery** is supplied by **both** the **right coronary artery** and the **circumflex artery,** then the coronary circulation is called **codominant.**

▶ **IMPORTANT POINTS**

- The **overwhelming majority** of the population is **right-dominant**, about 10% are left-dominant, and the remainder are codominant. A **left-dominant** coronary artery system is associated with an **increased risk of nonfatal myocardial infarction** and increased overall mortality.

- It is possible to perform an emergent CT scan that will allow for the simultaneous evaluation of **coronary artery disease, aortic dissection,** and **pulmonary thromboembolic disease,** the so-called **triple scan (triple rule-out)** for patients who

Fig. 4.15 CT Coronary Angiogram, Right Coronary Artery. The **right aortic sinus** (*black arrow*) gives rise to the **right coronary artery (RCA)** (*white arrow*), which courses between the right atrium and right ventricle to the inferior part of the septum. In most people, as here, the RCA continues to the **posterior descending artery.** *LV,* Left ventricle.

present with **acute chest pain.** Such scans have been shown to improve clinical decision making and allow for earlier discharge from the hospital.

CARDIAC MRI

- MRI can be used to obtain **anatomic** and **functional** images of the heart with a combination of ECG-gating and rapid acquisition of images. Respiratory motion, which would also contribute to blurring the image, can be reduced by having patients hold their breath for short periods of time while the images are acquired. (eVideo 4.2)
- **Cardiac MRI** can depict scarring from a myocardial infarction, perfusion of the heart, anatomic defects or masses and can assess the function of the valves and cardiac chambers.
- Cardiac MRI can be performed without intravenous contrast or with intravenous contrast (**Gadolinium: see Chapter 21**). Cardiac MRI is particularly useful in children as a way of evaluating congenital heart disease after other studies (e.g., echocardiography) produce inconclusive or conflicting information.

Normal Cardiac MRI Anatomy

- One of the benefits of MRI is that its images can be displayed in **any** plane. Besides the axial, sagittal, and coronal planes, several additional views are typically used in cardiac MRI that allow for the best visualization of the heart. They are called the **horizontal long axis** (otherwise known as the **four-chamber view**), **vertical long axis**, **short axis**, and **three-chamber views.**
- The anatomy of the heart in the **axial, sagittal, and coronal** planes is the same as that seen on CT (Fig. 4.16).
- The **horizontal long axis (four-chamber) view** resembles an axial view and is best used for evaluating the left ventricle's septal and lateral walls and apex, the right ventricular free

Fig. 4.16 Cardiac MRI, Axial, Coronal, and Sagittal Planes. These three planes produce images the same as those on CT (see **Fig. 3.12).** (A) The axial view at this level shows the **right (RV) and left ventricles (LV)** and the **descending aorta** (*arrow*). (B) This coronal image demonstrates the **right atrium** (*solid arrow*), **left ventricle (LV), aorta (Ao),** and **main pulmonary artery** (*dotted arrow*). (C) The sagittal image at this level shows the **right ventricle (RV), pulmonary artery (PA), left atrium (LA),** and **aorta (Ao).** In all of these images, the blood is depicted as "bright" (white).

Fig. 4.17 Cardiac MRI, Horizontal Long Axis View. This is another standard view of the heart with MRI called the **horizontal long axis** or **four-chamber view**. The **right (RV)** and **left ventricles (LV)** are separated by the **interventricular septum** (*solid white arrow*). Posterior to each of them are the **right atrium (RA)** and **left atrium (LA)**, separated by the regions of the **tricuspid** (*dotted white arrow*) and **mitral valves** (*solid black arrow*), respectively. *A,* Anterior; *P,* posterior.

Fig. 4.18 Cardiac MRI, Vertical Long Axis View. The **vertical long axis** or **two-chamber view** demonstrates the **left ventricle (LV)** separated from the more posterior **left atrium (LA)** by the **mitral valve area** (*black arrow*). **Pulmonary veins** drain into the left atrium (*white arrow*). The **aorta (Ao)** sits atop the **pulmonary artery (PA)**. *A,* Anterior; *P,* posterior.

wall, and for the size of the cardiac chambers. The mitral and tricuspid valves are especially well visualized in this view (Fig. 4.17).

- The **vertical long axis view** resembles a sagittal view and is best used in the evaluation of the anterior and inferior walls and apex of the left ventricle (Fig. 4.18).
- The **short axis view** depicts the left and right ventricles in a way that is useful for making **volumetric measurements** (Fig. 4.19).
  - Because MR images of the heart are already obtained with three-dimensional volumes in both end-systole and end-diastole, computer-based measurements of **ventricular mass, end-diastolic volume** and **end-systolic volume** can be made, and from them, **stroke volume** and **ejection fraction** can be calculated without intervention.
- The **three-chamber view,** which is similar to a coronal view, is particularly helpful in assessing the mitral and aortic valves, left atrial size, and the walls of the left ventricle (Fig. 4.20).
- Depending on the MRI pulse sequence used to obtain the images, **blood** can be depicted as either **black** (usually using something called a *spin echo* pulse sequence) and **most often used for anatomic evaluation** or **bright** (i.e., **white**, usually using something called a *gradient echo* pulse sequence), most often used for **functional evaluation** (Fig. 4.21).

Fig. 4.19 Cardiac MRI, Short Axis View. This is a standard view of the heart with MRI called the **short axis view**. The **right ventricle (RV)** lies anterior to the **left ventricle (LV)**, separated by the **interventricular septum** (*solid white arrow*). Note the normally thicker wall of the left ventricle (*dotted white arrow*) than the right ventricle. *A,* Anterior; *P,* posterior.

Fig. 4.20 Cardiac MRI, Three-Chamber View. The **three-chamber view** is similar to a coronal view and shows the **aorta (Ao), left ventricular outflow tract (LVOT), left ventricle (LV), left atrium (LA), pulmonary veins (PV)**, the **anteroseptal wall (ASW)**, and **inferolateral wall (ILW)** of the left ventricle (which are abnormally thickened in this person).

Fig. 4.21 Cardiac MRI, *Bright Blood* and *Black Blood* Images. With different imaging algorithms, MRI is capable of displaying the same tissues with differing appearances. (A) and (B) are both axial sections through the heart, showing the **right ventricle** (*solid white arrows*), the **left ventricle** (*dotted white arrows*), and the **aorta (Ao)**. (A) The **bright blood** technique is used to assess **cardiac function,** whereas (B) the **black blood** technique is usually better at depicting **cardiac morphology**. *A,* Anterior; *P,* posterior.

TAKE HOME POINTS

- In adults, a quick assessment of heart size can be made with the **cardiothoracic ratio**, which is the ratio of the widest transverse diameter of the heart compared with the widest internal diameter of the rib cage. In normal adults, the cardiothoracic ratio is usually less than 50%.
- The normal contours of the heart are reviewed.
- The ventricles respond to obstruction to their outflow by first undergoing hypertrophy rather than dilatation. On plain films, **cardiomegaly** is primarily produced by **ventricular enlargement.** The most marked chamber enlargement will occur from **volume overload** rather than pressure overload.
- Normal CT anatomy of the major structures is described at six levels in the chest (from top to bottom): five-vessel view, aortic arch, aortopulmonary window, main pulmonary artery, upper cardiac, and lower cardiac levels.
- **Cardiac CT** scanning uses a fast, multislice CT scanner, usually with intravenous iodinated contrast and ECG-gated acquisition to reduce motion artifact.
- Cardiac CT scanning is used to evaluate the coronary arteries, the presence of cardiac masses, abnormalities of the aorta (including aortic dissection), and pericardial diseases.
- Normal coronary artery anatomy is described. The artery that supplies the posterior descending artery determines **coronary artery dominance.** The overwhelming majority of the population is **right-dominant.**

- For patients who present with **acute chest pain**, it is possible to perform an emergent CT scan for the simultaneous evaluation of **coronary artery disease, aortic dissection,** and **pulmonary thromboembolic** disease *(triple rule-out scan).*
- MRI can be used to obtain anatomic and functional images of the heart. Cardiac MRI can show scarring from a myocardial infarction; depict perfusion of the heart, anatomic defects, or masses; and can assess the function of the valves and cardiac chambers.
- Several specific views that are typically used in cardiac MRI that allow for the best visualization of the heart are described. They are called: the **horizontal long axis** (otherwise known as the **four-chamber view**), **vertical long axis, short axis,** and **three-chamber** views.
- **Cardiac function** is usually evaluated with MRI sequences producing **bright blood** images, which are so-called because the blood is depicted with increased signal intensity.
- **Cardiac morphology** is usually evaluated with MRI sequences producing **"black blood"** images. These images allow for anatomic assessment of the cardiac structures without interference from the bright blood signal.

 More information on recognizing normal cardiac anatomy is available to registered users online.

5

Recognizing Airspace Versus Interstitial Lung Disease

We have reviewed the normal imaging anatomy of the heart and lungs in the previous two chapters. Make sure to come back to them for a brush-up whenever needed. Recognizing the difference between normal anatomy and what is abnormal is critical to your ability to make the correct diagnosis. In this chapter, we are going into the realm of the abnormal to examine the major patterns of parenchymal lung disease.

CLASSIFYING PARENCHYMAL LUNG DISEASE

- Diseases that affect the lung parenchyma **can be arbitrarily divided into two main categories** based, in part, on their **pathology** and, in part, on the **pattern** they typically produce on a chest imaging study.
  - **Airspace (alveolar) disease**
  - **Interstitial (infiltrative) disease**
- Why learn the difference?
  - Although many diseases produce abnormalities that display both patterns, recognition of these two patterns frequently helps **narrow** the disease possibilities so that you can form a reasonable **differential diagnosis** (Box 5.1).

CHARACTERISTICS OF AIRSPACE DISEASE

- Airspace disease characteristically produces opacities in the lung that can be described as **fluffy, cloudlike, or hazy.**
- The **margins of airspace disease are indistinct,** meaning it is frequently difficult to identify a clear demarcation point between the disease and the adjacent normal lung.
- These fluffy opacities also tend to be **confluent,** meaning they blend into one another with **imperceptible margins.**

BOX 5.1 Classification of Parenchymal Lung Diseases

Airspace Diseases	Interstitial Diseases
Acute	*Reticular*
Pneumonia	Pulmonary interstitial edema
Pulmonary alveolar edema	Interstitial pneumonia
Hemorrhage	Scleroderma
Aspiration	Sarcoid
Near-drowning	
	Nodular
Chronic	Bronchogenic carcinoma
Adenocarcinoma (subtype formerly called bronchoalveolar carcinoma)	Metastases
	Silicosis
Alveolar cell proteinosis	Miliary tuberculosis
Sarcoidosis	Sarcoid
Lymphoma	

- Airspace disease may be **distributed throughout the lungs,** as in pulmonary edema (Fig. 5.1), or it may **appear more localized** as in a segmental or lobar pneumonia (Fig. 5.2).

Fig. 5.1 Diffuse Airspace Disease of Pulmonary Alveolar Edema. Opacities are seen throughout both lungs, primarily involving the upper lobes, which can be described as **fluffy, hazy, or cloudlike and are confluent and poorly marginated**, all pointing to airspace disease. This is a typical example of pulmonary alveolar edema (caused by a heroin overdose in this patient).

Fig. 5.2. Right Lower Lobe Pneumonia. An area of increased opacification is seen in the right mid-lung field (*solid black arrow*) that has indistinct margins (*solid white arrow*), characteristic of airspace disease. The minor fissure (*dotted black arrow*) appears to bisect the disease, localizing this pneumonia to the **superior segment** of the **right lower lobe.** The right heart border and the right hemidiaphragm are still visible because the disease is not in anatomic contact with either of those structures.

- Airspace disease may contain **air bronchograms.**
  - The **visibility of air in the bronchus because of surrounding airspace disease** is called an *air bronchogram.*
  - An air bronchogram is almost always a **sign of airspace disease.**
    - Bronchi are **normally not visible** because their walls are **very thin,** they **contain air,** and they are **surrounded by air.** When something like fluid or soft tissue replaces the air normally surrounding the bronchus, then the air inside of the bronchus becomes visible as **a series of black, branching tubular structures**—this is called an *air bronchogram* (Fig. 5.3).
  - What can fill the airspaces besides air?
    - **Fluid,** such as occurs in pulmonary edema
    - **Blood** (e.g., pulmonary hemorrhage)
    - **Gastric juices** (e.g., aspiration)
    - **Inflammatory exudate** (e.g., pneumonia)
    - **Water** (e.g., near-drowning)

> ▶▶ **IMPORTANT POINTS**
>
> - Airspace disease may also demonstrate the *silhouette sign* (Fig. 5.4).

- The silhouette sign occurs when two objects **of the same radiographic density** (e.g., water and soft tissue) **touch each other, which results in the loss of the edge or margin between them.** It will be impossible to tell where one object begins and the other ends. **The *silhouette sign* is valuable not only in the chest but as an aid in the analysis of imaging studies throughout the body.**
- The characteristics of airspace disease are summarized in Box 5.2.

SOME CAUSES OF AIRSPACE DISEASE

- There are many causes of airspace disease, three of which will be highlighted here. Each is described in greater detail later in the text.
- **Pneumonia (see also Chapter 9)**
  - About 90% of the time, community-acquired lobar or segmental pneumonia is caused by *Streptococcus pneumoniae* (Fig. 5.5). Pneumonia usually manifests as patchy, segmental

or lobar airspace disease. Pneumonias may contain air bronchograms. **Clearing** usually occurs **in fewer than 10 days** (pneumococcal pneumonia may clear within 48 hours).

- **Pulmonary alveolar edema (see also Chapter 12)**
  - Acute, pulmonary alveolar edema classically produces **bilateral, perihilar airspace disease,** sometimes described as having a *bat-wing* or *angel-wing configuration* (Fig. 5.6).
  - It is usually **bilateral,** but may be **asymmetric.** Pulmonary edema that is **cardiac** in origin is frequently associated with **pleural effusions** and fluid that thickens the **major** and **minor fissures.**
  - Because pulmonary edema fluid fills not only the airspaces but the bronchi themselves, **no air bronchograms** are usually seen in pulmonary alveolar edema. Classically, **pulmonary edema clears rapidly** after treatment (<48 hours).
- **Aspiration (see also Chapter 9)**
  - Aspiration tends to affect whatever part of the lung is **most dependent** at the time the patient aspirates and its manifestations depend on the substance(s) aspirated. For most bedridden patients, aspiration usually occurs into either the **lower lobes** or the **posterior portions of the upper lobes.**

Fig. 5.3 Air Bronchograms Demonstrated on CT Scan. Numerous black, branching structures (*black arrows*) represent air that is now visible inside the bronchi because the surrounding airspaces are filled with inflammatory exudate in this patient with an obstructive pneumonia from a bronchogenic carcinoma.

> **BOX 5.2   Characteristics of Airspace Disease**
>
> - Produces opacities in the lung, which can be described as **fluffy, cloudlike, and hazy.**
> - The **margins** of airspace disease are fuzzy and **indistinct.**
> - The **opacities** tend to be **confluent,** merging into one another.
> - **Air bronchograms** or the **silhouette sign** may be present.

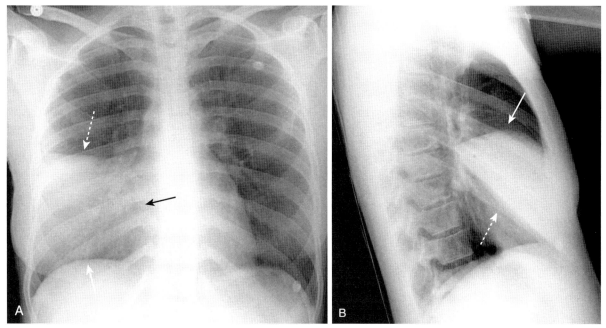

Fig. 5.4 Silhouette Sign, Right Middle Lobe Pneumonia. (A) A homogeneous area of increased density is seen to the right of the heart. It obscures the right heart border (*solid black arrow*). Called the **silhouette sign,** it establishes that the disease (1) is in contact with the right heart border (which lies anteriorly in the chest) and (2) that the disease is the same radiographic density as the heart (in this case, fluid or soft tissue). The disease does not obscure the right hemidiaphragm (*solid white arrow*). It is also bounded superiorly by the minor (horizontal) fissure (*dotted arrow*), placing it in the **right middle lobe.** (B) The area of the consolidation is indeed anterior, located in the right middle lobe, which is bounded by the major fissure below (*dotted white arrow*) and the minor fissure above (*solid white arrow*).

Fig. 5.6 Acute Pulmonary Alveolar Edema. Fluffy, bilateral, perihilar airspace disease with indistinct margins, sometimes described as having a **bat-wing** or **angel-wing** configuration, is present (*white arrows*). No air bronchograms are seen. The heart is enlarged. This represents pulmonary alveolar edema secondary to congestive heart failure.

Fig. 5.5 Right Upper Lobe Pneumococcal Pneumonia. Close-up view of the right upper lobe demonstrates confluent airspace disease with air bronchograms (*dotted white arrow*). The inferior margin of the pneumonia is more sharply demarcated because it is in contact with the minor fissure (*solid white arrow*). This patient had *Streptococcus pneumoniae* cultured from the sputum.

- Because of the course and caliber of the right main bronchus, **aspiration occurs more often in the right lower lobe** than the left lower lobe (Fig. 5.7).
- Depending on what is aspirated and whether it becomes infected determines the radiographic appearance of aspiration and how quickly the airspace disease resolves. **Aspiration of** bland (neutralized) gastric juice or **water usually clears rapidly** within 24 to 48 hours, whereas aspiration that becomes **infected** can take **weeks** to resolve.

CHARACTERISTICS OF INTERSTITIAL LUNG DISEASE

- The lung's interstitium consists of **connective tissue, lymphatics, blood vessels, and bronchi.** These are the structures that surround and support the airspaces.
- Interstitial lung disease (sometimes referred to as *infiltrative lung disease*) has the following characteristics:

> ### ⟫ IMPORTANT POINTS
>
> - Interstitial lung disease produces what can be thought of as **discrete "particles" of disease** which develop in the abundant interstitial network of the lung. These "particles" of disease can be further characterized as having three patterns of presentation (Fig. 5.8).

- **Reticular interstitial disease** appears as a network of lines (Fig. 5.8A).
- **Nodular interstitial disease** appears as an assortment of dots (Fig. 5.8B).
- **Reticulonodular interstitial disease** contains both lines and dots (Fig. 5.8C).

- These "particles" or "packets" of interstitial disease tend to be **inhomogeneous,** separated from each other by visible areas of normally aerated lung.
- The **margins of interstitial lung disease are sharper** than are the margins of airspace disease, whose boundaries tend to be indistinct.

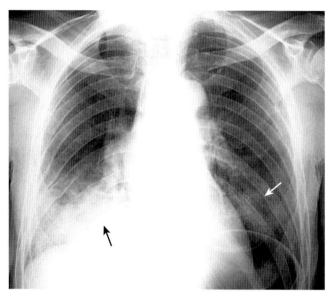

Fig. 5.7 Aspiration, Right and Left Lower Lobes. An area of opacification in the right lower lobe is fluffy and confluent with indistinct margins characteristic of airspace disease (*black arrow*). To a much lesser extent, there is a similar density in the left lower lobe (*white arrow*). The **bibasilar distribution** of this disease should raise the suspicion of aspiration as an etiology. This patient had a recent stroke and aspiration was demonstrated on a video swallowing study.

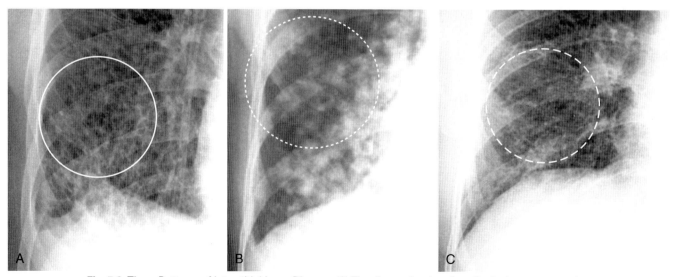

Fig. 5.8 Three Patterns of Interstitial Lung Disease. (A) The disease is primarily **reticular** in nature, consisting of crisscrossing lines (*solid white circle*). This patient had advanced sarcoidosis. (B) The disease is predominantly **nodular** (*dotted white circle*). The patient was known to have thyroid carcinoma, and these nodules represent innumerable, small metastatic foci in the lungs. (C) **Reticulonodular** interstitial disease of the lung. Most interstitial diseases of the lung have a mixture of both a reticular (lines) and nodular (dots) pattern, as does this case, which is a close-up view of the right lower lobe in another patient with sarcoidosis (*dashed white circle*).

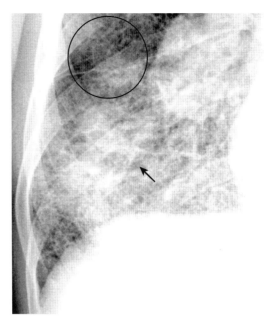

Fig. 5.10 The Edge of the Lesion. Notice how a portion of this disease appears confluent, like airspace disease, because of the superimposition of all of the tissues of the lung upon each other (*black arrow*). Always look at the peripheral margins of parenchymal lung disease to best determine the nature of the "packets" of abnormality. At the periphery of this disease (*black circle*), this is more clearly seen to be reticular and interstitial, not airspace disease.

Fig. 5.9 Varicella Pneumonia. Innumerable calcified granulomas, which occur in the lung interstitium, are seen here as small, discrete, nodules in the right lung (*white circles*). This patient had a history of varicella (chicken pox) pneumonia years earlier. Varicella pneumonia heals with multiple small calcified granulomas remaining.

- Interstitial lung disease **can be focal** (as in a solitary pulmonary nodule) **or diffusely distributed** in the lungs (Fig. 5.9).
- **Usually no air bronchograms are present,** as there may be with airspace disease.

! DIAGNOSTIC PITFALLS

- Sometimes, so much interstitial disease is present that the overlapping elements of disease may **superimpose** and mimic airspace disease on conventional chest radiographs. Superimposition of all of the lung's content on radiographs may make the tiny packets of interstitial disease seem **coalescent** and more like airspace disease.
- **Solutions:** Look at the **periphery** of such confluent shadows in the lung to help in determining whether they are, in fact, caused by airspace disease or a superimposition of numerous reticular and nodular densities (Fig. 5.10).
- Obtain a CT scan of the chest for even better characterization of the disease.

BOX 5.3   Characteristics of Interstitial Lung Disease

- Interstitial lung disease has discrete **reticular, nodular, or reticulonodular** patterns.
- "Packets" of disease are separated by normal-appearing, aerated lung.
- Margins of "packets" of interstitial disease are usually **sharp and discrete.**
- Disease may be **focal** or **diffusely distributed** in the lungs.
- Usually, **no air bronchograms** are present.

» IMPORTANT POINTS

- Keep in mind that **many diseases have patterns that overlap and many interstitial lung diseases have mixtures of both reticular and nodular changes (i.e., reticulonodular disease).**

- The characteristics of interstitial lung disease are summarized in Box 5.3.

SOME CAUSES OF INTERSTITIAL LUNG DISEASE

- Just as with the airspace pattern, many diseases produce an interstitial pattern in the lung. Several will be discussed briefly here. They are roughly divided into those diseases that are predominantly **reticular** and those that are predominantly **nodular.**

Predominantly Reticular Interstitial Lung Diseases

- **Pulmonary interstitial edema**
  - Pulmonary interstitial edema can occur because of increased capillary **pressure** (congestive heart failure), increased capillary **permeability** (allergic reactions), or decreased fluid **absorption** (lymphangitic blockade from metastatic disease).
  - Considered the precursor of alveolar edema, pulmonary interstitial edema classically manifests **four key radiologic findings: fluid in the fissures (major and minor),**

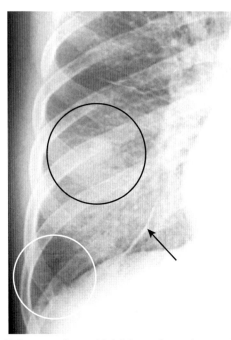

Fig. 5.11 Pulmonary Interstitial Edema Secondary to Congestive Heart Failure. A close-up view of the right lung shows an accentuation of the pulmonary interstitial markings (*black circle*). [The nodular density in the center of the circle is the superimposed nipple.] There are multiple Kerley B lines (*white circle*) representing fluid in thickened interlobular septa. Fluid is seen in the inferior accessory fissure (*black arrow*).

Fig. 5.12 Usual Interstitial Pneumonia (UIP). An axial CT scan of the chest shows abnormalities at the lung bases, in a subpleural location, the typical distribution for UIP. There are small cystic spaces called **honeycombing** (*white ovals*) with evidence of **bronchiectasis**, as manifest by thickened bronchial walls (*dotted white arrows*).

Fig. 5.13 Nonspecific Interstitial Pneumonia (NSIP). A **ground-glass opacity** is seen in a subpleural location on the right (*white circle*). Ground-glass opacities are nonspecific abnormal areas of the lung that have increased attenuation (are whiter) in which the vascular markings and bronchi mostly appear intact. They can be associated with both benign and malignant diseases. Also present is bronchiectasis in both lungs (*white arrows*). The patient was known to have scleroderma.

peribronchial cuffing (from fluid in the walls of bronchioles), pleural effusions, and Kerley B lines (Fig. 5.11).

- Classically, patients may have **few physical findings** in the lungs (rales) even though their chest radiograph demonstrates considerable pulmonary interstitial edema, because almost all of the fluid is in the interstitium of the lung, rather than in the airspaces.
- With appropriate therapy, pulmonary interstitial edema usually clears rapidly (<48 hours).
- **Interstitial pneumonia**
  - There are many forms of interstitial pneumonia, the most common being **usual interstitial pneumonia.** Another form, called **nonspecific interstitial pneumonia** is a pattern of disease that does not fall easily into any of the other categories.
  - **Usual interstitial pneumonia (UIP)**
    - UIP is sometimes used to mean *idiopathic interstitial fibrosis.* UIP is more **common in older men** and has associations with **cigarette smoking** and **gastroesophageal reflux.**
    - Chest radiographs may be **normal** in UIP. The earliest manifestation on chest radiographs consists of a **fine reticular pattern, particularly at the lung bases.** The pattern then becomes coarser as the disease progresses and ends with a pattern that, for obvious reasons, is called **honeycomb lung** (other diseases also produce the honeycomb pattern). There may also be **progressive volume loss.**
    - Imaging diagnosis is made on CT scans of the chest where **honeycombing, subpleural reticular opacities** and **traction bronchiectasis** are present, especially at the lung bases (Fig. 5.12).

- **Idiopathic pulmonary fibrosis** is considered the end-stage disease along the spectrum of these interstitial pneumonias.
- **Nonspecific interstitial fibrosis (NSIP)**
  - NSIP is a pattern of lung injury that is seen in a large percentage of patients with **connective tissue diseases,** such as **scleroderma,** who have pulmonary findings.
  - Patients with a pattern of NSIP, in general, have a **better prognosis** than patients with UIP.
  - Imaging diagnosis is made on CT scans of the chest where basilar "**ground-glass**" opacities are present and **traction bronchiectasis** is seen in advanced cases (Fig. 5.13).
- **Lymphangitic carcinoma (see "Metastases to the lung" in next section)**

Fig. 5.14 **Adenocarcinoma, Right Upper Lobe.** A mass is seen in the right upper lobe (*white arrow*). Its margin is slightly indistinct along the superolateral border (*black arrow*). CT scan of the chest confirmed the presence of the mass and also demonstrated paratracheal and right hilar adenopathy. The mass was biopsied and was an adenocarcinoma, primary to the lung. Adenocarcinoma of the lung most commonly presents as a peripheral nodule.

Predominantly Nodular Interstitial Diseases

- **Bronchogenic carcinoma (see Chapter 11)**
  - The four major cell types of bronchogenic carcinoma are **adenocarcinoma, squamous cell carcinoma,** and **small cell** and **large cell carcinoma.**
  - Adenocarcinomas, in particular, can present as a **solitary peripheral pulmonary nodule.**
  - As a rule, on conventional chest radiographs, nodules or masses in the lung are more **discrete** than airspace disease, producing a relatively clear demarcation between the nodule and the surrounding normal lung tissue.
  - CT scans may demonstrate **spiculation** or **irregularity** of the lung nodule itself that may not be apparent on conventional radiographs (Fig. 5.14).
- **Metastases to the lung**
  - Metastases to the lung can be divided into three categories depending on the pattern of disease demonstrated in the lung.
  - **Hematogenous metastases** arrive via the bloodstream and usually produce two or more **nodules** in the lungs that, when they achieve a large size, are sometimes called *cannonball metastases.* Primary tumors that classically produce nodular metastases in the lung include **breast, colorectal, renal cell, bladder and testicular, head and neck carcinomas, soft-tissue sarcomas,** and **malignant melanoma** (Fig. 5.15A).
  - The second form of tumor dissemination is **lymphangitic spread.** The pathogenesis of lymphangitic spread to the lungs is somewhat controversial, but most likely involves blood-borne spread to the pulmonary capillaries and then invasion of adjacent lymphatics. An alternative means of lymphangitic spread is obstruction of central lymphatics, usually in the hila, with retrograde dissemination through the lymphatics in the lung.
    - Regardless of the mode of transmission, lymphangitic spread to the lung tends to **resemble pulmonary interstitial edema from congestive heart failure** except, unlike congestive heart failure, it tends to be **localized to a lung segment or involve only one lung.**

Fig. 5.15 Metastases to the Lung, CT Scans. (A) Multiple **discrete nodules of varying size** appear throughout both lungs (*white arrows*). The diagnosis of exclusion is metastatic disease whenever multiple nodules are found in the lungs. In this case, the metastases were from colon carcinoma. (B) The interstitial markings in the right lung are prominent (*black oval*), there are thickened septal lines (*white oval*), fluid in the fissure (*white arrow*), and lymphadenopathy (*solid black arrow*) representing **lymphangitic spread of a bronchogenic carcinoma.** (C) In this case, the lung cancer has grown through the chest wall (*white arrow*) and invaded it by direct extension. The pleura usually serves as a strong barrier to the direct spread of tumor.

- Findings include **Kerley lines, fluid in the fissures, and pleural effusions** (Fig. 5.15B).
- Primary tumors that classically produce the lymphangitic pattern of metastases in the lung include **breast, lung, stomach, pancreatic, and, infrequently, prostate carcinoma.**
- **Direct extension** is the least common form of tumor spread involving the lungs because the **pleura** is surprisingly **resistant to the spread of malignancy** through direct violation of its layers. Direct extension would most likely produce a **localized subpleural mass** in the lung, frequently with **adjacent rib destruction** (Fig. 5.15C).

Mixed Reticular and Nodular Interstitial Disease (Reticulonodular Disease)

- **Sarcoidosis**
  - In addition to the **bilateral hilar** and **right paratracheal adenopathy** characteristic of this disease, about half of patients with thoracic sarcoid also demonstrate **interstitial lung disease.** The interstitial lung disease is frequently a mixture of both **reticular** and **nodular** components.
  - A progression of disease in sarcoid tends to start with adenopathy (**Stage I**), proceed to a combination of both interstitial lung disease and adenopathy (**Stage II**), and then progress to a stage in which the adenopathy regresses whereas the interstitial lung disease remains (**Stage III**).
  - Most patients with parenchymal lung disease from sarcoidosis will undergo complete resolution of the disease (Fig. 5.16).

Mixed Airspace and Interstitial Disease

- Not all diseases follow the rule of producing **either** airspace **or** interstitial disease. Some produce a mixture of **both** at the same time or may initially present as airspace disease followed in time by interstitial disease. **Tuberculosis** is one such disease.

Tuberculosis

- Up to a third of the world's population is believed to have been infected with *Mycobacterium tuberculosis* (TB). Although the incidence of TB is decreasing in the United States, it has been increasing in developing countries. Most infections cause no symptoms but about one in ten go on to active tuberculosis.

Primary Pulmonary Tuberculosis

- Relatively few patients with primary TB have clinical manifestations. The **upper lobes** are affected slightly more than the lower. Classical manifestations include **lobar pneumonia** (Fig. 5.17), especially with associated **adenopathy**, unilateral **hilar or mediastinal adenopathy without parenchymal disease** (more common in children), and **large and typically asymptomatic pleural effusions** (more common in adults) (Fig. 5.18). **Cavitation is rare.**

Postprimary Tuberculosis ("Reactivation TB")

- Most cases of TB in adults occur as reactivation of a primary focus of infection acquired in childhood. The infection is limited mainly to the **apical and posterior segments of the upper lobes and the superior segments of the lower lobes.** **Caseous necrosis** and the **tubercle** (accumulations of mononuclear macrophages, Langerhans giant cells surrounded by lymphocytes and fibroblasts) are the pathologic hallmarks of post-primary TB.
- **Healing** typically occurs with **fibrosis** and **contraction.**

Patterns of Distribution of Postprimary Tuberculosis

- Bilateral upper lobe **cavitary disease** is very common. The cavity is usually **thin walled, smooth on the inner margin, and contains no air-fluid level** (Fig. 5.19).
- It may present as **pneumonia.**
- **Transbronchial spread** may occur from one upper lobe to the **opposite** lower lobe or to another lobe in either lung (Fig. 5.20).
- **Bronchiectasis:** usually asymptomatic (Fig. 5.21).

Fig. 5.16 Sarcoidosis. A frontal radiograph of the chest reveals bilateral hilar (*solid black arrows*) and right paratracheal adenopathy (*dotted black arrow*), a classic distribution for the adenopathy in sarcoidosis. In addition, the patient has diffuse, bilateral interstitial lung disease (*black circle*) that is **reticulonodular** in nature. In some patients with this stage of disease, the adenopathy regresses while the interstitial disease remains.

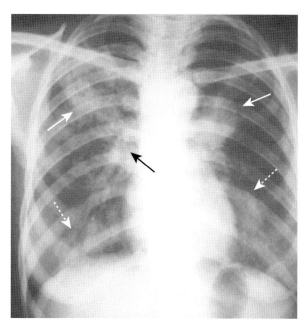

Fig. 5.17 Primary Tuberculosis. The prominence seen of the right hilum is caused by adenopathy (*solid black arrow*). Unilateral hilar adenopathy may be the only manifestation of primary infection with *Mycobacterium tuberculosis,* especially in children. When it produces pneumonia, primary TB affects the upper lobes (*solid white arrows*) slightly more than the lower (*dotted white arrows*).

Fig. 5.18 Tuberculous Effusion. A large, left pleural effusion is present (*white arrow*). Tuberculous effusions are **exudates** that can occur in either primary or postprimary forms of the disease but are **more common in the primary form.** They are usually **unilateral** and have a tendency to loculate **(see Chapter 8).** They may grow large, as in this case, while the patient is still relatively symptom-free.

Fig. 5.19 Postprimary Tuberculous Cavity. There is a thin-walled upper lobe cavity with no air-fluid level (*white arrow*). The characteristics are consistent with tuberculosis. In the presence of a cavity, activity is best excluded on a **clinical basis.** This patient had clinical findings of active tuberculosis.

Fig. 5.20 Postprimary TB With Transbronchial Spread. Pneumonia is seen in both upper lobes (*solid white arrows*). Numerous lucencies (cavities) are seen in the airspace disease in both upper lobes (especially, *solid black arrow* on the left). **A cavitary upper lobe pneumonia is presumptively TB**, until proved otherwise. In addition, there is airspace disease in the lingula (*dotted white arrow*), another finding suggestive of TB, a disease that can spread via a **transbronchial route** to the opposite lower lobe or another lobe in the same lung.

Fig. 5.21 Tuberculous Bronchiectasis. Bronchiectasis secondary to tuberculosis, both primary and postprimary, is relatively common. It may occur as a result of endobronchial infection or adjacent fibrosis *(traction bronchiectasis)*. The apical and posterior segments of the upper lobes are the most common sites. Multiple, small cystic structures creating an appearance that resembles a *honeycomb* may be seen (*white circle*).

Fig. 5.22 Miliary Tuberculosis. Innumerable small, round nodules are present in this axial CT scan of the chest in a patient with miliary tuberculosis (*white circle*). At the start of the disease, the nodules are so small they are frequently difficult to detect on conventional radiographs. When they reach about 1 mm or more in size, they begin to become visible. Miliary tuberculosis represents the widespread hematogenous dissemination of the tubercle bacillus.

- Bronchostenosis due to fibrosis and stricture. Fibrosis may cause distortion of a bronchus and atelectasis many years after the initial infection, producing what is called **"middle lobe syndrome."**
- Solitary pulmonary nodules—the **tuberculoma**—may occur in either primary or postprimary disease. These **round** or **oval** lesions are frequently associated with small, discrete shadows in the immediate vicinity of the lesion, which are called **satellite** lesions.
- Formation of a **pleural effusion in postprimary TB** almost always means direct spread of the disease into the pleural cavity and should be regarded as an **empyema**, which carries a **graver prognosis** than the pleural effusion of the **primary form.**

Miliary Tuberculosis

- The onset of miliary TB is insidious. **Fever, chills, and night sweats are common.** It may take weeks between the time of dissemination and the radiographic appearance of disease. Miliary TB may occur as a manifestation of **either primary TB** or **postprimary TB**, although the clinical appearance of miliary TB may not occur for many years after the initial infection.
- When first visible, the miliary nodules **measure about 1 mm in size**; they can grow to 2 to 3 mm if left untreated. When treated, clearing is rapid. **Miliary TB seldom, if ever, heals with calcifications** (Fig. 5.22).

⌂ TAKE HOME POINTS

- Parenchymal lung disease can be divided into **airspace (alveolar)** and **interstitial (infiltrative)** patterns.
- Recognizing the pattern of disease can help in reaching the correct diagnosis.
- Characteristics of **airspace disease** include fluffy, confluent densities that are indistinctly marginated and may demonstrate air bronchograms.
- An **air bronchogram** is typically a sign of airspace disease; it occurs when something other than air (e.g., inflammatory exudate or blood) surrounds the bronchus allowing the air inside the bronchus to become visible.
- When two objects of the **same** radiographic density are in **contact** with each other, the normal edge or margin between them will disappear. The loss of the margin between these two objects is called the **silhouette sign,** which is useful throughout radiology in identifying either the **location** or the **radiographic density** of the abnormality in question.

- Examples of airspace disease include pulmonary alveolar edema, pneumonia, and aspiration.
- Characteristics of **interstitial lung disease** include discrete "particles" or "packets" of disease with distinct margins that tend to occur in a pattern of **lines (reticular), dots (nodular)** or, very frequently, a combination of **lines and dots (reticulonodular).**
- Examples of interstitial lung disease include pulmonary interstitial edema, interstitial pneumonia, bronchogenic carcinoma, metastases to the lung, pulmonary fibrosis, and sarcoidosis.
- **Tuberculosis** is an example of a disease process that can demonstrate both airspace and interstitial lung patterns.

 More information on recognizing airspace versus interstitial lung disease is available to registered users online.

6

Recognizing the Causes of an Opacified Hemithorax

- Mrs. Smith, a 66-year-old female, comes into the emergency department with increasing shortness of breath. This is her frontal chest radiograph (Fig. 6.1). Would your preliminary recommendation be bronchoscopy for **atelectasis,** thoracentesis for a large **pleural effusion,** or a course of antibiotics for her extensive **pneumonia?**
  - To be able to treat her correctly, you have to determine the cause of the opacification and the answer to that question is demonstrated on the radiograph if you know how to approach the problem.
- **The three major causes of an opacified hemithorax** (plus one other that is less common) are:
  - **Atelectasis of the entire lung**
  - **A very large pleural effusion**
  - **Pneumonia of an entire lung**
  - And a fourth cause:
    - Pneumonectomy: removal of an entire lung

ATELECTASIS OF THE ENTIRE LUNG

- **Atelectasis of an entire lung** usually results from **complete obstruction of the right or left main bronchus.** With bronchial obstruction, no air can enter the lung. The remaining air in the lung is absorbed into the bloodstream through the pulmonary capillary system. This leads to **loss of volume** of the affected lung.
- In an older individual, atelectasis might be caused by an **obstructing neoplasm,** like a bronchogenic carcinoma. In younger individuals, **asthma** may produce **mucous plugs** that

obstruct the bronchi. A **foreign body** may be aspirated (in children, peanuts are a frequent culprit) that also leads to bronchial obstruction. Critically ill patients also develop atelectasis from **mucous plugs**.

- In **obstructive atelectasis,** even though there is volume loss within the affected lung, **the visceral and parietal pleura almost never separate from each other.** That is an important fact about atelectasis, and it is sometimes confusing to beginners who try to picture **atelectasis** and a **pneumothorax** as both producing collapse of a lung without understanding why they look completely different radiographically (Fig. 6.2 and Table 6.1).

Fig. 6.2 Obstructive Atelectasis Versus a Pneumothorax: Two Different Causes of Lung Collapse and the Difference in Their Radiologic Appearance. (A) There is **atelectasis** of the entire right lung (*solid black arrow*) from an obstructing endobronchial lesion. The **visceral and parietal pleura remain in contact** with each other. Other mobile structures in the mediastinum, such as the trachea and right main bronchus (*dotted black arrows*), shift toward the atelectasis. The left lung over-expands and crosses the midline (*solid white arrow*). (B) This patient has a large right-sided **pneumothorax.** Air (*solid white arrow*) interposes between the visceral (*dotted white arrows*) and parietal pleura, causing the lung to undergo passive atelectasis (*solid black arrow*). There is a chest tube in the right hemithorax (*arrowhead*) that had been removed from suction.

Fig. 6.1 This is the frontal chest radiograph of Mrs. Smith. Would your preliminary recommendation be bronchoscopy for **atelectasis,** thoracentesis for a large **pleural effusion,** or a course of antibiotics for her extensive **pneumonia?** The answer can be found on the image (and in this chapter).

TABLE 6.1   Pneumothorax Versus Obstructive Atelectasis

Feature	Pneumothorax	Obstructive Atelectasis
Pleural space	Air in the pleural space **separates** the visceral from the parietal pleura.	The visceral and parietal pleura **do not separate** from each other.
Density	The pneumothorax itself will appear "black" (air density). The hemithorax may appear more lucent than normal.	Atelectasis is the absence of air in the lung. The hemithorax will appear more opaque ("whiter") than normal.
Shift	There is **never** a shift of the heart or trachea **toward** the side of a pneumothorax.	There is almost **always** a shift of the heart and trachea **toward** the side of the atelectasis.

TABLE 6.2   Recognizing a "Shift" in Atelectasis/Pneumonectomy

Structure	Normal Position	Right-Sided Atelectasis or Pneumonectomy	Left-Sided Atelectasis or Pneumonectomy
Heart	Midline	Heart moves rightward; left heart border may come to lie near left side of spine	Heart moves leftward; right heart border overlaps the spine
Trachea	Midline	Shifts toward right	Shifts toward left
Hemidiaphragm	Right slightly higher than left	Right hemidiaphragm moves upward and may disappear (silhouette sign)	Left hemidiaphragm moves upward and may disappear (silhouette sign)

- Because the visceral and parietal pleura **do not separate** from each other in atelectasis, mobile structures in the thorax are **"pulled toward"** the side of the atelectasis producing a *shift* (movement) of these mobile thoracic structures **toward the side of opacification.**
- The most visible mobile structures in the thorax are the **heart,** the **trachea,** and the **hemidiaphragms. In obstructive atelectasis,** one or all of these structures will **shift toward the side of opacification (toward side of volume loss)** (Fig. 6.3).
- Table 6.2 summarizes the movement of the mobile structures in the thorax in patients with obstructive atelectasis.

MASSIVE PLEURAL EFFUSION

- If fluid, whether blood, an exudate or a transudate, fills the pleural space so as to opacify almost the entire hemithorax, then the **fluid may act like a mass** compressing the underlying lung tissue. A pleural effusion compresses the lung beneath it, but that finding is usually not visible on conventional chest radiographs.

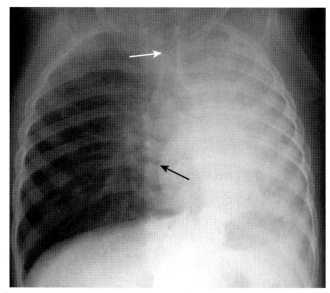

Fig. 6.3 Atelectasis. Frontal chest radiograph shows opacification of the entire left hemithorax. There is a shift of the heart toward the left such that the right heart border no longer projects to the right of the spine. The heart now overlies the spine (*black arrow*). The trachea (*white arrow*) has moved leftward from the midline **toward** the side of the opacification. These findings are characteristic of volume loss from atelectasis of the entire lung. The child had asthma. Bronchoscopy was performed and a large mucous plug that was obstructing the left main bronchus was removed.

▶ IMPORTANT POINTS

- When enough pleural fluid accumulates, the **large effusion "pushes" mobile structures away** and the heart and trachea **shift away from the side of opacification** (Fig. 6.4).

- Massive pleural effusions are frequently the result of malignancy, either in the form of a **bronchogenic carcinoma** or secondary to **metastases to the pleura** from a distant organ. Trauma can produce a **hemothorax** and **tuberculosis** is notorious for causing large, clinically silent effusions (see Fig. 5.18). The effusions from **congestive heart failure,** although very common, are most often *bilateral (but asymmetric)* and they **rarely** grow large enough to **occupy an entire hemithorax.**

! DIAGNOSTIC PITFALLS

- At times, there may be a perfect **balance** between the **push** of a large malignant effusion and the **volume loss** caused by underlying obstructive atelectasis secondary to the malignancy itself.
- In an adult patient with an **opacified hemithorax, no air bronchograms,** and **little or no shift** of the mobile thoracic structures, it is important to suspect an **obstructing bronchogenic carcinoma,** perhaps with metastases to the pleura. A CT scan of the chest will reveal the abnormalities (Fig. 6.5).

- Table 6.3 summarizes the movement of the mobile structures in the thorax in patients with a large pleural effusion.

Fig. 6.4 Large Pleural Effusion. There is complete opacification of the right hemithorax. The trachea is deviated to the left (*black arrow*) and the apex of the heart is also displaced to the left, close to the lateral chest wall (*white arrow*). These findings are characteristic of a **large pleural effusion** that is producing a mass effect. Almost two liters of serosanguinous fluid were removed at thoracentesis. The fluid contained malignant cells from a primary bronchogenic carcinoma.

Fig. 6.5 Effusion and Atelectasis in Balance. There is a balance between a large **pleural effusion** (E) and **atelectasis** of the right lung (*black arrow*) so that there is **no significant resultant shift** of the mobile midline structures. The heart essentially remains in its normal position (*white arrow*). This combination of findings is highly suggestive of a central bronchogenic malignancy with a malignant effusion.

TABLE 6.3	Recognizing a "Shift" in Pleural Effusion		
Structure	**Normal Position**	**Right-Sided Effusion**	**Left-Sided Effusion**
Heart	Midline	Heart moves leftward; apex may lie near the left lateral chest wall	Heart moves rightward; more of heart protrudes to right of spine
Trachea	Midline	Shifts toward left	Shifts toward right
Hemidiaphragm	Right higher than left	Right hemidiaphragm disappears on chest radiograph (silhouette sign)	Left hemidiaphragm disappears on chest radiograph (silhouette sign)

TABLE 6.4	Recognizing a "Shift" in Pneumonia		
Structure	Normal Position	Right-Sided Pneumonia	Left-Sided Pneumonia
Heart	Midline	There is usually no shift of the heart from its normal position	There is usually no shift of the heart from its normal position
Trachea	Midline	Midline	Midline
Hemidiaphragm	Right higher than left	Right hemidiaphragm may disappear on chest radiograph (silhouette sign)	Left hemidiaphragm may disappear on chest radiograph (silhouette sign)

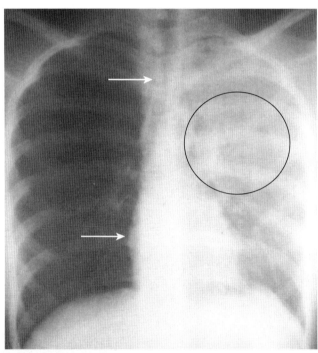

Fig. 6.6 Pneumonia of the Left Upper Lobe. There is near-complete opacification of the left hemithorax with **no shift** of the heart and little shift of the trachea (*white arrows*). There are air bronchograms suggested within the upper area of opacification (*circle*). These findings suggest a pneumonia rather than atelectasis or pleural effusion. The patient had *Streptococcus pneumoniae* present in the sputum and improved quickly on antibiotics.

Fig. 6.7 Postpneumonectomy Right Hemithorax, Day 1. This postoperative radiograph was obtained less than 24 hours after this patient underwent a pneumonectomy on the right side for a bronchogenic carcinoma. There are surgical clips in the region of the right hilum (*black arrows*) and the right fifth rib has been surgically removed in order to perform the pneumonectomy. Over the next several weeks, the **right hemithorax will fill with fluid** followed by a gradual shift of the heart and mediastinal structures **toward** the side of the pneumonectomy.

PNEUMONIA OF AN ENTIRE LUNG

- With pneumonia, inflammatory exudate fills the air spaces causing consolidation and opacification of the lung.

> **IMPORTANT POINTS**
>
> - The hemithorax becomes opaque because the lung no longer contains air, but there is **neither a pull toward** the side of the pneumonia by volume loss **nor a push** away from the side of the pneumonia by a large effusion. There is **no shift of the heart or trachea.**

- **Air bronchograms** may be present (Fig. 6.6).
- Table 6.4 summarizes the movement of the mobile structures in the thorax in patients with pneumonia of the entire lung.

POSTPNEUMONECTOMY

- Pneumonectomy means the removal of an entire lung.
- For this procedure to be performed, e**ither the fifth or sixth rib on the affected side is almost always removed.** In most cases, **metallic surgical clips will be visible in the region of the hilum** on the pneumonectomized side.
- For about 24 hours after the surgery, only air occupies the hemithorax from which the lung has been removed (Fig. 6.7).
- Over the course of the next 2 weeks, the hemithorax gradually **fills with fluid.**
- By about 4 months after surgery, the pneumonectomized hemithorax should be **completely opaque.**
- Eventually, **fibrous tissue forms in the pneumonectomized hemithorax** and, in most patients, the **entire hemithorax is forever completely opaque.** The heart and trachea shift **toward** the side of opacification.

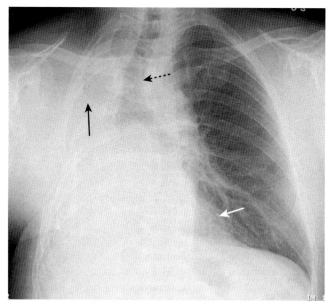

Fig. 6.8 One Year After Pneumonectomy. There is complete opacification of the right hemithorax. The right fifth rib (*solid black arrow*) is surgically absent. The heart (*solid white arrow*) and trachea (*dotted black arrow*) are deviated **toward** the side of opacification. These signs are characteristic of **volume loss**. The surgery had been performed one year earlier for a bronchogenic carcinoma. The fluid which gradually filled the right hemithorax immediately following the pneumonectomy has probably fibrosed leading to a permanent shift toward the pneumonectomized side.

Fig. 6.9 Mrs. Smith's Frontal Chest Radiograph. There is opacification of the entire left hemithorax. There is also a shift of the trachea **away** from the side opacified toward the right (*solid black arrow*) and the heart is displaced to the right as well (*dotted black arrow*). Both of these mobile structures have moved **away** from the side of opacification. These signs are characteristic of a **very large plural effusion**. Given its size and unilateral, left-sided location, an underlying malignancy was suspected. Thoracentesis revealed malignant cells from a left-sided bronchogenic carcinoma.

- The chest examination looks **identical** to that of a patient with atelectasis of the entire lung. To tell the difference, look for the missing 5th or 6th rib and for the surgical clips in the hilum to indicate a pneumonectomy has been performed (Fig. 6.8).
- Return to the frontal radiograph of Mrs. Smith with the opacified hemithorax, who has been waiting patiently in the emergency department while you finished reading this chapter.
  - Now, how would you proceed with her abnormality?

- You will notice a shift of the heart and trachea away from the side of opacification (Fig. 6.9). This is characteristic of a very large pleural effusion. Because of her age (66), an underlying malignancy should be suspected.
- Mrs. Smith had a CT scan performed that showed the large effusion and multiple pleural metastases from a bronchogenic carcinoma. She subsequently underwent bronchoscopy and a squamous cell carcinoma of her bronchus was found.

🏠 TAKE HOME POINTS

- The differential possibilities for an opacified hemithorax should include atelectasis of the entire lung, a very **large pleural effusion, pneumonia of the entire lung, or postpneumonectomy.**
- The trachea, heart and hemidiaphragms are mobile structures that have the capability of moving **(shifting)** if there is either something pushing on them or something pulling them.
- With **atelectasis,** there is a shift **toward** the side of the opacified hemithorax because of volume loss in the affected lung.
- With a **large pleural effusion**, there is a shift **away** from the side of opacification because the large pleural effusion can act as if it were a mass.

- With **pneumonia** of most or the entire lung, there is usually **no shift**, but air bronchograms may be present.
- Occasionally, the shift of a malignant effusion may be balanced by the opposite shift of atelectasis caused by an underlying, obstructing bronchogenic carcinoma, so that the hemithorax will be completely opaque but there will be no shift of the midline structures.
- In the **postpneumonectomy** patient, there is eventually volume loss on the side from which the lung has been removed, and the clues to such surgery may include surgical **absence of the 5th or 6th rib** on the affected side or **metallic surgical clips** in the hilum.

 More information on differentiating the causes of an opacified hemithorax is available to registered users online.

Recognizing Atelectasis

WHAT IS ATELECTASIS?

- Common to all forms of atelectasis is a **loss of volume in some or all of the lung, usually leading to increased density of the lung involved.**
  - The lung normally appears "black" on a chest radiograph because it contains air. When something of fluid or soft-tissue density is substituted for that air or when the air in the lung is resorbed (as it can be in atelectasis), that part of the lung becomes **whiter (more dense or more opaque).**
- Unless mentioned otherwise, statements in this chapter that refer to "atelectasis" are referring to *obstructive atelectasis.* This might be a good time to review the chart from *Chapter 6: Recognizing the Causes of an Opacified Hemithorax* (see Table 6.1) highlighting the markedly different appearances of a large pneumothorax versus atelectasis of the entire lung (see Fig. 6.2).

SIGNS OF ATELECTASIS

- **Displacement (shift) of the interlobar fissures** (major and minor) **toward** the area of atelectasis.
- **Increase in the density of the affected lung** (Fig. 7.1).
- **Displacement (shift) of the mobile structures of the thorax.** The **mobile structures** are those capable of movement due to changes in lung volume. They include:
  - **Trachea**
    - **Normally midline in location** and centered on the spinous processes of the vertebral bodies (also midline structures) on a nonrotated, frontal chest x-ray There is always a **slight rightward deviation** of a portion of the trachea at the site of the **left-sided aortic knob.**
  - With atelectasis, especially of the upper lobes, the trachea may shift **toward** the side of the volume loss (Fig. 7.2).

Fig. 7.1 Right Middle Lobe Atelectasis. Frontal (A) and lateral (B) views of the chest show an area of increased density (*solid white arrow*), which is silhouetting the normal right heart border (*solid black arrow*) indicating its anterior location in the right middle lobe. On the lateral view (B), the minor fissure is displaced downward (*dotted white arrow*) and the major fissure is displaced slightly upward (*dotted black arrow*).

Fig. 7.2 Right Upper Lobe Atelectasis. A fan-shaped area of increased density is seen on the frontal projection (A) representing the airless right upper lobe. The minor fissure is displaced upward (*white arrow*). The trachea is shifted to the right (*black arrow*). The lateral view (B) demonstrates a similar wedge-shaped density near the apex of the lung. There is a band-like density formed by the atelectatic upper lobe (*black* and *white arrows*). This is a child with asthma that led to formation of a mucous plug obstructing the right upper lobe bronchus.

Fig. 7.3 Atelectasis of the Left Lung. There is complete opacification of the left hemithorax with shift of the trachea (*solid black arrow*) and the esophagus (marked here by a nasogastric tube) (*dotted black arrow*) toward the side of the atelectasis. The right heart border, which should project about a centimeter to the right of the spine, has been pulled to the left side and is no longer visible. The heart itself is not visible because it is no longer bordered by an air-filled lung. The patient had an obstructing bronchogenic carcinoma in the left main bronchus.

Fig. 7.4 Atelectasis of the Right Lung. There is complete opacification of the right hemithorax with a shift of the trachea (*black arrow*) toward the side of the atelectasis. The left heart border is displaced far to the right and now almost overlaps the spine (*white arrow*). This patient had an endobronchial metastasis in the right main bronchus from her left-sided breast cancer. Did you notice the left breast was surgically absent?

- **Heart**
  - **At least 1 cm of the right heart border normally projects to the right of the spine** on a nonrotated, frontal radiograph.
  - With atelectasis, especially of the **lower lobes,** the heart may shift to one side or the other. When the heart shifts toward the **left,** the right heart border will overlap the spine (Fig. 7.3). When the heart shifts toward the **right,** the left heart border will approach the midline (Fig. 7.4).
- **Hemidiaphragm**
  - The **right hemidiaphragm is almost always higher than the left** by about half the interspace distance between two adjacent ribs. In about 10% of individuals, the left hemidiaphragm is higher than the right.

- In the presence of lobar atelectasis, the hemidiaphragm on the affected side will usually be **displaced upward** (Fig. 7.5).
- **Overinflation of the unaffected ipsilateral lobes or the contralateral lung**
  - The greater the volume loss and the longer its presence, the more the lung on the side **opposite** the atelectasis or

the **unaffected lobe(s) in the ipsilateral lung** will attempt to **overinflate** to compensate for the volume loss. This may be especially noticeable on the lateral projection by an **increase in the size of the retrosternal clear space** and on the frontal projection by **extension of the overinflated contralateral lung across the midline** (Fig. 7.6).

- The signs of atelectasis are summarized in Box 7.1.

Fig. 7.5 Left Upper Lobe Atelectasis. (A) On the frontal projection there is a hazy density surrounding the left hilum (*white arrow*) and a soft-tissue mass in the left hilum (*black arrow*). Notice how **the left hemidiaphragm has been pulled up to the same level as the right**. (B) The lateral projection shows a band-like zone of increased density (*white arrows*) representing the atelectatic left upper lobe sharply demarcated by the major fissure, which has been pulled anteriorly. The patient had a squamous cell carcinoma of the left upper lobe bronchus that was producing complete obstruction of that bronchus.

Fig. 7.6 Left-Sided Pneumonectomy. (A) Complete opacification of the left hemithorax is most likely from a fibrothorax produced following complete removal of the lung. There is associated marked volume loss with shift of the trachea and cardiac silhouette to the left (*dotted black arrows*). The left fifth rib was surgically removed during the pneumonectomy (*white arrow*). (B) The **right lung has herniated** across the midline in an attempt to "fill up" the left hemithorax, which is seen by the increased lucency behind the sternum (*white arrow*). Notice that because only the right hemithorax has an aerated lung remaining, only the right hemidiaphragm is visible on the lateral projection (*black arrow*). The left hemidiaphragm has been silhouetted by the airless hemithorax above it.

BOX 7.1 **Signs of Atelectasis**

- Displacement of the MAJOR or minor fissure[a]
- Increased density of the atelectatic portion of lung
- Shift of the mobile structures in the thorax (i.e., the heart, trachea, and/or hemidiaphragms)
- [a]Compensatory overinflation of the unaffected segments, lobes, or lung

[a]**Toward** the atelectasis.

TYPES OF ATELECTASIS

- **Subsegmental atelectasis** (also called **discoid atelectasis** or **plate-like atelectasis**) (Fig. 7.7)

Fig. 7.7 Subsegmental Atelectasis. Close-up view of the lung bases demonstrates several linear densities extending across all segments of the lower lobes, paralleling the diaphragm (*black arrows*). This is a characteristic appearance of *subsegmental atelectasis*, sometimes also called *discoid atelectasis* or *plate-like atelectasis*. The patient was postoperative from abdominal surgery and was unable to take a deep breath. The atelectasis disappeared within a few days after surgery.

- **Subsegmental atelectasis produces linear densities of varying thickness usually parallel to the diaphragm,** most commonly **at the lung bases.** It does not produce a sufficient amount of volume loss to cause a shift of the mobile thoracic structures.
- It occurs **mostly in patients who are "splinting"** (i.e., not taking a deep breath), such as **postoperative patients** or patients with **pleuritic chest pain.**
    - **Subsegmental atelectasis is not caused by bronchial obstruction.** It is most likely related to **deactivation of surfactant,** which leads to collapse of airspaces in a nonsegmental or nonlobar distribution.

! DIAGNOSTIC PITFALLS

- On a single study, without prior examinations for comparison, subsegmental atelectasis and **chronic, linear scarring can look identical.** Subsegmental atelectasis **typically disappears within a matter of days** with resumption of normal, deep breathing, whereas **scarring remains.**

- **Compressive atelectasis**
    - Loss of volume due to **passive compression of the lung** can be caused by:
        - A poor inspiratory effort in which there is passive atelectasis of the lung at the bases (Fig. 7.8A).
        - A **large pleural effusion, large pneumothorax,** or a **space-occupying lesion** (e.g., a large mass in the lung) (Fig. 7.8B).

A   B

Fig. 7.8 Compressive (Passive) Atelectasis. (A) Passive compression of the lung can occur either from a poor inspiratory effort, and is manifest as increased density at the lung bases (*solid white arrow*) or is secondary to a large pleural effusion or pneumothorax. (B) Axial CT scan of the chest showing only the left hemithorax demonstrates a large left pleural effusion (*solid black arrow*). The left lower lobe (*dotted black arrow*) is atelectatic, having been compressed by the pleural fluid surrounding it.

! DIAGNOSTIC PITFALLS

- When caused by a poor inspiratory effort, passive atelectasis may **mimic airspace** disease at the bases. Suspect compressive atelectasis if the patient has taken **fewer than an eight posterior-rib** breath. Check the lateral projection to confirm the presence of real airspace disease at the base.

- When caused by a large effusion or pneumothorax, the loss of volume associated with compressive atelectasis may **balance** the increased volume produced by either fluid (as in pleural effusion) or air (as in pneumothorax). In an adult patient with an **opacified hemithorax, no air bronchograms,** and **little or no shift of the mobile thoracic structures,** it is important to **suspect an obstructing bronchogenic carcinoma,** perhaps with metastases to the pleura (Fig. 7.9).
- **Round atelectasis**
  - This form of compressive atelectasis is **usually seen at the periphery of the lung base** and develops from a **combination of prior pleural disease** (e.g., from asbestos exposure or tuberculosis) **and the formation of a pleural effusion that produces adjacent compressive atelectasis.**

! DIAGNOSTIC PITFALLS

- When the pleural effusion recedes, the underlying pleural disease leads to a portion of the **atelectatic lung becoming "trapped."** This **produces a mass-like lesion** that can be confused for a tumor.

  - On CT scan of the chest, the bronchovascular markings characteristically lead from the **round atelectasis** back to the hilum producing a *comet-tail* appearance (Fig. 7.10).
- **Obstructive atelectasis** (see Fig. 7.3)
  - Obstructive atelectasis is associated with the **resorption of air from the alveoli,** through the pulmonary capillary bed, **distal to an obstructing lesion** of the bronchial tree.
  - The rate at which air is absorbed and the lung collapses depends on its gas content at the time the bronchus is occluded. It takes about **18 to 24 hours for an entire lung to collapse** with the patient breathing room air but **less than an hour** with the patient breathing near 100% oxygen.
  - The **affected segment, lobe, or lung collapses** and becomes more opaque (whiter) because it contains no air. The **collapse leads to volume loss** in the affected segment/lobe/lung. Because the visceral and parietal pleura invariably remain in contact with each other as the lung loses volume, there is a *pull* on **the mobile structures of the thorax toward the area of atelectasis.**
- The types of atelectasis are summarized in Table 7.1.

Patterns of Collapse in Lobar Atelectasis

- Obstructive atelectasis produces **consistently recognizable patterns of collapse,** depending on the location of the atelectatic segment or lobe and the degree to which such factors as collateral airflow between lobes and obstructive pneumonia allow the affected lobe to collapse.

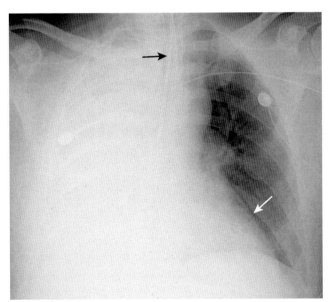

Fig. 7.9 Atelectasis and Effusion in Balance, an Ominous Combination. There is complete opacification of the right hemithorax. There are neither air bronchograms to suggest pneumonia nor any shift of the trachea (*black arrow*) or heart (*white arrow*). The absence of any shift suggests the possibility of **atelectasis and pleural effusion** in balance, a combination that should raise suspicion for a central bronchogenic carcinoma (producing obstructive atelectasis) with metastases (producing a large pleural effusion).

Fig. 7.10 Round Atelectasis, Left Lower Lobe. A mass-like density is seen in the left lower lobe (*dotted black arrow*). The patient has underlying pleural disease in the form of pleural plaques from asbestos exposure (*solid black arrows*). **Comet-tail** shaped bronchovascular markings emanate from the "mass" and extend back to the hilum (*solid white arrow*). This combination of findings is characteristic of round atelectasis and should not be mistaken for a tumor.

TABLE 7.1 Types of Atelectasis

Type	Associated With	Remarks
Subsegmental atelectasis	Splinting, especially in postoperative patients and those with pleuritic chest pain	May be related to deactivation of surfactant; does not usually lead to volume loss; disappears in days
Compressive atelectasis	Passive external compression of the lung from poor inspiration, pneumothorax, or pleural effusion	Volume loss of compressive atelectasis can balance volume increase from effusion or pneumothorax resulting in no shift; *round atelectasis* is a form of compressive atelectasis
Obstructive atelectasis	Obstruction of a bronchus from malignancy or mucous plugging	Visceral and parietal pleura maintain contact; mobile structures in the thorax are pulled toward the atelectasis

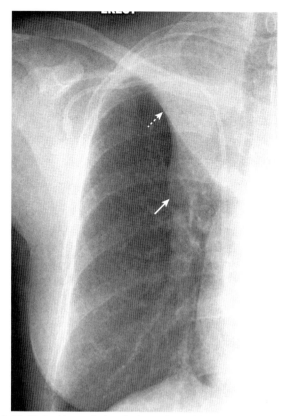

Fig. 7.11 Right Upper Lobe Atelectasis and Hilar Mass: *S Sign of Golden.* A soft-tissue mass in the right hilum (*solid white arrow*) is causing opacification of the right upper lobe from atelectasis. The minor fissure is displaced upward toward the area of increased density (*dotted white arrow*) indicating right upper lobe volume loss. The shape of the curved edge formed by the mass and the elevated minor fissure comprise what is called the **reverse S sign of Golden**. The patient had a large squamous cell carcinoma obstructing the right upper lobe bronchus.

- In general, lobes collapse in a **fan-like** configuration with the **base** of the fan-shaped triangle **anchored at the pleural surface** and the **apex of the triangle anchored at the hilum.**
- Other, unaffected lobes will undergo compensatory hyperinflation in an attempt to "fill" the affected hemithorax and this hyperinflation may limit the amount of shift of the mobile chest structures.

❗ DIAGNOSTIC PITFALLS

- The **more atelectatic a lobe or segment becomes** (i.e., the smaller its volume), the **less visible it becomes on the chest radiograph.** This can lead to the false assumption that improvement has occurred when, in fact, the atelectasis is worsening. This can usually be resolved with a careful analysis of the study to check for the degree of displacement of the interlobar fissures or hemidiaphragms or with a CT scan of the chest.

- **Right upper lobe atelectasis** (see Fig. 7.2)
  - On the frontal radiograph:
    - There is an **upward** shift of the **minor fissure**
    - There is a **rightward** shift of the **trachea**
  - On the lateral radiograph:
    - There is an **upward** shift of the **minor fissure** and **forward** shift of the **major fissure.**

- If there is a large enough mass in the right hilum producing right upper lobe atelectasis, the combination of the **hilar mass** and the **upward shift of the minor fissure** produces a characteristic appearance on the frontal radiograph called the *S sign of Golden* (Fig. 7.11).
- **Left upper lobe atelectasis** (see Fig. 7.5)
  - On the frontal radiograph:
    - There is a hazy area of increased density surrounding the left hilum.
    - There is a **leftward** shift of the **trachea.**
    - There may be elevation with **"tenting"** (peaking) of the **left hemidiaphragm.**
    - Compensatory **overinflation** of the **lower lobe** may cause the superior segment of the left lower lobe to extend to the apex of the thorax on the affected side.
  - On the lateral radiograph:
    - There is **forward** displacement of the **major fissure** and the opacified upper lobe forms a band of increased density running roughly parallel to the sternum.

Fig. 7.12 Left Lower Lobe and Right Lower Lobe Atelectasis. (A) A fan-shaped area of increased density behind the heart is sharply demarcated by the medially displaced major fissure (*solid black arrows*) representing the characteristic appearance of left lower lobe atelectasis. The medial portion of the left hemidiaphragm has been silhouetted by the airless lobe above it (*dotted black arrow*). (B) On the lateral view, the major fissure (*white arrows*) is displaced posteriorly. The small triangular density in the posterior costophrenic sulcus is in the characteristic location for left lower lobe atelectasis on the lateral projection. (C) In a different patient a fan-shaped triangular density is seen in the right lower lobe bounded superiorly by the major fissure (*white arrow*). Notice how the unaerated lower lobe silhouettes the right hemidiaphragm (*black arrow*).

- **Atelectasis of either lower lobe** (Fig. 7.12A,B)
  - On the frontal radiograph:
    - Both the right and left lower lobes collapse to form a **triangular density** that extends from its apex at the hilum to its base at the medial portion of the affected hemidiaphragm.
    - There is **elevation** of the **hemidiaphragm** on the affected side.
    - The heart may shift **toward** the side of the volume loss.
    - There is a **downward** shift of the **major fissure** (Fig. 7.12C).
  - On the lateral radiograph:
    - There is both **downward** and **posterior** displacement of the **major fissure** until the completely collapsed lower lobe forms a small triangular density at the posterior costophrenic angle (Fig. 7.12B).

▶▶ **IMPORTANT POINTS**

- **In the critically ill patient, atelectasis occurs most frequently in the left lower lobe.**
- Always check the visibility of the left hemidiaphragm to be sure it is seen in its entire extent through the heart shadow because left lower lobe atelectasis will manifest by disappearance (silhouetting) of all or part of the left hemidiaphragm (see Fig. 7.12A).

- **Right middle lobe atelectasis** (see Fig. 7.1)
- On the frontal radiograph:
  - There is a triangular density with its base silhouetting the right heart border and its apex pointing toward the lateral chest wall.
  - The **minor fissure** is displaced **downward**.

- On the lateral radiograph:
  - There is a triangular density with its base directed anteriorly and its apex at the hilum.
  - The **minor fissure** may be displaced **inferiorly** and the **major fissure superiorly.**
- **Endotracheal tube too low** (Fig. 7.13)
  - If the tip of an endotracheal tube enters the right lower lobe bronchus, only the right lower lobe tends to be aerated and remains expanded. Within a short time, atelectasis of the **entire left lung** and sometimes the right upper and middle lobes will develop.
  - Once the tip of the endotracheal tube is withdrawn above the carina, the atelectasis usually clears quite rapidly.
- **Atelectasis of the entire lung** (see Figs. 7.3 and 7.4)
  - On the frontal radiograph:
    - There is **opacification of the atelectatic lung** due to loss of air.
    - The **hemidiaphragm** on the side of the atelectasis will be **silhouetted** by the nonaerated lung above it.
    - There is a **shift** of all of the mobile structures of the thorax **toward** the side of the atelectatic lung.
  - On the lateral radiograph:
    - The **hemidiaphragm on the side of the atelectasis will be silhouetted by the nonaerated lung above it.** Look closely and you will see **only one hemidiaphragm** on the lateral image, instead of two.

HOW ATELECTASIS RESOLVES

- Depending in part on the rapidity with which the segment, lobe, or lung became atelectatic, atelectasis has the capacity to **resolve within hours or last for many days once the obstruction has been removed.**

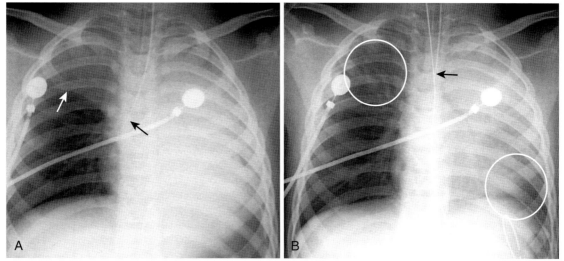

Fig. 7.13 Right Upper Lobe and Left Lung Atelectasis From an Endotracheal Tube. (A) The tip of the endotracheal tube extends beyond the carina into the bronchus intermedius (*black arrow*), which aerates only the right middle and lower lobes. The right upper lobe and entire left lung are opaque from atelectasis. The minor fissure is elevated (*white arrow*). (B) One hour later, the tip of the endotracheal tube has been retracted above the carina (*black arrow*) and the right upper lobe and a portion of the left lower lobe are again aerated (*white circles*).

TABLE 7.2 Most Common Causes of Obstructive Atelectasis

Cause	Remarks
Tumors	Includes bronchogenic carcinoma (especially squamous cell), endobronchial metastases, carcinoid tumors
Mucous plug	Especially in bedridden individuals; postoperative patients; those with asthma, cystic fibrosis
Foreign body aspiration	Especially peanuts, toys; following a traumatic intubation
Bronchial stenosis	As in scarring caused by tuberculosis

- Slowly resolving lobar or whole-lung atelectasis may manifest patchy areas of airspace disease surrounded by progressively increasing zones of aerated lung until the atelectasis has completely cleared.
- The most common causes of obstructive atelectasis are summarized in Table 7.2.

🏠 TAKE HOME POINTS

- Common to all forms of atelectasis is **volume loss,** but the radiographic appearance of atelectasis will differ, depending on the **type** of atelectasis.
- The three most commonly observed types of atelectasis are subsegmental atelectasis (also known as **discoid** or **plate-like atelectasis**), compressive or passive atelectasis, and obstructive atelectasis.
- **Subsegmental atelectasis** usually occurs in patients who are not taking a deep breath (splinting) and produces linear densities, usually at the lung bases.
- **Compressive atelectasis** occurs passively when the lung is collapsed by a poor inspiration (at the bases) or from a large, adjacent pleural effusion or pneumothorax. When the underlying abnormality is removed, the lung usually expands.
- **Round atelectasis** is a type of passive atelectasis in which the lung does not reexpand when a pleural effusion recedes, usually due to preexisting

pleural disease. Round atelectasis may simulate a mass-like lesion on chest radiographs, mimicking a tumor.
- **Obstructive atelectasis** occurs distal to an occluding lesion of the bronchial tree because of reabsorption of the air in the distal airspaces via the pulmonary capillary bed.
- Obstructive atelectasis produces consistently recognizable **patterns** of collapse based on the assumptions that the visceral and parietal pleura invariably remain in contact with each other and every lobe of the lung is anchored at or near the hilum.
- **Signs of obstructive atelectasis** include displacement of the fissures, increased density of the affected lung, shift of the mobile structures of the thorax toward the atelectasis, and compensatory overinflation of the unaffected ipsilateral or contralateral lung.
- Atelectasis tends to resolve quickly if it occurs acutely; the more chronic the process, the longer it usually takes to resolve.

 More information on recognizing atelectasis is available to registered users online.

8

Recognizing a Pleural Effusion

NORMAL ANATOMY AND PHYSIOLOGY OF THE PLEURAL SPACE

- **Normal anatomy**
  - The **parietal pleura lines the inside of the thoracic cage** and the **visceral pleura adheres to the surface of the lung** parenchyma including its interface with the mediastinum and diaphragm (**see Chapter 3**).
  - The **enfolds of the visceral pleura form the interlobar fissures**–the **major (oblique)** and **minor (horizontal)** on the right, only the major on the left. The space between the visceral and parietal pleura (i.e., the **pleural space**) is a **potential space** normally containing only **about 2 to 5 mL of pleural fluid.**
- **Normal physiology**
  - Normally, several hundred milliliters of pleural fluid are produced and reabsorbed each day. Fluid is **produced primarily at the parietal pleura** from the pulmonary capillary bed and is **resorbed at both the visceral pleura and by lymphatic drainage through the parietal pleura.**

MODALITIES FOR DETECTING PLEURAL EFFUSIONS

- **Conventional radiography** is usually the first step in detecting a pleural effusion. Other modalities used include **CT** and **ultrasound (US)**. CT and US are both sensitive in detecting small amounts of fluid. CT is best in evaluating the disease underlying the effusion or in complete opacification of the hemithorax by effusion. Ultrasound can be especially helpful in guiding an intervention to remove the pleural fluid. The fundamental appearances of pleural effusion are similar regardless of the modality.

CAUSES OF PLEURAL EFFUSIONS (TABLE 8.1)

- Fluid accumulates in the pleural space when the rate at which the fluid **forms** exceeds the rate by which it is **cleared.**
  - The **rate of formation** may be increased by:
    - **Increasing hydrostatic pressure,** as in left heart failure
    - **Decreasing colloid osmotic pressure,** as in hypoproteinemia
    - **Increasing capillary permeability,** as can occur in toxic disruption of the capillary membrane in pneumonia or hypersensitivity reactions

TABLE 8.1 Some Causes of Pleural Effusions

Cause	Examples
Excess formation of fluid	Congestive heart failure
	Hypoproteinemia
	Parapneumonic effusions
	Hypersensitivity reactions
Decreased resorption of fluid	Lymphangitic blockade from tumor
	Elevated central venous pressure
	Decreased intrapleural pressure
Transport from peritoneal cavity	Ascites

- The **rate of resorption** can **decrease** by:
  - **Decreased absorption** of fluid **by lymphatics, either from lymphangitic blockade by tumor or from increased venous pressure,** which decreases the rate of fluid transport via the thoracic duct.
  - **Decreased pressure in the pleural space,** as in atelectasis of the lung owing to bronchial obstruction.
- Pleural effusions can also form when there is **transport of peritoneal fluid from the abdominal cavity** through openings in the diaphragm or via lymphatics from a subdiaphragmatic process.

TYPES OF PLEURAL EFFUSIONS

- Pleural effusions are divided into **exudates** or **transudates,** depending on their **protein content** and their **LDH (lactate dehydrogenase) concentrations.**
- **Transudates** tend to form when there is **increased capillary hydrostatic pressure or decreased osmotic pressure.** Causes include:
  - **Congestive heart failure,** primarily left-heart failure, is the most common cause of a transudative pleural effusion.
  - **Hypoalbuminemia**
  - **Cirrhosis**
  - **Nephrotic syndrome**
- **Exudates** tend to be the result of inflammation.
  - **The most common cause of an exudative pleural effusion is malignancy.**
  - An **empyema** is an exudate containing pus.
  - In a **hemothorax,** the fluid has a hematocrit that is greater than 50% of the blood hematocrit.
  - A **chylothorax** contains increased triglycerides or cholesterol.

SIDE-SPECIFICITY OF PLEURAL EFFUSIONS

- Certain diseases tend to produce bilateral pleural effusions, and some are more often unilateral.
- Diseases that usually produce **bilateral effusions:**
  - **Congestive heart failure** usually produces about the same amount of fluid in each hemithorax, sometimes slightly more on the right than on the left side. With **markedly** different amounts of fluid in each hemithorax, suspect a **parapneumonic effusion** or malignancy on the side with the significantly greater volume of fluid.
  - **Lupus erythematosus** usually produces bilateral effusions, but when unilateral it is usually **left-sided.**
- Diseases that can produce **effusions on either side (but are usually unilateral):**
  - **Tuberculosis** and other exudative effusions associated with infectious agents, including viruses.
  - **Pulmonary thromboembolic disease**
  - **Trauma**
- Diseases that usually produce only **left-sided effusions:**
  - **Pancreatitis**
  - **Distal thoracic duct obstruction**
  - **Dressler's syndrome** (Box 8.1, Fig. 8.1)

- Diseases that mostly produce only **right-sided effusions:**
  - **Abdominal disease related to the liver or ovaries.** Some ovarian tumors can be associated with a right pleural effusion and ascites *(Meigs' syndrome).*
  - **Rheumatoid arthritis,** which can produce an effusion that remains unchanged for years.
  - **Proximal thoracic duct obstruction.**

RECOGNIZING THE DIFFERENT APPERANCES OF PLEURAL EFFUSIONS

- Forces that influence the appearance of pleural fluid on a chest radiograph depend on the **position** of the patient, the force of **gravity,** the **amount** of fluid, and the degree of **elastic recoil** of the lung. The descriptions that follow, unless otherwise indicated, assume the patient is in the upright position.

Subpulmonic Effusions

- It is believed that **almost all pleural effusions first collect in a subpulmonic location beneath the lung** between the parietal pleura lining the superior surface of the diaphragm and the visceral pleura lining the lower lobe.
- If the effusion remains entirely subpulmonic in location, it may be difficult to detect on conventional radiographs, except for contour alterations in what appears to be the hemidiaphragm but is actually the interface between the pleural fluid and the lung.
- The different appearances of subpulmonic effusions are summarized in Table 8.2.

BOX 8.1 Dressler's Syndrome

- Also known as *postpericardiotomy/postmyocardial infarction syndrome.*
- Typically occurs 2 to 3 weeks after a transmural myocardial infarct producing fever, chest pain, a left pleural effusion, pericardial effusion, and patchy airspace disease at the left lung base.
- Associated with chest pain and fever, it usually responds to high-dose aspirin or steroids.

▶ **IMPORTANT POINTS**

- Subpulmonic does not mean loculated.
- **Most subpulmonic effusions flow freely** as the patient changes position.

A   B

Fig. 8.1 Dressler's Syndrome (Postpericardiotomy/Postmyocardial Infarction Syndrome). (A) A left pleural effusion is present *(solid black arrows* in both A and B). This patient had coronary artery bypass surgery several weeks earlier. The patient has a dual lead pacemaker in place and, on the lateral projection (B), the leads are seen in the region of the right atrium *(dotted black arrow)* and right ventricle *(arrowhead).*

TABLE 8.2 Recognizing a Subpulmonic Effusion

RIGHT-SIDED FINDINGS (FIG. 8.2)		LEFT-SIDED FINDINGS (FIG. 8.3)	
Frontal View	**Lateral View**	**Frontal View**	**Lateral View**
The highest point of the **apparent hemidiaphragm**[a] is displaced more laterally than the highest point of a normal hemidiaphragm (which is usually in the middle). More difficult to recognize than left-sided subpulmonic effusions because the liver below is the same density as the pleural fluid above it.	Posteriorly, the **apparent hemidiaphragm**[a] has a curved arc but as it meets the junction with the major fissure, the apparent hemidiaphragm[a] assumes a flat edge that drops sharply to the anterior chest wall.	Increased distance between the stomach bubble and the **apparent left hemidiaphragm**[a] (should normally be only about 1 cm from top of stomach bubble to bottom of aerated left lower lobe). The highest point of the apparent hemidiaphragm[a] is displaced more laterally than the highest point of a normal hemidiaphragm.	Posteriorly, the **apparent hemidiaphragm**[a] has a curved arc, but as it meets the junction with the major fissure, the apparent hemidiaphragm[a] assumes a flat edge that drops sharply to the anterior chest wall.

[a]**Apparent hemidiaphragm** is the term used because the shadow being cast is actually from the **subpulmonic fluid** interfacing with the lung. The **actual hemidiaphragm** is **not visible**, silhouetted by the soft tissue in the abdomen below it and the pleural fluid above it.

Fig. 8.2 Right-Sided Subpulmonic Effusion. (A) In the frontal projection, the *apparent right hemidiaphragm* appears to be elevated (*black arrow*). The edge to which this arrow points represents the interface between the effusion and the base of the lung, not the hemidiaphragm which has been rendered invisible by the pleural fluid that has accumulated above it. Thus the term "apparent hemidiaphragm." There is blunting of the right costophrenic sulcus (*white arrow*). (B) On the lateral projection, there is blunting of the posterior costophrenic sulcus (*white arrow*). The apparent hemidiaphragm is **rounded posteriorly,** but then characteristically has a **flatter anterior** contour as the effusion interfaces with the major fissure on the left side (*black arrow*).

Fig. 8.3 Left-Sided Subpulmonic Effusion. (A) In the frontal projection, more than 1 cm distance is seen between the air in the stomach and the apparent left hemidiaphragm (*double black arrow*). The *dotted white arrow* represents the edge between the aerated lung and the effusion. The actual hemidiaphragm is not visible. There is blunting of the costophrenic sulcus (*solid white arrow*) on both projections. (B) On the lateral projection, the apparent hemidiaphragm is rounded posteriorly but then flattens anteriorly as the effusion interfaces with the major fissure (*solid black arrow*).

Blunting of the Costophrenic Angles

- As the subpulmonic effusion grows in size, it first fills and thus *blunts* the **posterior costophrenic sulcus (angle),** visible on the lateral view of the chest. This occurs with approximately **75 mL of fluid** (Fig. 8.4).

- **When the effusion reaches about 300 mL in size, it blunts the lateral costophrenic angle,** visible on the frontal chest radiograph (Fig. 8.5).

Fig. 8.4 Normal and Blunted Posterior Costophrenic Sulci, Lateral Projection. When approximately 75 mL of fluid has accumulated in the pleural space, the fluid will typically ascend in the thorax and blunt the posterior costophrenic sulcus (angle) first. (A) Normal, acutely angled, posterior costophrenic sulcus (*dotted arrow*). (B) A few months later during an episode of congestive heart failure, the same patient has small, bilateral pleural effusions as demonstrated by blunting of the same costophrenic sulci (*solid arrow*).

Fig. 8.5 Normal and Blunted Right Lateral Costophrenic Sulcus. (A) The hemidiaphragm usually makes a sharp and acute angle as it meets the lateral chest wall on the frontal projection to produce the lateral costophrenic sulcus (*black arrow*). Notice how aerated lung normally extends to the inner margin of each of the ribs (*white arrows*). (B) When an effusion reaches about 300 mL in volume, the lateral costophrenic sulcus loses its acute angulation and becomes **blunted** (*black arrow*).

! **DIAGNOSTIC PITFALLS**

- **Pleural thickening** caused by **fibrosis** can also produce blunting of the costophrenic angle. One helpful clue is that scarring sometimes produces a characteristic **ski-slope appearance**, unlike the meniscoid appearance of a pleural effusion (Fig. 8.6). Also, pleural thickening will **not** change in location with a change in patient position, as most effusions will.

The Meniscus Sign

- Because of the natural elastic recoil of the lungs, **pleural fluid appears to rise higher along the lateral margin of the thorax than it does medially** in the frontal projection. This produces a characteristic *meniscus* shape to the effusion, higher on the sides, lower in the middle.

▶▶ **IMPORTANT POINTS**

- In the lateral projection, the fluid assumes a U shape, usually ascending equally high both anteriorly and posteriorly (Fig. 8.7). **Identifying an abnormal thoracic density that demonstrates a meniscoid-shape is strongly suggestive of a pleural effusion.**

- **Effect of patient positioning on the appearance of pleural fluid:**
  - In the **upright position,** pleural fluid descends to the **base** of the thoracic cavity because of the force of gravity. In the **supine position,** the same free-flowing effusion will layer along the **posterior** pleural space and produce a homogeneous "haze" over the entire hemithorax when viewed en face (Fig. 8.8).
  - When the patient is **semirecumbent,** pleural fluid will layer in a way that it forms a density of varying thickness

at the lung base with the **apex,** or **thinnest part,** of the triangle ascending to varying heights in the thorax, depending on how recumbent the patient is and how much fluid is present.

Fig. 8.6 Scarring Producing Blunting of the Left Costophrenic Angle. Scarring from such things as previous infection, surgery, or blood in the pleural space sometimes produces a characteristic "**ski-slope appearance**" of blunting (*black arrows*), unlike the **meniscoid** appearance of a pleural effusion. This scarring will not change in appearance or location with a change in the patient's position, unlike a free-flowing pleural effusion.

Fig. 8.7 Meniscus Sign, Right Pleural Effusion. (A) On the frontal projection in the upright position, an effusion typically ascends more laterally (*white arrow*) than it does medially (*black arrow*). (B) On the lateral projection in this patient, the effusion again demonstrates a meniscoid shape, rising slightly higher posteriorly than anteriorly (*dotted black arrows*). The U shape of the effusion is called the ***meniscus sign***.

Fig. 8.8 Effect of Patient Positioning on the Appearance of a Pleural Effusion. (A) In the recumbent position, this right-sided effusion layers in the posterior pleural space and produces a "haze" over the entire hemithorax that is densest at the base and less dense toward the apex of the lung (*black arrow*). (B) In the same patient x-rayed a few minutes later in a more upright position, pleural fluid falls to the base of the pleural space owing to the force of gravity (*white arrow*). This simple change in position can produce the mistaken impression that an effusion has lessened or worsened when there has actually been no change in the amount of pleural fluid.

Fig. 8.9 Decubitus Views of the Chest. (A) In a **right lateral decubitus** view of the chest, the film is exposed with the patient lying on the right side on the examining table while a horizontal x-ray beam is directed posteroanteriorly (PA). Because the patient's right side is dependent, any free-flowing pleural fluid will layer along the right side (*solid black arrows*), forming a band-like density. Notice how the fluid flows into the minor fissure (*dotted black arrow*). (B) In a **left lateral decubitus** view of the chest, the patient lies on the table with the left side down and free fluid on the left side layers along the left lateral chest wall (*solid black arrows*). (A) and (B) are the same patient who had bilateral pleural effusions from lymphoma.

! DIAGNOSTIC PITFALLS

- Depending on the patient's degree of recumbence, the upper lung fields may appear clearer (blacker) if the patient is more upright because the fluid settles to the base of the thorax or the upper lung fields may appear denser (whiter) as the patient becomes more recumbent and the effusion begins to **layer posteriorly.** This change in appearance can occur with the **same** volume of pleural fluid simply redistributed in the pleural space because of patient positioning. In the best of all worlds, each portable chest radiograph would be exposed with the patient in the same position.

- **The lateral decubitus view of the chest**
  - The effect of patient positioning on the location of pleural fluid can be used for diagnostic advantage by having the patient lie on the side containing the effusion while a chest

exposure is taken using an x-ray beam directed horizontally (parallel to the floor). If the patient lies on the right side, it is called a *right lateral decubitus* and if lying on the left side, it is called a *left lateral decubitus* view of the chest.

- **Decubitus views can be used to:**
  - **Confirm** the **presence of a pleural effusion**
  - **Determine whether a pleural effusion flows freely** in the pleural space or not, **an important factor to know before attempting to drain** pleural fluid
  - "**Uncover" a portion of the underlying lung** hidden by the effusion
- If a pleural effusion can **flow freely** in the pleural space, the fluid will produce a characteristic **band-like increased density** along the inner margin of the chest cage on the dependent side of the body (Fig. 8.9).

- There may be pleural fluid that **does not flow freely** in the pleural space, **if adhesions are present,** which might impede the free flow of the fluid (see "Loculated Effusions," later).
- **Decubitus views** of the chest **can demonstrate effusions as small as 15 to 20 mL,** but CT scans of the chest have largely supplanted decubitus views in detecting very small amounts of pleural fluid (Fig. 8.10).
- If the entire hemithorax is opacified, conventional decubitus views are of little value because the underlying lung will be no more visible in the decubitus position than it was with the patient upright. CT scan of the chest is a better means of evaluating the underlying lung if the hemithorax is opacified.

Opacified Hemithorax

- When the **hemithorax of an adult contains about 2 L of fluid,** the **entire hemithorax will be opacified** (Fig. 8.11).
- As fluid fills the pleural space, the lung tends to undergo passive collapse (atelectasis) **(see Chapter 7).**
- **Large effusions are sufficiently opaque** on conventional chest radiographs **to envelop and mask whatever disease may be present in the underlying lung. CT is the modality usually used** to visualize the lung rendered impenetrable by a large effusion (Fig. 8.12).
- **Large effusions** can act like a mass and **displace the heart and trachea away** from the **side of opacification** (see Fig. 8.11).
- For more on the opacified hemithorax, go to **Chapter 6.**

Loculated Effusions

- **Adhesions in the pleural space,** caused most often by old infection or hemothorax, **may limit the normal mobility of a pleural effusion,** so that it remains in the same location no matter what position the patient assumes. This produces a

loculated effusion. Fluid with restricted movement in the pleural space may affect the treatment strategy for draining the effusion.
- **Imaging findings of loculated effusions:**
  - Loculated effusions **can be suspected when an effusion has an unusual shape or location in the thorax** (e.g., the

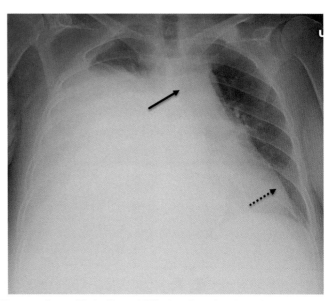

Fig. 8.11 Large Right Pleural Effusion. The right hemithorax is almost completely opacified and there is a shift of the mobile mediastinal structures such as the trachea (*solid black arrow*) and the heart (*dotted black arrow*) *away* from the side of opacification. This is characteristic of a large pleural effusion, which can act like a mass. In most adults, it requires about 2 L of fluid to fill or almost fill the entire hemithorax such as this. This patient had a right-sided bronchogenic carcinoma.

Fig. 8.10 Small Pleural Effusion Seen on CT. Here a small right pleural effusion (*white arrows*) collects in the dependent portion of the hemithorax (the patient is supine in the CT scanner). This effusion would probably not be visible on conventional chest radiographs as it would be obscured by the liver (L) on the frontal projection and the spine (S) on the lateral projection.

Fig. 8.12 Large Hemothorax on CT. A large fluid collection (F) on the right is causing complete compressive atelectasis of the right lung (*solid white arrow*) and a shift of the heart away from the side of the collection (*dotted white arrow*). On careful inspection, the fluid is denser (whiter) at the bottom of the collection (*solid black arrows*) than at the top, a **fluid-fluid** level that raises suspicion for the separation of blood products as would occur in a **hemothorax**. This patient was bleeding heavily from a lacerated intercostal artery.

effusion defies gravity by remaining at the nondependent part of the thorax when the patient is upright on a conventional radiograph or in the supine position on a CT scan of the chest) (Fig. 8.13).

- **Loculation of pleural fluid has therapeutic importance** because such collections tend to be traversed by multiple

Fig. 8.13 Loculated Pleural Effusions. These bilateral fluid collections (*white and black arrows*) have unusual shapes and seem to defy gravity, because they are trapped in the pleural space, usually by adhesions. Loculated effusions can be suspected when an effusion has something other than a meniscoid shape or collects in a location other than the base of the lung; for example, the effusion remains at the apex of the hemithorax even though the patient is upright. Pleural-based metastases were accounting for the loculated fluid in this patient.

adhesions, which makes it difficult to drain the noncommunicating pockets of fluid with a single pleural drainage tube in the same way free-flowing effusions can be drained.

- For more on the use of **ultrasound** in pleural effusions, see Chapter 20.

Fissural Pseudotumors

- *Pseudotumors* (also called *vanishing tumors*) are **sharply marginated collections of pleural fluid** contained either between the layers of an **interlobar pulmonary fissure** or in a subpleural location just beneath the fissure. They are **transudates,** which **almost always occur in patients with congestive heart failure (CHF).**
- The imaging findings of a pseudotumor are characteristic so that they should not be mistaken for an actual tumor (from which they derive their name).
  - They are **lenticular in shape,** most often occur in the **minor fissure (75%)** and frequently have **pointed ends on each side** where they insinuate into the fissure, much like the shape of a *lemon.* They **do not tend to flow freely** with a change in patient positioning.
  - They **disappear when the underlying condition (usually CHF) is treated,** but they **tend to recur in the same location** each time the patient's heart failure recurs (Fig. 8.14).

Laminar Effusions

- A laminar effusion is a form of pleural effusion in which the fluid assumes a **thin, band-like density along the lateral chest**

Fig. 8.14 Pseudotumor in the Minor Fissure, Frontal (A) and Lateral (B) Projection. (A) A sharply marginated collection of pleural fluid contained between the layers of the minor fissure produces a characteristic **lenticular shape** (*solid black arrows* in A and B) that frequently has pointed ends on each side where it insinuates into the fissure so that pseudotumors look like a *lemon* on frontal (A) or lateral (B) chest radiographs (*dotted black arrow* on A and *dotted white arrow* on B). Pseudotumors always occur along the course of a fissure which, along with their shape, helps distinguish them from an actual tumor of the lung.

Fig. 8.15 Normal Chest Versus Laminar Pleural Effusion. (A) Here is a normal patient in whom the normally aerated lung extends to the inner margin of each of the ribs (*white arrows*). The costophrenic sulcus is sharp (*black arrow*). (B) A thin band of increased density (*white arrow*) extends superiorly from the lung base, but does not appear to cause blunting of the costophrenic angle (*black arrow*). This is the appearance of a **laminar pleural effusion**. This patient was in congestive heart failure.

wall, especially near the costophrenic angle. The lateral costophrenic angle tends to maintain its acute angle with a laminar effusion, unlike the blunting that occurs with a usual pleural effusion.

- Laminar effusions are **almost always the result of** elevated left atrial pressure, as in **congestive heart failure** or secondary to **lymphangitic spread of malignancy.** They are **usually not free-flowing.**
- The imaging appearance of a laminar effusion is described in Fig. 8.15.

Hydropneumothorax

- The presence of *both* abnormal amounts of **fluid** in the pleural space (effusion or hydrothorax) *and* **air** in the pleural space (pneumothorax) is called a *hydropneumothorax.*
- Some of the more common causes of a hydropneumothorax are **trauma, surgery,** or a **recent thoracentesis to remove pleural fluid** in which air entered the pleural space.
  - *Bronchopleural fistula,* an abnormal and relatively uncommon connection between the bronchial tree and the pleural space, which is most often caused by tumor, surgery, or infection, can also produce both air and fluid in the pleural space.
- The imaging appearance of a hydropneumothorax is shown in Fig. 8.16.
  - CT is frequently necessary to distinguish between some presentations of **hydropneumothorax** and a large, **lung abscess,** both of which may have a similar appearance on conventional chest radiographs.

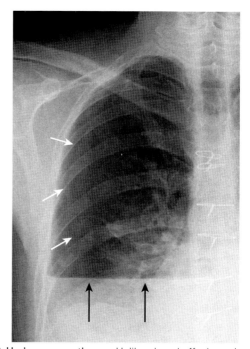

Fig. 8.16 Hydropneumothorax. Unlike pleural effusions alone, whose meniscoid shape is governed by the elastic recoil of the lung, hydropneumothorax produces an **air-fluid level** marked by a straight edge and a sharp, air-over-fluid interface (*black arrows*) when the exposure is made with a horizontal x-ray beam. This person was stabbed in the right side and there is a moderately large pneumothorax as shown by the visceral pleural white line (*white arrows*). This actually represents a **hemopneumothorax** but, unlike the CT in Fig. 8.12, conventional radiography is unable to distinguish between blood and any other fluid.

TAKE HOME POINTS

- Pleural effusions collect in the **potential space** between the visceral and parietal pleura and are either **transudates** or **exudates,** depending on their protein content and LDH concentration.
- Normally, a few milliliters of fluid are present in the pleural space; about **75 mL** are required to **blunt** the **posterior costophrenic sulcus** (seen on the lateral view) and about **200 to 300 mL** to **blunt** the **lateral costophrenic sulcus** (seen on the frontal view); approximately **2 L** of fluid will cause opacification of the **entire hemithorax** in an adult.
- Whether an effusion is unilateral or bilateral, mostly right-sided or mostly left-sided, can be an important clue as to its etiology.
- Most pleural effusions begin life collecting in the pleural space between the hemidiaphragm and the base of the lung; these are called **subpulmonic effusions.**
- As the amount of fluid increases, it forms a **meniscus** shape on the upright frontal chest radiograph owing to the natural elastic recoil properties of the lung.

- Very large pleural effusions may act like a **mass** and produce a shift of the mobile mediastinal structures (e.g., the heart) **away** from the side of the effusion.
- In the absence of pleural adhesions, effusions will **flow freely** and change location with a change in the patient's position; with pleural adhesions (usually from old infection or hemothorax), the fluid may assume unusual appearances or occur in atypical locations; such effusions are said to be **loculated.**
- A **pseudotumor** is a type of effusion that occurs in the fissures of the lung (mostly the minor fissure) and is most frequently secondary to CHF; it clears when the underlying heart failure is treated.
- **Laminar effusions** are best recognized at the lung base just above the costophrenic angles on the frontal projection and most often occur as a result of either CHF or lymphangitic spread of malignancy.
- A **hydropneumothorax** consists of both air and increased fluid in the pleural space and is recognizable on an upright view of the chest by a straight, air-fluid interface rather than the typical meniscus shape of pleural fluid alone.

 More information on pleural effusions is available to registered users online.

9

Recognizing Pneumonia

GENERAL CONSIDERATIONS

- Pneumonia can be **defined as consolidation of the lung produced by inflammatory exudate, usually as a result of an infectious agent.**
- **Most pneumonias produce airspace disease, either lobar or segmental.** Other pneumonias demonstrate **interstitial disease** and some produce findings in both the airspaces and the interstitium.
- Most microorganisms that produce pneumonia are **spread to the lungs via the tracheobronchial tree, either through inhalation or aspiration** of the organisms.
- In some instances, microorganisms are spread via the bloodstream and, in even fewer cases, by direct extension.
- Because many different microorganisms can produce similar imaging findings in the lungs, it is **difficult to identify with certainty the causative organism from the radiographic presentation alone.** However, **certain patterns** of disease **are very suggestive** of a particular causative organism (Table 9.1).
- Some use the term "infiltrate" synonymously with pneumonia, but many diseases, from amyloid to pulmonary fibrosis can *infiltrate* the lung.

GENERAL CHARACTERISTICS OF PNEUMONIA

- Because **pneumonia** fills the involved airspaces or interstitial tissues with some form of fluid or inflammatory exudate, pneumonias **appear denser (whiter) than the surrounding, normally aerated lung.**
- **Pneumonia may contain air bronchograms** if the bronchi themselves are not filled with inflammatory exudate or fluid (see Fig. 5.3).
  - Air bronchograms are **much more likely to be visible when the pneumonia involves the central portion** of the lung around the hilum. Near the periphery of the lung, the bronchi are usually too small to be visible (Fig. 9.1).
- Remember that anything of fluid or soft-tissue density that replaces the normal gas in the airspaces may also produce this sign so an **air bronchogram is not specific for pneumonia** (see Chapter 5: Recognizing Airspace versus Interstitial Lung Disease).

Fig. 9.1 Left Upper Lobe Pneumonia. Several black, branching structures appear in this left upper lobe pneumonia (*white arrows*) that represent typical **air bronchograms** seen in airspace disease. This patient had pneumococcal pneumonia. The disease is homogeneous in density, except for the presence of the air bronchograms. Because this is airspace disease, its outer edges are poorly marginated, indistinct, and fluffy (*black arrow*).

TABLE 9.1 Patterns That Might Suggest a Causative Organism	
Pattern of Disease	**Likely Causative Organism**
Upper lobe cavitary pneumonia with spread to the opposite lower lobe	*Mycobacterium tuberculosis* (TB)
Upper lobe lobar pneumonia with bulging interlobar fissure	*Klebsiella pneumoniae*
Lower lobe cavitary pneumonia	*Pseudomonas aeruginosa* or anaerobic organisms (*Bacteroides*)
Perihilar interstitial disease or perihilar airspace disease	*Pneumocystis carinii (jiroveci)*
Thin-walled upper lobe cavity	*Coccidioides* (Coccidiomycosis), TB
Airspace disease with effusion	*Streptococci, staphylococci,* TB
Diffuse nodules	*Histoplasma, Coccidioides, Mycobacterium tuberculosis* (histoplasmosis, coccidiomycosis, TB)
Soft-tissue, finger-like shadows in upper lobes	*Aspergillus* (allergic bronchopulmonary aspergillosis)
Solitary pulmonary nodule	*Cryptococcus* (Cryptococcosis)
Spherical soft-tissue mass in a thin-walled upper lobe cavity	*Aspergillus* (Aspergilloma)

Fig. 9.2 Lingular Pneumonia. Airspace disease is seen in the lingular segments of the left upper lobe. The disease is of homogeneous density. The disease is in contact with the left lateral border of the heart, which is **silhouetted** by the fluid density of the consolidated lingula in contact with the soft-tissue density of the heart (*black arrow*). Because the pneumonia and the heart are the same radiographic density, the border between them disappears.

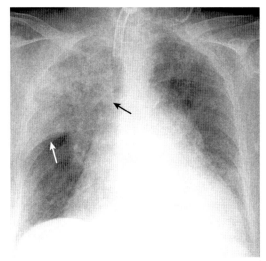

Fig. 9.3 Right Upper Lobe Pneumococcal Pneumonia. Airspace disease is seen in the right upper lobe that occupies the entire lobe. Because lobes are bounded by interlobar fissures, in this case the minor or horizontal fissure, the inferior margin of the pneumonia is sharply marginated (*white arrow*). Where the disease contacts the ascending aorta (*black arrow*), the border of the aorta is silhouetted by the fluid density of the pneumonia.

- Pneumonia that involves the airspaces **appears fluffy** and its **margins are indistinct.**
  - **Where pneumonia abuts a pleural surface,** such as an interlobar fissure or the chest wall, **it will be sharply marginated.**
- **Interstitial** pneumonia, on the other hand, may produce prominence of the interstitial markings in the affected part of the lung or may spread to adjacent airways and resemble airspace disease.
- Except for the presence of air bronchograms, airspace **pneumonia is usually homogeneous in density** (Fig. 9.2).
- In some types of pneumonia (e.g., bronchopneumonia), **the bronchi as well as the airspaces contain inflammatory exudate.** This can lead to **atelectasis associated with the pneumonia.**
- Box 9.1 summarizes the keys to recognizing pneumonia.

PATTERNS OF PNEUMONIA

- Pneumonias may be distributed in the lung in several patterns described as *lobar, segmental, interstitial, round,* and *cavitary* (Table 9.2).
- Remember, these are terms that simply describe the distribution of the disease in the lungs; they are not diagnostic of pneumonia because many other diseases can produce similar patterns of disease distribution in the lung.

LOBAR PNEUMONIA

- The **prototypical lobar pneumonia is pneumococcal pneumonia** caused by *Streptococcus pneumoniae* (Fig. 9.3).
- Although it is called lobar pneumonia, the patient may present before the disease involves the entire lobe. In its most classical form, the disease fills most or all of a lobe of the lung.

BOX 9.1 Recognizing a Pneumonia: Key Signs

- More **opaque** than surrounding normal lung.
- In airspace disease, the margins may be **fluffy** and **indistinct,** except when they abut a pleural surface, such as the interlobar fissures, where the margin will be sharp.
- Interstitial pneumonias will cause prominence of the interstitial tissues of the lung in the affected area; in some cases, the disease can spread to the alveoli and resemble airspace disease.
- Pneumonia tends to be **homogeneous** in density.
- Lobar pneumonias may contain **air bronchograms.**
- Pneumonias may be associated with **atelectasis** in the affected portion of the lung.

TABLE 9.2 Patterns of Appearance of Pneumonias

Pattern	Characteristics
Lobar	Homogeneous consolidation of affected lobe with air bronchogram
Segmental (bronchopneumonia)	Patchy airspace disease frequently involving several segments simultaneously; no air bronchogram; atelectasis may be associated
Interstitial	Reticular interstitial disease usually diffusely spread throughout the lungs early in the disease process; may progress to airspace disease
Round	Spherically shaped pneumonia usually seen in the lower lobes of children; may resemble a mass
Cavitary	Produced by numerous microorganisms, chief among them being *Mycobacterium tuberculosis*

- Because lobes are bound by interlobar fissures, **one or more of the margins of a lobar pneumonia may be sharply marginated.** Where the disease is not bound by a fissure, it will have an **indistinct** and **irregular margin.**
- Lobar pneumonias almost always produce a *silhouette sign* where they come in contact with the heart, aorta, or diaphragm and they almost always contain *air bronchograms* if they involve the central portions of the lung.

SEGMENTAL PNEUMONIA (BRONCHOPNEUMONIA)

- The **prototypical bronchopneumonia is that caused by *Staphylococcus aureus.*** Many gram-negative bacteria, such as *Pseudomonas aeruginosa*, can produce the same picture.
- Brochopneumonias are spread centrifugally via the tracheobronchial tree to **many foci in the lung at the same time.** Therefore, **they frequently involve several segments** of the lung simultaneously.
- Because lung segments are not bound by fissures, all of the **margins of segmental pneumonias tend to be fluffy and indistinct** (Fig. 9.4).
- Unlike lobar pneumonia, **segmental bronchopneumonias produce exudate that fills the bronchi.** Therefore, **air bronchograms are usually not present** and frequently some **volume loss (atelectasis)** is associated with bronchopneumonia.

INTERSTITIAL PNEUMONIA

- The **prototypes** for **interstitial pneumonia** are **viral pneumonia** and ***Mycoplasma pneumoniae*** as well as ***Pneumocystis pneumonia*** in patients with acquired immunodeficiency syndrome (AIDS).
- Interstitial pneumonias tend to involve the airway **walls** and **alveolar septa** and may produce, especially early in their course, a **fine, reticular pattern in the lungs.**
- Most **interstitial pneumonias eventually spread to the adjacent alveoli** and produce patchy or confluent airspace disease

making the original interstitial nature of the pneumonia **impossible to recognize** radiographically.

> ## ▶▶ IMPORTANT POINTS
>
> - ***Pneumocystis carinii (jiroveci)* pneumonia (PCP)**
>   - PCP is the **most common** clinically recognized infection in patients with AIDS.
>   - It classically presents as a **perihilar, reticular interstitial pneumonia**, or as **airspace disease that may mimic the central distribution pattern of pulmonary edema** (Fig. 9.5).
>   - Other presentations, such as unilateral airspace disease or widespread, patchy airspace disease, are less common.
>   - Usually **no pleural effusions** and **no hilar adenopathy are seen.**
>   - Opportunistic infections **usually occur with CD4 counts under 200** per cubic mL of blood.

ROUND PNEUMONIA

- Some pneumonias, mostly in children, can assume a **spherical shape** on chest radiographs. These *round pneumonias* are almost always **posterior** in the lungs, usually **in the lower lobes.**
- Causative agents include *Haemophilus influenzae, Streptococcus,* and *Pneumococcus.*
- A round pneumonia could be confused with a tumor mass, except that symptoms associated with infection usually accompany the pulmonary findings and tumors are uncommon in children (Fig. 9.6).

CAVITARY PNEUMONIA

- The prototypical organism producing cavitary pneumonia is *Mycobacterium tuberculosis.* Tuberculosis (TB) is discussed in Chapter 5: Recognizing Airspace versus Interstitial Disease.
- **Other infectious agents** that produce cavitary disease:
  - **Staphylococcal pneumonia** can cavitate and produce thinwalled **pneumatoceles.**

Fig. 9.5 *Pneumocystis carinii (jiroveci)* Pneumonia (PCP). There is bilateral, centrally located interstitial lung disease that is primarily reticular in nature. Without the additional history that this patient had acquired immunodeficiency syndrome (AIDS), this could be mistaken for pulmonary interstitial edema or for a chronic, fibrotic process such as sarcoidosis. However, no pleural effusions are present, as might be expected with pulmonary interstitial edema, and there is no evidence of hilar adenopathy, as might occur in sarcoid.

Fig. 9.4 Staphylococcal Bronchopneumonia. Multiple, irregularly marginated patches of airspace disease are seen in both lungs (*white arrows*). This is a characteristic distribution and appearance of **bronchopneumonia.** Staphylococcal pneumonia is more common in children, hospitalized patients, and debilitated adults. It also can develop in young adults after a bout of influenza. Methicillin-resistant *Staphylococcus aureus* (MRSA) pneumonia may be particularly difficult to treat.

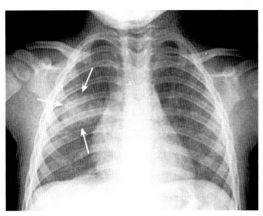

Fig. 9.6 Round Pneumonia. There is a soft tissue density in the right mid lung field, which has a rounded appearance (*white arrows*). This is a 2-year-old who had a cough and fever. Round pneumonia is rare after the age of 12 years and tumors are rare in children, so the differential diagnosis favors pneumonia in someone of this age.

Fig. 9.7 Cavitary Pneumonia. A nonenhanced axial CT image through the upper lobes demonstrates bilateral airspace disease (*solid white arrows*) containing multiple lucencies representing cavities (*dotted white arrows*). The cavities contain no air-fluid levels. Upper lobe cavitary pneumonia is presumptively tuberculosis (TB), until proved otherwise. This patient had postprimary TB (reactivation tuberculosis).

> ### ▶▶ IMPORTANT POINTS
>
> - **Cavitation is common in postprimary TB (re-activation TB), but rare in primary TB.** The cavities are usually located in the upper lobes, are **bilateral and thin-walled,** have a **smooth inner margin** and **no air-fluid level** (Fig. 9.7). **Transbronchial spread** (from one upper lobe to the opposite lower lobe, or to another lobe in the same lung) should make you think of infection with *Mycobacterium tuberculosis.*

- *Streptococcal* pneumonia, *Klebsiella* pneumonia, and coccidiomycosis can also produce cavitating pneumonias.

ASPIRATION

- There are many causes of aspiration of foreign material into the tracheobronchial tree, among them neurologic disorders (stroke, traumatic brain injury), altered mental status (anesthesia, drug overdose), gastroesophageal reflux, and postoperative changes from head and neck surgery.
- **Acute aspiration** will produce radiographic findings of **airspace disease.** Its **location,** the **rapidity** with which it appears, and the group of patients **predisposed** to aspirate are clues to its etiology (Fig. 9.8).

Fig. 9.8 Aspiration, Both Lower Lobes. Single, axial CT image of the lungs demonstrates bilateral lower lobe airspace disease (*black arrows*) in a patient who had aspirated. Aspiration usually affects the most dependent portions of the lung. In the upright position, the lower lobes are affected. In the supine position, the superior segments of the lower lobes and the posterior segments of the upper lobes are most involved. Aspiration of water or neutralized gastric acid will usually clear in 24 to 48 hours, depending on the volume aspirated.

TABLE 9.3 Three Patterns of Acute Aspiration

Pattern	Characteristics
Bland gastric acid or water	Rapidly appearing and rapidly clearing airspace disease in dependent lobe(s); not a pneumonia
Infected aspirate (aspiration pneumonia)	Usually lower lobes; frequently cavitates and may take months to clear
Nonneutralized stomach acid (chemical pneumonitis)	Almost immediate appearance of dependent airspace disease that frequently becomes secondarily infected

> ### ▶▶ IMPORTANT POINTS
>
> - **Recognizing the different types of aspiration (Table 9.3)**
>   - The clinical and radiologic course of aspiration depends on **what** was aspirated.
>   - **Aspiration of bland (neutralized) gastric juices or water**
>   - This is technically **not a pneumonia** because it does not involve an infectious agent, is handled by the lungs as if it were pulmonary edema fluid and **classically remains for only a day or two before clearing** through resorption.
>   - **Aspiration that produces pneumonia owing to microorganisms in the lung**
>   - Although **we routinely aspirate numerous microorganisms present in the normal oropharyngeal flora,** there are some patients in whom these microorganisms can develop into pneumonia, including those who are immunocompromised, elderly, debilitated, or have underlying lung disease.
>   - **Pneumonia** caused by aspiration is usually secondary to **anaerobic organisms,** such as *Bacteroides*. These organisms produce **lower lobe airspace disease** that **frequently cavitates.** They may take **months to resolve.**
>   - **Aspiration of nonneutralized stomach acid *(Mendelson's Syndrome)***
>   - When large quantities of nonneutralized gastric acid are aspirated, **chemical pneumonitis develops** producing dependent lobe airspace disease or diffuse **pulmonary edema.** The disease may appear quickly, within a few **hours** of the aspiration. Clearing may take **days or longer** and the chemical pneumonitis is prone to become **secondarily infected.**

LOCALIZING PNEUMONIA

- Although it is true that an antibiotic will travel to every lobe of the lung without regard for which lobe actually harbors the pneumonia, determining the location of a pneumonia may provide clues to the **causative organism** (e.g., if in the upper lobes, think of TB) and the presence of **associated pathology** (e.g., if in lower lobes, think of recurrent aspiration).
- **On conventional radiographs,** it is always **best to localize any disease with two views taken at 90° to each other** (*orthogonal views*), such as a frontal and lateral chest radiograph. CT may further localize and characterize the disease as well as demonstrate associated pathology, such as pleural effusions or cavities too small to see on conventional radiographs.
- Sometimes, only a frontal radiograph may be available, as with critically ill or debilitated patients who require a portable bedside examination. Nevertheless, it is still frequently **possible to localize the pneumonia with only the frontal radiograph** by analyzing which structure's margins are obscured by the disease (i.e., the silhouette sign) (Table 9.4).

TABLE 9.4 Using the Silhouette Sign on the Frontal Chest Radiograph

Structure That Is No Longer Visible	Disease Location
Ascending aorta	Right upper lobe
Right heart border	Right middle lobe
Right hemidiaphragm	Right lower lobe
Descending aorta	Left upper or lower lobe
Left heart border	Lingula of left upper lobe
Left hemidiaphragm	Left lower lobe

- **Silhouette sign** (see also Chapter 5, section Characteristics of Airspace Disease)
  - If two objects of the **same** radiographic density **touch** each other, then the **edge between them disappears (see Fig. 9.2).** The silhouette sign is valuable in localizing and identifying tissue types throughout the body, not just the chest.

> ### ▶▶ IMPORTANT POINTS
>
> - The *spine sign* (Fig. 9.9)
>   - On the lateral chest radiograph, the **thoracic spine normally appears to get darker (blacker) as you survey it from the shoulder girdle to the diaphragm.**
>   - The reason is that the x-ray beam normally needs to penetrate more tissue (more bones, more muscle) around the shoulders than it does just above the diaphragm, where it needs to pass through only the heart and aerated lungs.
>   - **When disease** of soft tissue or fluid density **involves** the **posterior portion of the lower lobe,** more of the x-ray beam will be absorbed by the new, added density and **the spine will appear to become "whiter" (more opaque) just above the posterior costophrenic sulcus.**
>   - This is called the *spine sign* and it provides another way to localize disease in the lungs.
>   - The lower lobe disease **may not be apparent** on the **frontal projection,** if it lies **deep in the posterior costophrenic sulcus.** Therefore the *spine sign* **may indicate** the presence of lower lobe **disease,** such as lower lobe pneumonia, **which may be otherwise invisible on the frontal projection.**

- Fig. 9.10 is a composite of the characteristic appearances of lobar pneumonia as seen on a frontal chest radiograph.

Fig. 9.9 The Spine Sign. Frontal and lateral views of the chest demonstrate airspace disease on the lateral film (B) in the right lower lobe (*white arrow*) that may not be immediately apparent on the frontal film (you can see the pneumonia in the right lower lobe in [A] [*black arrow*]). In this case, a right lower lobe pneumonia superimposed on the lower spine on the lateral view makes the spine appear "whiter" (more dense) just above the diaphragm. This is called the *spine sign* (see also Figs. 3.3 and 3.4).

Fig. 9.10 Composite Appearances of Lobar Pneumonias. (A) **Right upper lobe.** The disease obscures (silhouettes) the ascending aorta. Where it abuts the minor fissure, it produces a sharp margin (*white arrow*). (B) **Right middle lobe.** The disease silhouettes the right heart border (*solid black arrow*). Where it abuts the minor fissure, it produces a sharp margin (*solid white arrow*). (C) **Right lower lobe.** The disease silhouettes the right hemidiaphragm (*solid black arrow*). It spares the right heart border (*dotted black arrow*). (D) **Left upper lobe.** The disease is poorly marginated (*solid white arrow*) and obscures the aortic knob (*solid black arrow*). (E) **Lingula.** The disease silhouettes the left heart border (*solid black arrow*), but spares the left hemidiaphragm (*dotted black arrow*). (F) **Left lower lobe.** The disease obscures the left hemidiaphragm (*dotted black arrow*) but spares the left heart border (*solid black arrow*).

Fig. 9.11 Resolving Pneumonia. Pneumonia can resolve in several days if the organism is sensitive to the antibiotic administered, especially pneumococcal pneumonia. Most pneumonias, like that in the radiographs of the left lung taken four days apart (A) and (B), typically resolve from within **(vacuolize),** gradually disappearing in a patchy fashion over days or weeks.

HOW PNEUMONIA RESOLVES

- Pneumonia can resolve in 2 to 3 days if the organism is sensitive to the antibiotic administered, especially pneumococcal pneumonia.
- **Most pneumonias typically resolve from within** *(vacuolize)*, gradually disappearing in a patchy fashion over days or weeks (Fig. 9.11).

- If a pneumonia **does not** resolve in several weeks, consider the presence of an underlying **obstructing lesion**, such as a **neoplasm**, that is preventing adequate drainage from that portion of the lung. A CT scan of the chest may help to demonstrate the obstructing lesion.

🏠 TAKE HOME POINTS

- Pneumonia is more opaque than the surrounding normal lung; its margins may be **fluffy** and **indistinct,** except for where it abuts a pleural margin; it tends to be **homogeneous** in density; it may contain **air bronchograms;** it may be associated with **atelectasis.**
- Although there is considerable overlap in the patterns of pneumonia different organisms produce, some appearances are highly suggestive of particular etiologies.
- **Lobar pneumonia** (prototype: pneumococcal pneumonia) tends to be homogeneous, occupies most or all of a lobe, has air bronchograms centrally, and produces the **silhouette sign.**
- **Segmental pneumonia** (prototype: staphylococcal pneumonia) tends to be multifocal, does not have air bronchograms, and can be associated with volume loss because the bronchi are also filled with inflammatory exudate.
- **Interstitial pneumonia** (prototype: viral pneumonia or PCP) tends to involve the airway walls and alveolar septa and may produce, especially early in its course, a fine, reticular pattern in the lungs; later in its course, it may produce airspace disease.

- **Round pneumonia** (prototype: *Haemophilus*) usually occurs in **children** in the lower lobes **posteriorly** and can resemble a mass, the clue being that actual masses in children are uncommon.
- **Cavitary pneumonia** (prototype: tuberculosis) contains lucent cavities produced by lung necrosis as its hallmark; **postprimary tuberculosis** usually involves the upper lobes; it can spread via a transbronchial route that can infect the opposite lower lobe or another lobe in the same lung.
- **Aspiration** occurs in the most dependent portion of the lung at the time of the aspiration, usually the lower lobes or the posterior segments of the upper lobes; aspiration can be bland and clear quickly, can be infected and take months to clear, or be from a chemical pneumonitis, which can take weeks to clear.
- Pneumonia can be localized with the **silhouette sign** and the **spine sign** as aids.
- Pneumonias frequently resolve by "breaking up" so that they contain patchy areas of newly aerated lung within the confines of the previous pneumonia **(vacuolization).**

 More information on recognizing pneumonia is available to registered users online.

10

Recognizing the Correct Placement of Lines and Tubes And Their Potential Complications: Critical Care Radiology

- Patients in the critical or intensive care units (ICU) are monitored on a frequent basis with portable chest radiography, both to check on the position of their multiple assistive devices and to assess their cardiopulmonary status.
- Diseases commonly seen in critically ill patients are discussed in other chapters (Table 10.1).
- In this chapter, you will get practical advice for evaluating the successful (or unsuccessful) insertion and ultimate position of multiple tubes, lines, catheters, and other supportive apparatus used in the ICU. **Information for even more devices can be found online for registered users.**
- Most times, a conventional radiograph is obtained **after** the insertion or attempted insertion of one of these devices to check on its position and to rule out any unintended complications.
- Therefore, **for each tube or device, you will learn:**
  - **Why** they are used
  - **Where** they belong when properly placed
  - **How** such devices can be malpositioned and **what** complications may occur from the device

ENDOTRACHEAL AND TRACHEOSTOMY TUBES

Endotracheal Tubes (ETT)

- **Why endotracheal tubes are used**
  - Assist ventilation
  - Isolate the trachea to permit control of the airway
  - Prevent gastric distension
  - Provide a direct route for suctioning
  - Administer medications

TABLE 10.1 Common Diseases in Critically Ill Patients

Finding or Disease	Discussed in
Adult respiratory distress syndrome	Chapter 12
Aspiration	Chapter 9
Atelectasis	Chapter 7
Congestive heart failure (pulmonary edema)	Chapter 12
Pleural effusion	Chapter 8
Pneumomediastinum	Chapter 25
Pneumonia	Chapter 9
Pneumothorax	Chapter 25
Pulmonary embolic disease	Chapter 11

- **Correct placement of an ETT** (Box 10.1)
  - Endotracheal tubes are usually **wide-bore tubes** (about 1 cm) with a **radio-opaque marker stripe** and **no side holes. The tip is frequently diagonally shaped.**
  - With the patient's head in the **neutral** position (i.e., bottom of mandible is at the level of C5-C6), the **tip of ETT should be about 3 to 5 cm from the carina.** This is roughly **half the distance between the medial ends of clavicles and the carina** (Fig. 10.1).

BOX 10.1 Endotracheal Tubes

- The tip should be about 3 to 5 cm above the carina.
- The inflated cuff should not distend the lumen of the trachea.
- The tip is most commonly malpositioned in the right main or right lower lobe bronchus.
- If positioned with its tip in the neck, damage to vocal cords can occur.

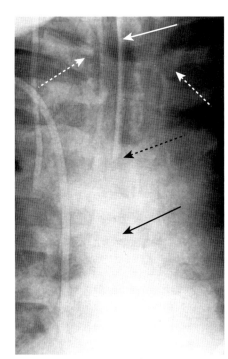

Fig. 10.1 Endotracheal Tube in Satisfactory Position. Endotracheal tubes (ETT) have a radiopaque marker stripe (*solid white arrow*). The tip is diagonally angled (*dotted black arrow*). In adults, they usually have an inflatable cuff. Most endotracheal tubes are inserted via the oral, rather than the nasal, route. With the patient's head in the neutral position, the tip of ETT should be roughly half the distance between the medial ends of clavicles (*dotted white arrows*) and the carina (*solid black arrow*).

Fig. 10.2 Endotracheal Tube With Cuff Overinflated. The inflated balloon (*white arrows*) of the endotracheal tube (*black arrow*) is wider than the diameter of the trachea. The cuff should not distend the trachea. Prolonged compression on the tracheal wall by an overinflated cuff can result in necrosis of the wall and tracheal stenosis.

- Ideally **the diameter of the endotracheal tube should be one-half to two-thirds the width of trachea.** An inflated cuff (balloon), if present, may fill, but should not distend, the lumen of the trachea (Fig. 10.2).

> **IMPORTANT POINTS**
>
> - **How to find the carina on a frontal chest radiograph**
>   - Follow the **right** or **left** main bronchus backward until either meets the opposite main bronchus. The carina projects over the T5, T6, or T7 vertebral bodies in 95% of people.

- **Movement of tip with flexion and extension**
  - Neck **flexion** may cause **2 cm of descent** of the tube tip. This is why the tip should be 3 to 5 cm above the carina.
  - Neck **extension** from neutral **may cause 2 cm of ascent** of the tip.
  - A helpful sentence to remember the direction of movement of the tip of an ETT compared with movement of the

Fig. 10.3 Endotracheal Tube Too High. The tip of the tube (*white arrow*) should not be placed in or near the larynx or pharynx as it can produce damage to these structures if it remains in this position. High placement can also predispose to aspiration. This patient also has a nasogastric tube (*dotted white arrow*) and several overlying cardiac monitor leads (*black arrows*).

head: "The tip of the **hose** (ETT) follows the tip of the **nose**."

- **Incorrect placement and complications of an ETT**
  - **Most common malposition** results because of the shallower angle and wider diameter of the **right main bronchus** or bronchus intermedius; the **tip of the ETT will tend to slide into the right-sided bronchial tree** preferentially to the left.
    - This can lead to **atelectasis** (especially of the nonaerated right upper lobe and left lung) (**see Fig. 7.13**).
    - Intubation of the right main bronchus could also lead to a **right-sided tension pneumothorax.**
  - Inadvertent **esophageal intubation** will produce a grossly dilated stomach.
  - The tip of the tube should not be positioned in the larynx or pharynx; the tip should be at least 3 cm distal to the level of the vocal cords or **the tube can damage the vocal chords or lead to aspiration** (Fig. 10.3).

Tracheostomy Tubes

- **Why tracheostomies are used**
  - In patients with airway obstruction at or above the level of the larynx
  - In respiratory failure requiring long-term intubation (>21 days)
  - For airway obstruction during sleep apnea
  - When there is paralysis of the muscles that affect swallowing or respiration

Fig. 10.4 Tracheostomy Tube in Correct Position. The tip (*solid black arrow*) is about half-way between the stoma in which the tracheostomy tube was inserted (*dotted white arrow*) and the carina (*solid white arrow*). This is usually around the level of T3. The tip of a tracheostomy tube is not affected by flexion and extension of the neck.

- **Correct placement of a tracheostomy tube**
  - The **tip** should be **about half-way between the stoma** in which the tracheostomy tube was inserted **and the carina.** This is usually around the **level of T3** (Fig. 10.4).
  - Unlike an ETT, the placement of the tip of a tracheostomy tube is not affected by flexion and extension of the head.
  - **The width of the tracheostomy tube should be about two-thirds the width of trachea.**
- **Incorrect placement and complications of a tracheostomy tube** (Box 10.2)
  - Immediately after insertion, **look for signs of** inadvertent **perforation of the trachea,** such as pneumomediastinum, pneumothorax, and subcutaneous emphysema.
  - If the tracheostomy tube is equipped with a **cuff,** the cuff should generally be inflated to a diameter that **fills,** but **does not distend, the normal tracheal contour.**

BOX 10.2 Tracheostomy Tubes

- The tip should be halfway between the entrance stoma and the carina.
- If so equipped, the cuff is generally not inflated to a size greater than the tracheal lumen.
- Short-term complications may include perforation of trachea.
- Tracheal stenosis is the most common long-term complication, usually at the site of the entrance stoma.

BOX 10.3 Central Venous Catheters

- The tip should lie in the superior vena cava.
- All bends in the catheter should be smooth curves, not sharp kinks.
- Most common malpositions are the **right atrium** and **internal jugular vein** (for subclavian-inserted catheters).
- Always **check for pneumothorax** after successful or unsuccessful insertion attempt.

✳ IMAGE-GUIDED INTERVENTION

This is a 55-year-old with known history of kidney failure presenting with intractable shortness of breath. How might an image-guided procedure benefit in this case? See the answer in Chapter 29.

- **Long-term complication of tracheostomies:**
  - **Tracheal stenosis is the most common late-occurring complication** of a tracheostomy tube; it can occur at the entrance stoma, level of the cuff, or at the tip of tube, but is **most common at the stoma.**

INTRAVASCULAR CATHETERS

Central Venous (Pressure) Catheters (CVC, CVP)
- **Why they are used**
  - For venous access to instill chemotherapeutic and hyperosmolar agents not suitable for peripheral venous administration
  - To measure central venous pressure
  - To maintain and monitor intravascular blood volume
- **Correct placement of central venous catheters** (Box 10.3)
  - **Central venous catheters** have a **small diameter** (3 mm) and are **uniformly opaque without a marker stripe.**

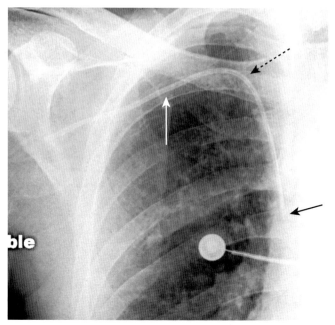

Fig. 10.5 Subclavian Central Venous Catheter in Correct Position. A central venous catheter is in place on the right (*solid white arrow*) which passes over the medial end of the clavicle (*dotted black arrow*) before descending to the right of the spine with its tip in the superior vena cava (*solid black arrow*).

Fig. 10.6 Central Venous Catheter Malpositioned in Internal Jugular Vein. Central venous catheters, especially those placed by the subclavian route (*dotted white arrow*), are frequently malpositioned. They are most often malpositioned with their tips in the right atrium or the internal jugular vein, as in this case (*solid white arrow*). The catheter was removed and repositioned.

- They are usually inserted either by the **subclavian** or **internal jugular** route. The internal jugular veins join the subclavian veins to form the brachiocephalic (innominate) veins which, in turn, drain into the superior vena cava. The junctions of the subclavian and brachiocephalic veins generally occur **posterior** to the **medial ends** of the clavicles.
- The path of a central venous catheter should reach the **medial end of the clavicle before descending.**
- The catheter should **descend lateral to the right side of the spine** and the **tip should lie in the superior vena cava at its junction with the right atrium** (Fig. 10.5). The junction of the superior vena cava and the right atrium usually lies at the level of the fifth or s thoracic vertebral body or about two vertebral bodies **below** the level of the carina.
- **All bends in the catheter should be smooth curves,** without any kinks. A kink in the catheter may interfere with its function and may signal perforation of a vessel.
- **Incorrect placement and complications of central venous catheters**
  - Central venous catheters, more frequently those placed by the subclavian route, can be malpositioned.
  - They are **most often malpositioned** with their tips **in the right atrium or internal jugular vein** (if inserted via the subclavian vein) (Fig. 10.6). **In the right atrium,** they can produce **cardiac arrhythmias.** When central venous catheters are malpositioned, they may provide **inaccurate central venous pressure readings.**
  - **Pneumothorax** can occur in up to 5% of CVC insertions, more often with the subclavian approach than via the internal jugular route.

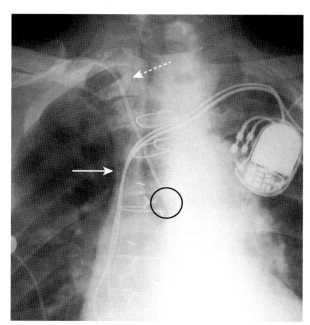

Fig. 10.7 Arterial Placement of Central Venous Catheter. Sometimes, central lines may be inadvertently inserted in the subclavian **artery** rather than the subclavian **vein.** Note that this catheter does not reach the medial end of the clavicle (*dotted white arrow*) before descending and its tip (*black circle*) is directed **over** the spine, away from the location of the superior vena cava (*solid white arrow*). Suspect arterial placement if the return flow is pulsatile or bright red.

- **Occasionally CVCs may perforate the vein** and lie outside of the blood vessel. Look for sharp bends/kinks in the catheter as a clue to a potential perforation.
- Sometimes, they may **inadvertently be inserted in the subclavian artery** rather than the subclavian vein. Suspect **arterial placement** if the **blood return is pulsatile** and the course of the catheter **parallels the aortic arch** or **fails to descend to the right of the spine** (Fig. 10.7).

>> IMPORTANT POINTS

- **Two or more attempts at inserting a CVC**
  - A frontal chest radiograph is obtained following placement of a CVC. **Should initial placement fail**, it is customary to **obtain a chest radiograph before trying insertion on the other side** to avoid the possibility of producing bilateral pneumothoraces.

PERIPHERALLY INSERTED CENTRAL CATHETERS: PICC

- **Why they are used**
  - For long-term venous access (months)
    - To administer medications such as chemotherapy or antibiotics
    - For frequent blood sampling
      - Because of their small size, they can be introduced via an antecubital vein.
- **Correct placement of peripherally inserted central catheters** (Box 10.4)
  - The **tip** should lie **within** the **superior vena cava,** but may be placed in an axillary vein. Because the lines are so small, they may be difficult to visualize (Fig. 10.8).
- **Incorrect placement and complications of peripherally inserted central catheters**
  - Tips may become **malpositioned** over time, rather than on initial insertion.
  - **Thrombosis** of the line may occur because of its small lumen size.

Pulmonary Artery Catheters: Swan-Ganz Catheters

- **Why are they used**
  - To monitor hemodynamic status of critically-ill patients
  - To help in differentiating cardiac from noncardiac pulmonary edema
- **Correct placement of Swan-Ganz catheters** (also known as *pulmonary capillary wedge pressure catheters*)
  - Swan-Ganz catheters **have the same appearance as central venous catheters, but are longer.**
  - Inserted via the subclavian vein or internal jugular vein, their tips are floated out into the proximal right or proximal left pulmonary artery. The **tip of the Swan-Ganz catheter should be no more than about 2 cm from the hila** (Fig. 10.9).
  - A balloon at the catheter's tip is temporarily inflated only when pressure measurements are made and should then be deflated.

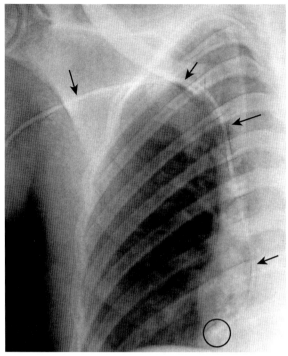

Fig. 10.8 Peripherally Inserted Central Catheter (PICC) line in right atrium. A PICC (*black arrows*) is inserted in the upper forearm or lower arm and fed through the axillary vein to the superior vena cava (SVC) or junction between the SVC and right atrium. In this case, the tip extends to the region of the right atrium (*black circle*).

Fig. 10.9 Swan-Ganz Catheter in Correct Position. A Swan-Ganz catheter (*black arrow*) is a multilumen catheter that has the same appearance as a central venous line but its tip (*black circle*) is "floated" out into the pulmonary arteries through inflation of a balloon at the tip. If the tip is "wedged" in a small pulmonary vessel, a measurement called **pulmonary capillary wedge pressure** can be made. In the presence of a normal mitral valve, this measurement reflects left atrial pressure.

BOX 10.4   Peripherally Inserted Central Catheters

- The tip should lie in the superior vena cava or axillary vein.
- PICCs may be difficult to visualize because of their small size.
- Thrombosis of the line may occur over time.

BOX 10.5   Pulmonary Artery Catheters (Swan-Ganz Catheters)

- Tip should be about 2 cm from the hilum in either the right or left pulmonary artery.
- Balloon should be inflated only when pressure measurements are performed.
- The tip of the catheter should not lie within a peripheral pulmonary artery.

BOX 10.6   Multiple Lumen Catheters

- The tip should either be in the superior vena cava or right atrium. Some catheters are designed with separate lumens so that one tip is in the superior vena cava and the other is in the right atrium.
- The **right internal jugular vein** has the lowest incidence of clotting so it is the preferred access route.
- **Complications** include pneumothorax, thrombosis, and infection.

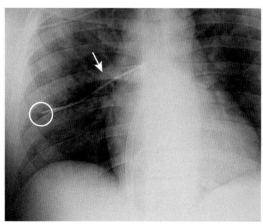

Fig. 10.10 Swan-Ganz Catheter With Tip Too Peripheral. The tip of this Swan-Ganz catheter (*white circle*) is located near the periphery of the right lung, too far from the right pulmonary artery (*white arrow*). The tip of a Swann-Ganz catheter should lie within 2 cm of the hilar shadow. The catheter was withdrawn because the tip in this location increases the risk of a complication, such as **pulmonary infarction** or **pseudoaneurysm** formation.

- **Incorrect placement and complications of Swan-Ganz catheters** (Box 10.5)
  - **Serious complications are uncommon.**
  - The most common significant complication is **pulmonary infarction** from occlusion of a pulmonary artery by the catheter itself or from emboli arising from the catheter.
  - Peripherally placed catheters may produce a localized, confined blood vessel perforation or *pseudoaneurysm* that can be recognized by **consolidation** or a **mass** that forms at the **site of the catheter tip** in a critical-care patient who also develops **hemoptysis.**
  - **Make sure the catheter tip does not lie in a distal branch of a pulmonary artery** as this increases the risk of complication (Fig. 10.10).

MULTIPLE LUMEN CATHETERS: "QUINTON CATHETERS," HEMODIALYSIS CATHETERS

- **Why are multiple lumen catheters used** (Box 10.6)?
  - Hemodialysis
  - Simultaneous ports for administration of medication and blood sampling
- **Correct placement of multiple lumen catheters for hemodialysis**
  - These are **large-bore catheters** that are **typically marked with a central stripe.**
  - There are many variations in design among different commercial brands, but all have at least two lumens arranged

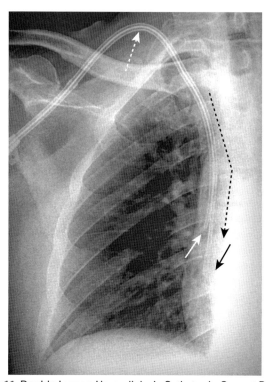

Fig. 10.11 Double Lumen Hemodialysis Catheter in Correct Position. These large-bore catheters with at least two lumens are typically marked with a central stripe (*dotted white arrow*). Because the direction of blood flow is as indicated by the dotted black arrow, to minimize immediate recirculation, the tip from which blood is **withdrawn** from the patient (*solid white arrow*) is more **proximal** than the tip through which blood is **returned** to the patient (*solid black arrow*).

coaxially inside a single catheter with the goal to **minimize the amount of recirculation** that occurs between the two internal ports.
- The **"arterial" port** from which blood is **withdrawn from the patient is proximal to the "venous" port** through which blood is **returned to the patient** to minimize recirculation of blood. Some catheters are designed as two separate single-lumen catheters with one catheter tip in the superior vena cava and the other catheter tip in the right atrium (Fig. 10.11).
- The **right internal jugular route is most often used for access.**
- **Incorrect placement and complications of multiple lumen catheters**
  - **Immediate complications** can include **pneumothorax, malposition,** or **perforation of the tip.**
  - **Long-term complications** include **infection** and **thrombosis** of the vein containing the catheter or **occlusion** of the catheter itself.

PLEURAL DRAINAGE TUBES (CHEST TUBES, THORACOTOMY TUBES)

- **Why are thoracotomy tubes used?**
  - To remove either air or abnormal collections of fluid from the pleural space
- **Correct placement of pleural drainage tubes** (Box 10.7)
  - Chest tubes are **wide-bore tubes with a radio-opaque stripe** used as a marker. The stripe is **discontinuous** at the site of a **side-hole.**
  - Ideal position is **anterosuperior for evacuating a pneumothorax** and **posteroinferior for draining an effusion,** but chest tubes usually work well no matter where positioned (Fig. 10.12).
  - **None of the side-holes should lie outside of the thoracic wall** (Fig. 10.13).

> ## BOX 10.7 Pleural Drainage Tubes (Chest Tubes)
>
> - In general, chest tubes work well no matter where they are positioned, but malpositioning can result in ineffective drainage.
> - For pleural effusions, they work best with their tip placed **posteriorly** and **inferiorly.**
> - For pneumothorax, they work best with their tip placed **anteriorly** and **superiorly.**
> - Rapid drainage of a large pleural effusion or large pneumothorax can produce **reexpansion pulmonary edema** in the underlying lung.

- **Incorrect placement and complications of pleural drainage tubes**
  - Most malpositions lead to **inadequate drainage** rather than serious complications. This includes malpositions in which the tube is inadvertently placed in the major fissure (Fig. 10.14).
  - If the **side-hole extends outside of the chest wall,** this can lead to an *air-leak* causing both inadequate drainage and subcutaneous emphysema.
  - **Serious complications are uncommon** and include:
    - **Bleeding secondary to laceration of intercostal artery**
    - **Laceration of liver or spleen on insertion**
    - **Rapid reexpansion of a collapsed lung** caused by either a large pneumothorax or a large pleural effusion may lead to unilateral, *re-expansion pulmonary edema* (see Fig. 12.12).

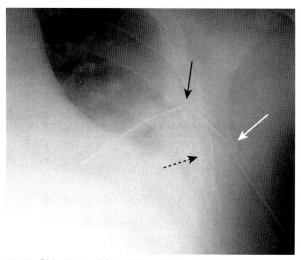

Fig. 10.13 Side-Hole of Chest Tube Extends Outside Thorax. Chest tubes typically have one or more side-holes marked by a discontinuity in the marker stripe (*solid white arrow*). None of the side-holes should lie **outside** the rib cage (*dotted black arrow*) as it does in this patient. An **air leak** can develop, leading to persistence of the underlying problem, in this case a pleural effusion. This tube is also **kinked** as it enters the chest (*solid black arrow*), which may further reduce its drainage efficiency.

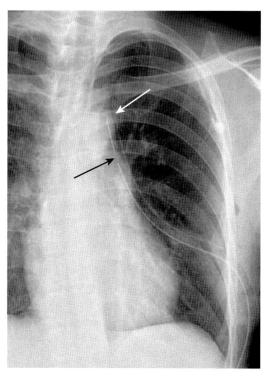

Fig. 10.12 Chest Tube in Correct Position. Chest tubes are wide-bore tubes with a radiopaque stripe used as a marker. The stripe "breaks" at the site of the side-hole (*black arrow*). The white arrow points to the tip. Chest tubes are inserted in an intercostal space as close to the superior rib margin as possible because the intercostal nerves and blood vessels course along the lower margin of each rib. This tube was inserted for a pneumothorax, which has been evacuated.

Fig. 10.14 Chest Tube in Major Fissure. Suspect insertion of a chest tube into one of the interlobar fissures when the tube is oriented along the course of the fissure. This tube lies within the right major fissure (white arrow on the frontal view [A] and black arrow on the lateral view [B]). Malpositions like this can lead to inefficient drainage.

Fig. 10.15 Dual-Lead Pacemaker in Correct Position. Pacemakers consist of a pulse generator (G) usually implanted in the left chest wall and one or more electrode leads inserted via the subclavian vein. This patient has a **dual-lead** pacemaker. One of the leads is in the apex of the right ventricle (*solid black arrow* in [A] and [B]), while the other lead is in the right atrium (*dotted black arrow* in [A] and [B]). Notice that the right ventricular lead (*solid black arrows*) normally projects to the left of the midline (A) and anteriorly (B), and the right atrial lead typically curls upward (A) and (B).

BOX 10.8   Pacemakers

- Usually placed in the left anterior chest wall; at least one lead should be in the right ventricular apex.
- Remember that the right ventricle projects to the left of the spine on the frontal view and anteriorly on the lateral view of the chest.
- Complications are infrequent, but include fractures in the lead wires and pneumothorax.
- Ectopically placed leads may result in failure of the pacemaker to function properly.

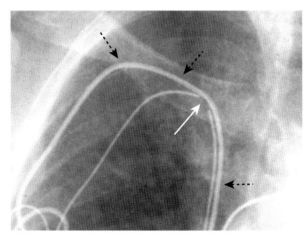

Fig. 10.16 Fractured Pacemaker Lead. Fractures of pacemaker or automatic implantable cardiac defibrillator (AICD) leads may occur at any of three places. In this patient, the break (*solid white arrow*) occurred at the point of insertion into the subclavian vein. The broken lead had been discovered earlier and a second, intact lead is already in place (*dotted black arrows*).

CARDIAC DEVICES: PACEMAKER, AUTOMATIC IMPLANTABLE CARDIAC DEFIBRILLATOR (AICD), INTRA-AORTIC BALLOON PUMP (IABP)

Pacemakers

- **Why are they used**
  - Used for cardiac conduction abnormalities
  - Certain conditions refractory to medical treatment (e.g., congestive heart failure)
- **Correct placement of cardiac pacemakers** (Box 10.8)
  - All **pacemakers consist of a pulse generator** usually implanted subcutaneously in the left anterior chest wall and **at least one lead (electrode)** inserted percutaneously most often via the subclavian vein.

⟫   IMPORTANT POINTS

- The **tip of one lead is almost always located in the apex of the right ventricle.** Remember that **in the frontal projection, the apex of the right ventricle lies to the left of the spine** and on the lateral film the **apex of the right ventricle is anterior** (Fig. 10.15).

- Some pacemakers have two leads (usually their tips are in the right atrium and right ventricle), whereas others may have three leads (with their tips usually in the right atrium, right ventricle, and coronary sinus).
- **All leads should have gentle curves.** There should be no sharp kinks in the electrodes.
- **Incorrect placement and complications of cardiac pacemakers**
  - **Pneumothoraces** are infrequent complications of either pacemaker or automatic implantable cardiac defibrillator (AICD) insertion.
  - **Fracture of the leads** may occur at any of three places: the generator itself, the site of venous access, or the tip of the lead. Breaks in the lead can be **recognized by discontinuity in the wire lead itself** (Fig. 10.16).

Fig. 10.17 Twiddler Syndrome. Some patients inadvertently "twiddle" with their subcutaneous pulse generator and, if the subcutaneous tissue allows, may rotate the generator many times on its own axis, curling the lead(s) around the device (*black arrow*). This can retract the tip of the electrode from the inner wall of the right ventricle, rendering the pacemaker useless. This lead has retracted to the superior vena cava (*white arrow*). "Twiddling" can also affect an AICD or chest infusion port.

- **Leads can perforate the heart,** producing cardiac tamponade. **Look for sharp bends** in leads secondary to perforation of a blood vessel.
- **Leads may retract from normal contact with the ventricular wall** because the patient *twists* or *twiddles* the pacemaker generator under the skin, unknowingly winding the leads around the generator and causing retraction of the tips (*Twiddler syndrome*) (Fig. 10.17) or from subcutaneous migration of the pacer.
- **Leads may be ectopically placed** (e.g., in the hepatic vein).

AUTOMATIC IMPLANTABLE CARDIAC DEFIBRILLATORS (AICD)

- **Why they are used**
  - To prevent sudden death, usually from tachyarrhythmias such as ventricular fibrillation or ventricular tachycardia
- **Correct placement of automatic implantable cardiac defibrillators** (Box 10.9)
  - AICDs can usually be **differentiated from pacemakers by the wider and more opaque segment of at least one of the electrodes** (Fig. 10.18). One electrode is usually placed

Fig. 10.18 Automatic Implantable Cardiac Defibrillator (AICD). The generator (G) for an AICD is placed in the subcutaneous tissue of the anterior chest wall (pectoral area). AICDs have a thicker segment that is part of the defibrillation coil or coils (*solid white and black arrows*). The electrodes are fed through the superior vena cava (*solid white arrow*) with their tips in the right atrium (*black circle*) and the apex of the right ventricle (*solid black arrow*). This AICD has a third lead that entered the coronary sinus (*dotted black arrow*).

> ### BOX 10.9 Automatic Implantable Cardiac Defibrillator
> - Automatic implantable cardiac defibrillators can be differentiated from pacemakers by the presence of a thicker section on at least one lead.
> - They may have one (right ventricle), two (right atrium and right ventricle), or three leads (right atrium, right ventricle, and coronary sinus).
> - Bends in the leads should be smooth curves, not sharp kinks.
> - Visible complications can include lead breakage and dislodgement.

in the superior vena cava or brachiocephalic vein. If another electrode is used, its tip is placed in the apex of the right ventricle.
  - **All bends in the leads should be smooth curves,** not sharp kinks.
- **Incorrect placement and complications of automatic implantable cardiac defibrillators**
  - Leads may **migrate** and become dislodged.
  - Leads may **fracture.**

INTRA-AORTIC COUNTERPULSATION BALLOON PUMP (IABP OR IACB)

- **Why are they used**
  - To improve cardiac output and improve perfusion of the coronary arteries following surgery or in patients with

---

BOX 10.10   **Intra-aortic Balloon Pumps**

- The tip has a metallic marker which should lie distal to the origin of the left subclavian artery.
- When inflated, the balloon may be visible as an air-containing, "sausage-like" structure in the thoracic aorta.
- Catheters placed too proximally may occlude the great vessels.
- Catheters placed too distally may be ineffective.

BOX 10.11   **Nasogastric Tube (Levin Tube)**

- The tip of a nasogastric tube should extend into the stomach about 10 cm past the esophagogastric (EG) junction.
- Nasogastric (NG) tubes are the most commonly malpositioned of all tubes; always check their positioning with a radiograph.
- When malpositioned, they most frequently coil in the esophagus.
- If inserted in the trachea, they can extend into a bronchus to the periphery of lung, more often on the right side.

Fig. 10.19 Intra-aortic Counterpulsation Balloon Pump (IABP). Inserted via the femoral artery, a long "hot dog-shaped" balloon is rhythmically inflated during early diastole and deflated during early systole. The tip can be identified by a small, linear metallic marker in the region of the descending thoracic aorta (*solid black arrow*). The tip should lie distal to origin of the left subclavian artery so as not to occlude it. This is usually about 2 cm from the top of the aortic arch (*solid white arrow*). A Swan-Ganz catheter is also in place in the right pulmonary artery (*dotted black arrow*).

cardiogenic shock or refractory ventricular failure. Placed in the proximal **descending** thoracic aorta, a long, cylindrical **balloon** is **inflated** in **diastole,** increasing blood flow to the coronary arteries, and is **deflated** in **systole,** which reduces the cardiac afterload.

- **Correct placement of intra-aortic balloon pumps** (Box 10.10)
  - **Tip can be identified by small, linear metallic marker** (Fig. 10.19).
    - **The tip should lie distal to the origin of the left subclavian artery** so as not to occlude it.
    - Metallic **marker may point slightly toward the right** in the region of the aortic arch.
  - When inflated, the sausage-shaped balloon may be visualized as an air-containing structure in the descending thoracic aorta.
- **Incorrect placement and complications of intra-aortic balloon pumps**
  - If the catheter is **too proximal, the inflated balloon may occlude the great vessels,** leading to **stroke.**
  - If the balloon is **too distal,** the **device has decreased effectiveness.**

- Aortic dissection and arterial perforation may occur infrequently.

GI TUBES AND LINES: NASOGASTRIC TUBES, FEEDING TUBES

Nasogastric Tubes (NGT)

- **Why are they used**
  - Short-term feeding
  - Gastric sampling and decompression through suction
  - Administering medication
- **Correct placement of nasogastric tubes** (Box 10.11)
  - **Nasogastric (NG) tubes** are **wide tubes** (about 1 cm) marked with a **radio-opaque stripe** that is **discontinuous** at a **side-hole,** usually about **10 cm from the tip.**
  - **The tip and any side-holes** of the tube should **extend about 10 cm into the stomach beyond the esophagogastric (EG) junction** to prevent aspiration from administration of a feeding into the esophagus. If the NGT is to be used only for suction, the position of the side-hole is less important (Fig. 10.20).

Fig. 10.20 Normal Esophagogastric Junction; Nasogastric Tube in Stomach. (A) This is a close-up view of the left lower thorax from an upper gastrointestinal series to illustrate the close proximity of the esophagogastric (EG) junction (*dotted white arrow*) to the junction of the left hemidiaphragm and the spine (*solid arrow*). *E* Esophagus; *G*, stomach. (B) In a different patient, a nasogastric tube enters the stomach at the EG junction (*dotted white arrow*) near the junction between the left hemidiaphragm and spine (*solid white arrow*) and extends around the greater curvature of the stomach almost to the pylorus. The "break" in the marker stripe (*solid black arrow*) marks the location of the side-hole, about 10 cm from the tip.

> ## IMPORTANT POINTS
>
> - **How to recognize the location of the EG junction**
>   - The **EG junction** is usually **located** near the **junction of the left hemidiaphragm** and the **left side** of the **thoracic spine** (see Fig. 10.20A).

- Incorrect placement and complications of nasogastric tubes
  - The **nasogastric tube is the most commonly malpositioned of all tubes and lines.**
    - **Coiling of the NG tube in the esophagus is the most common malposition.**
    - It may be **inadvertently inserted into the trachea** and enter a bronchus (Fig. 10.21).
    - **Perforation caused by an NG tube is rare** but, when it occurs, it usually occurs in the cervical esophagus.
    - A long-term, indwelling NG tube **can lead to gastroesophageal reflux** which may, in turn, produce **esophagitis** and **stricture.**
  - Always obtain a confirmatory radiograph before feeding the patient or administering any medication through the tube.

Feeding Tubes (Dobbhoff Tubes, DHT)

- **Why they are used**
  - Used for nutrition

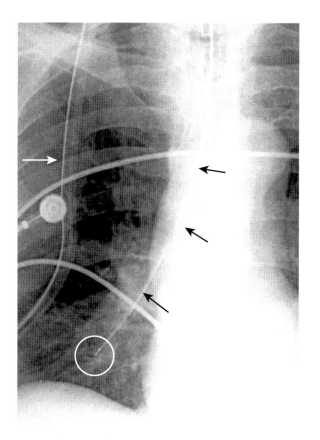

Fig. 10.21 Nasogastric Tube (NG) in Right Lower Lobe Bronchus. In this patient, the nasogastric tube (*black arrows*) is in the trachea instead of the esophagus and its tip extends to the right lower lobe (*white circle*). Rarely, the tube can perforate the lung and enter the pleural space. A radiograph to confirm positioning of a nasogastric tube is obtained before using it for feeding. A portion of the NG tube that lies outside the patient is superimposed on the chest (*white arrow*), as are several heart monitor leads.

Fig. 10.22 Dobbhoff Tube in Duodenum. Correctly placed, the tip of a Dobbhoff feeding tube should be in the duodenum so as to reduce risk of aspiration after feeding. The tip is usually recognizable by a weighted, metallic end (*solid white arrow*). This Dobbhoff tube enters the stomach (*solid black arrow*), courses around the duodenal sweep (*dotted black arrow*), and ends at the junction between the fourth portion of the duodenum and the jejunum, the location of the *ligament of Treitz* (*solid white arrow*).

Fig. 10.23 Dobbhoff Tube in Left and Right Lower Lobe Bronchi. In this case, the Dobbhoff tube inadvertently entered the trachea (*dotted black arrow*), and was advanced so that it looped back upon itself (*dotted white arrow*) to end in the right lower lobe bronchus (*solid white arrow*). It is important to obtain a confirmatory radiograph prior to using the tube for feedings.

BOX 10.12 Feeding Tubes (Dobbhoff Tubes)

- The tip should ideally be in the duodenum, although most lie in the stomach.
- The tip is recognizable by a metallic marker.
- If inadvertently inserted into the trachea, the tip may extend into the lung.
- Always obtain a confirmatory radiograph before using the tube for feedings.

- **Correct placement of feeding tubes** (Box 10.12)
  - The ideal position of the **tip of the feeding tube is considered to be postpyloric (i.e., in the duodenum or jejunum),** the rationale being to reduce the risk of aspiration after feeding (Fig. 10.22). In fact, placement in the stomach is very common.

- The tip of a DHT is recognizable by a weighted, metallic, linear density attached to the tip.
  - Did you know that the Dobbhoff tube was not named after a person called "Dobbhoff?" The tube is named after two physicians, Drs. Dobbie and Hoffmeister.
- **Incorrect placement and complications of feeding tubes**
  - **Placement in the trachea** rather than the esophagus may lead to the tip entering the lung. Always obtain a confirmatory radiograph before feeding the patient (Fig. 10.23).
  - **Perforation of the esophagus by the guidewire** is an uncommon complication.
    - Once the guidewire is removed, it is not reinserted.

🏠 TAKE HOME POINTS

Tube or Line[a]: Desired Position

Endotracheal tube (ETT):   Tip 3 to 5 cm from carina; usually, half the distance between the medial clavicles and carina

Tracheostomy tube tip: Halfway between stoma and carina

Central venous catheter (CVC):   Tip in superior vena cava

Peripherally inserted central catheter (PICC):   Tip in superior vena cava

Swan-Ganz catheter: Tip in proximal right or left pulmonary artery, within 2 cm from hilum

Double-lumen (Quinton) catheters: Tips in either superior vena cava or right atrium (or both) depending on type of catheter

Pleural drainage tube: Anterosuperior for pneumothorax; posteroinferior for pleural effusion

Pacemaker: Tip at apex of right ventricle; other lead(s) in right atrium and/or coronary sinus

Automatic implantable cardiac defibrillator (AICD):   One lead in superior vena cava; other lead(s) in right ventricle and/or coronary sinus

Intra-aortic balloon pump (IABP):   Tip about 2 cm from top of aortic arch in descending thoracic aorta

Nasogastric (Levin) tube (NGT):   Tip in stomach, 10 cm from esophagogastric junction

Feeding (Dobbhoff) tube (DHT):   Tip ideally in the duodenum, but more frequently in stomach

[a]Additional devices discussed online include: valve replacements, left ventricular assist devices, the Impella pump, left atrial occlusion clips, implantable loop recorders, coronary artery stents, tissue expanders, and percutaneous endoscopic gastrostomy tubes. See eFigs. 10.1 to 10.10.

📶 More information on recognizing the correct placement of lines and tubes and their potential complications: critical care radiology is available to registered users online.

11

Recognizing Other Diseases of the Chest

In this chapter, you will learn how to recognize mediastinal masses, benign and malignant pulmonary neoplasms, pulmonary thromboembolic disease, and selected airway diseases.

- Several chest abnormalities are discussed in other chapters (Table 11.1). A complete discussion of all of the abnormalities imaged in the chest is beyond the scope of this text. We will begin here with mediastinal masses and work our way outward to the lungs.

MEDIASTINAL MASSES

- The mediastinum is an area **whose lateral margins are defined by the medial borders of each lung,** whose **anterior margin** is the **sternum and anterior chest wall** and whose **posterior margin is the spine,** usually including the paravertebral gutters.
- The mediastinum can be arbitrarily subdivided into three compartments: *anterior, middle, and posterior* compartments and each contains its favorite set of diseases. The *superior mediastinum,* roughly the area above the plane of the aortic arch, is a division which is now usually combined with one of the other three compartments mentioned above (Fig. 11.1).

> **❗ DIAGNOSTIC PITFALLS**
>
> - Because these compartments have no true anatomic boundaries, **diseases from one compartment may extend into another compartment.** When a mediastinal abnormality becomes widespread or a mediastinal mass becomes quite large, it is often impossible to determine which compartment was its site of origin.

TABLE 11.1 **Chest Abnormalities Discussed Elsewhere in This Text**	
Topic	Appears in
Atelectasis	**Chapter 7**
Pleural effusion	**Chapter 8**
Pneumonia	**Chapter 9**
Pneumothorax, pneumomediastinum and pneumopericardium	**Chapter 25**
Cardiac and thoracic aortic abnormalities	**Chapter 12**
Chest trauma	**Chapter 25**

- **Differentiating a mediastinal from a parenchymal lung mass on frontal and lateral chest** radiographs can be difficult. Some helpful clues include:
  - If a **mass is completely surrounded by lung tissue in both the frontal and lateral projections, it lies within the lung,** not the mediastinum.
  - In general, **the margin of a mediastinal mass is sharper** than a mass originating in the lung.
  - Mediastinal masses frequently **displace, compress, or obstruct** other mediastinal structures (e.g., the trachea or esophagus).
- Ultimately, computed tomography (**CT**) **imaging** of the chest is **more accurate** in determining the location and nature of a mediastinal mass than conventional radiographs.

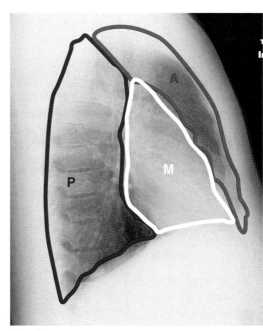

Fig. 11.1 The Mediastinal Compartments. The mediastinum is arbitrarily subdivided into three compartments: anterior, middle, and posterior. The anterior mediastinum extends from the back of the sternum to the anterior border of the heart and great vessels (A). The middle mediastinum extends from the anterior border of the heart and aorta to the posterior border of the heart and origins of the great vessels (M). The posterior mediastinum extends from the posterior border of the heart to the anterior border of the vertebral column (P). The posterior mediastinum includes the paravertebral gutters.

ANTERIOR MEDIASTINUM

- The **anterior mediastinum** is the compartment that extends from the **back of the sternum** to the **anterior border of the heart and great vessels.**
- A **differential diagnosis for anterior mediastinal masses** most often includes:
  - Substernal **thyroid masses**
  - **Lymphoma**
  - **Thymoma,** and
  - **Teratoma**
  - As a helpful way of remembering these four diseases, lymphoma is sometimes called "Terrible lymphoma" in this list so that all of the diseases "start" with the letter "T" (Table 11.2).

Thyroid Masses

- In **everyday practice, enlarged substernal thyroids** are the **most frequently encountered anterior mediastinal mass.** The vast majority of these masses are **multinodular goiters** and the mass is called a *substernal goiter, or a substernal thyroid or substernal thyroid goiter.*
- On occasion, the isthmus or lower pole of either lobe of the thyroid may enlarge, but project **downward** into the upper thorax rather than **anteriorly** into the neck. About three out of four thyroid masses extend anterior to the trachea; the remaining (almost all of which are right-sided) descend posterior to the trachea.

TABLE 11.2	Anterior Mediastinal Masses ("Four T's")
Mass	**What to Look for**
Thyroid goiter	The only anterior mediastinal mass that routinely deviates the trachea
Lymphoma (Lymphadenopathy)	Lobulated, polycyclic mass; frequently asymmetric; may occur in any compartment of the mediastinum
Thymoma	Look for a well-marginated mass that may be associated with myasthenia gravis
Teratoma	Well-marginated mass that may contain fat and calcium visible on CT scans

- Substernal goiters characteristically displace the trachea either to the left or right above the level of the aortic arch, a tendency the other anterior mediastinal masses do not typically demonstrate. Classically, **substernal goiters do not extend below the top of the aortic arch** (Fig. 11.2).

> ### »» IMPORTANT POINTS
>
> - Therefore, **think of an enlarged substernal thyroid** whenever you see an **anterior mediastinal mass that displaces the trachea**.

- Radioisotope **thyroid scans are the study of first choice** in confirming the diagnosis of a substernal thyroid as virtually all of them will display some uptake of the radioactive tracer which can be imaged and recorded with a special camera (**see online chapter: Nuclear Medicine: Understanding the Principles and Recognizing the Basics**).
- **On CT**, substernal thyroid masses are **contiguous with the thyroid gland; they frequently contain calcification** and avidly take up intravenous contrast, but **with a mottled, inhomogeneous appearance** (Fig. 11.3).

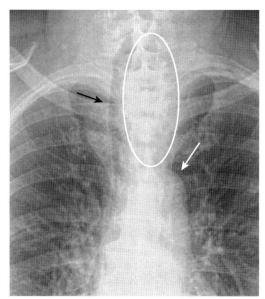

Fig. 11.2 Substernal Thyroid Mass. The left lobe of the thyroid is enlarged and projects downward into the upper thorax (*white oval*) displacing the trachea to the right (*black arrow*). Note the mass does not extend below the top of the aortic arch (*white arrow*). Most patients with palpable thyroid goiters are female and asymptomatic.

Fig. 11.3 CT of a Substernal Thyroid Goiter Without and With Contrast Enhancement. (A) Before administration of intravenous contrast, this substernal thyroid mass (*solid white arrow*) is well-defined and contains coarse calcifications (*dotted white arrow*). (B) After contrast administration and at the same level as before, the goiter avidly takes up intravenous contrast, frequently with a mottled appearance (*solid white arrow*). This mass is displacing the trachea (T) slightly to the left.

Lymphoma

- **Lymphadenopathy,** whether from lymphoma, metastatic carcinoma, sarcoid, or tuberculosis, is the most common cause of a mediastinal mass overall.
- **Anterior mediastinal lymphadenopathy is most common in Hodgkin lymphoma, especially the nodular sclerosing variety.** Hodgkin lymphoma is a malignancy of the lymph nodes, more common in females, which most often presents with painless, enlarged lymph nodes in the neck.
- Unlike teratomas and thymomas, which are presumed to expand outward from a single abnormal cell, lymphomatous masses are frequently composed of several contiguously enlarged lymph nodes. As such, **lymphadenopathy frequently presents with a border that is lobulated** or **polycyclic in contour** owing to the conglomeration of enlarged nodes that make up the mass.

> ### ⯈ IMPORTANT POINTS
>
> - On chest radiographs, this lobulation **may help differentiate lymphadenopathy from other mediastinal masses.**

- **Mediastinal lymphadenopathy** in **Hodgkin lymphoma** is usually **bilateral and asymmetric** (Fig. 11.4). In addition, **asymmetric hilar adenopathy** is associated with mediastinal adenopathy in many patients with Hodgkin lymphoma.
- In general, **mediastinal lymph nodes that exceed about 1 cm** measured along their **short axis** on CT scans of the mediastinum are **considered to be enlarged.**
- Lymphoma will **produce multiple, lobulated soft-tissue masses** or one **large, soft-tissue mass** from lymph node aggregation.
- The **mass is usually homogeneous** in density on CT but **may be heterogeneous** when it achieves a sufficient size to undergo **necrosis (areas of lower attenuation, i.e., blacker)** or **hemorrhage (areas of higher attenuation, i.e., whiter)** (Fig. 11.5).
- Some findings of lymphoma may **mimic** those of **sarcoid** because both produce thoracic adenopathy. Table 11.3 contains several key points to differentiate the two diseases.

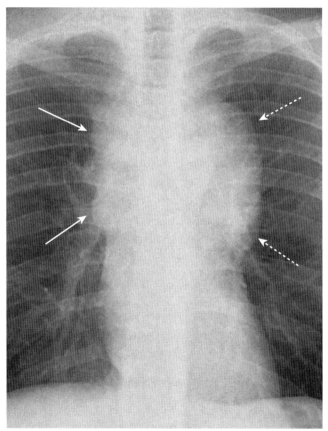

Fig. 11.4 Mediastinal Adenopathy From Hodgkin Lymphoma. Lymphadenopathy frequently presents with a lobulated or polycyclic border because of the conglomeration of enlarged nodes that produce the mass (*solid and dotted white arrows*). Hodgkin lymphoma is usually confined to nodes above the diaphragm. Pain in the affected lymph nodes after alcohol consumption is a classic, but uncommon, sign of the disease.

Fig. 11.5 CT of Anterior Mediastinal Adenopathy in Hodgkin Lymphoma. On CT, lymphadenopathy will produce multiple, lobulated soft-tissue masses or a large soft-tissue mass from lymph node aggregation (*white arrows*). The mass is usually homogeneous in density, as in this case. The superior vena cava (SVC) is compressed, but not occluded, by the nodes. *A,* Ascending aorta; *Ao,* descending aorta.

TABLE 11.3	**Sarcoidosis vs. Lymphoma**
Sarcoid	**Lymphoma**
Bilateral hilar and right paratracheal adenopathy are classic combination	More often mediastinal adenopathy is associated with asymmetric hilar enlargement
Enlarged bronchopulmonary nodes are more peripheral	Enlarged hilar nodes are more central
Pleural effusion in about 5%	Pleural effusion more common, in 30%
Anterior mediastinal adenopathy is uncommon	Anterior mediastinal adenopathy is common

Fig. 11.6 Thymoma: Chest Radiograph and CT Scan. (A) The chest radiograph shows a smoothly marginated anterior mediastinal mass (*black arrow*). (B) Contrast-enhanced CT scan confirms the anterior mediastinal location and homogeneous density of the mass (*white arrow*). Most thymomas are benign. The patient had myasthenia gravis and improved following resection of the thymoma. *A,* Ascending aorta; *Ao,* descending aorta; *PA,* main pulmonary artery; *SVC,* superior vena cava.

Thymic Masses

- **Normal thymic tissue can be visible on CT throughout life,** although the gland begins to **involute after age 20.**
- **Thymomas** are neoplasms of thymic epithelium and lymphocytes. They occur most often in **middle-aged adults,** generally at an **older** age than those with **teratomas.** Most thymomas are **benign.**

> ### ≫ IMPORTANT POINTS
>
> - Thymomas are **associated with myasthenia gravis about 35% of the time** they are present. Conversely, about **15% of patients with** clinical **myasthenia gravis will** be found to **have a thymoma.** The importance of identifying a thymoma in patients with myasthenia gravis lies in the more **favorable prognosis** for patients with myasthenia **after thymectomy.**

- On **CT scans, thymomas** classically present as **smooth or lobulated masses** that arise near the **junction of the heart and great vessels** and which, like teratomas, **may contain calcification** (Fig. 11.6).
- Other lesions can produce enlargement of the thymus, but they are rare and include thymic cysts, thymic hyperplasia, thymic lymphoma, carcinoma, or lipoma.

Teratoma

- Teratomas are **germinal tumors** that typically **contain all three germ layers** (ectoderm, mesoderm, and endoderm). Most teratomas are benign and occur earlier in life than thymomas. Usually **asymptomatic** and discovered serendipitously, about **30% of mediastinal teratomas are malignant** and have a poor prognosis.
- The most common variety of teratoma is **cystic;** it produces a **well-marginated mass** near the origin of the great vessels that characteristically **contains fat, cartilage, and possibly bone on CT examination** (Fig. 11.7).

Fig. 11.7 Mediastinal Teratoma. The most common variety of teratoma is cystic, which usually produces a well-marginated mass near the origin of the great vessels. On CT, they characteristically contain fat (*solid black arrow*), cartilage, and sometimes bone (*dotted white arrow*). They are usually benign, well-encapsulated with an enhancing rim, as in this case (*solid white arrows*). Treatment is surgical excision.

MIDDLE MEDIASTINAL MASSES

- The **middle mediastinum** is the compartment that extends from the **anterior border of the heart and aorta** to the **posterior border of the heart;** it **contains** the **heart,** the **origins of the great vessels, the trachea,** and the **main bronchi** along with **lymph nodes** (see Fig. 11.1).
- **Lymphadenopathy produces the most common mass in this compartment.** Although Hodgkin lymphoma is the most likely cause of mediastinal adenopathy, other malignancies and several benign diseases can produce such findings.
  - Other malignancies that produce mediastinal lymphadenopathy include **small cell lung carcinoma** and

Fig. 11.8 **Middle Mediastinal Lymphadenopathy.** Mediastinal adenopathy may be "reactive" (e.g., tuberculosis), malignant (e.g., lymphoma, small cell lung carcinoma and metastatic disease), or even occur with autoimmune diseases such as systemic lupus erythematosus. This patient has a mediastinal mass demonstrated on both the frontal (A) (*solid white arrows*) and lateral (B) views (*solid black arrow*). The mass is pushing the trachea forward on the lateral view (*dotted white arrow*). The biopsied lymph nodes in this patient demonstrated small cell carcinoma of the lung.

Fig. 11.9 **Neurofibromatosis.** A large, posterior mediastinal neurofibroma (*white arrows*) is seen in the right, paravertebral gutter on the frontal (A) and lateral (B) views. Neurofibromas can occur as an isolated tumor or as part of the **neurofibromatosis, type 1 (NF-1) syndrome,** as it did this case. NF-1 is autosomal dominant and features a myriad of signs and symptoms, including cutaneous, neural, and musculoskeletal abnormalities.

metastatic disease such as from primary **breast carcinoma** (Fig. 11.8).

- Benign causes of mediastinal lymphadenopathy include **infectious mononucleosis** and **tuberculosis,** the latter usually producing **unilateral mediastinal adenopathy.**

POSTERIOR MEDIASTINAL MASSES

- The **posterior mediastinum** is the compartment that extends from the **posterior border of the heart** to the **anterior border of the vertebral column.** For imaging purposes, however, it is **considered to extend to either side of the spine into the paravertebral gutters** (see Fig. 11.1).
- It contains the **descending aorta, esophagus, lymph nodes,** is the site of masses representing **extramedullary hematopoiesis** and, most importantly, is the home of **tumors of neural origin.**

Neurogenic Tumors

- Although neurogenic tumors produce the largest percentage of posterior mediastinal masses, none of these lesions is particularly common. Neurogenic tumors include such entities as **neurofibroma, Schwannoma, ganglioneuroma,** and **neuroblastoma.**
- **Nerve sheath tumors** (Schwannoma) are the **most common** and are almost always **benign.** They usually affect persons 20 to 50 years of age and, because they are slow growing, may produce no symptoms until late in their course.
- Neoplasms that arise from nerve elements **other than the sheath,** such as **ganglioneuromas** and **neuroblastoma,** are **usually malignant.**
- **Neurogenic tumors** will produce a soft-tissue **mass, usually sharply marginated,** in the paravertebral gutter (Fig. 11.9). Both benign and malignant tumors **may erode adjacent ribs**

Fig. 11.10 Rib-Notching and a Dumbbell-Shaped Neurofibroma. (A) Plexiform neurofibromas can produce erosions along the inferior borders of the ribs (where the intercostal nerves are located) and produce either notching or a wavy appearance called ***ribbon ribs*** (*solid white arrows*). (B) Another patient demonstrates a large neurofibroma that is enlarging the neural foramen, eroding half of the vertebral body (*solid black arrow*) and producing a dumb-bell shaped lesion that arises from the spinal canal, but projects through the foramen into the mediastinum (*dotted white arrow*).

(Fig. 11.10A). They may **enlarge neural foramina** producing ***dumbbell***-shaped lesions that arise from the spinal canal, but project through the neural foramen into the mediastinum (Fig. 11.10B).

- **Neurofibromas** most often occur as an **isolated tumor** arising from the Schwann cell of the nerve sheath **or as part of a syndrome** called ***neurofibromatosis, type 1 (NF1).*** As part of the latter, they are a component of a neurocutaneous bone dysplasia that can cause numerous abnormalities, including **subcutaneous nodules, erosion of adjacent bone (*rib notching*), scalloping** of the posterior aspect of the vertebral bodies (Fig. 11.11), **absence** of the **sphenoid wings, pseudarthroses,** and **sharp-angled kyphoscoliosis** at the thoracolumbar junction.

SOLITARY NODULE/MASS IN THE LUNG

- **The difference between a *nodule* and a *mass* is size:** in general, under 3 cm it is usually called a ***nodule*** and over 3 cm a ***mass.***
- Much has been written about the workup of a patient in whom a single nodular density is discovered in the lung on imaging of the thorax (i.e., the **solitary pulmonary nodule [SPN]).** It is estimated that as many as 50% of smokers have a nodule discovered by chest CT, yet a tiny percentage of small nodules show any malignant tendencies (growth or metastases) when followed for years.
- In evaluating a solitary pulmonary nodule, the **critical question** to be answered is: **Is the nodule most likely benign or most likely malignant?** If most likely benign, it can be watched in follow-up, whereas, if most likely malignant, it will almost certainly be treated aggressively with therapies which themselves carry some risk of morbidity and mortality.

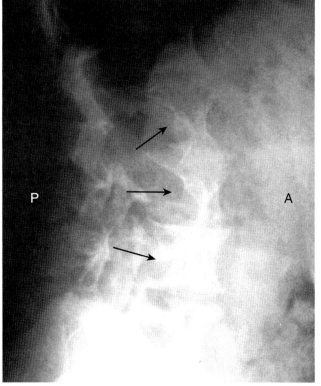

Fig. 11.11. Scalloping of the Vertebral Bodies in Neurofibromatosis. Many skeletal abnormalities are associated with neurofibromatosis, including scalloping of the posterior vertebral bodies (*black arrows*), especially in the thoracic or lumbar spine as shown here in this lateral view. This is produced by diverticula of the thecal sac caused by dysplasia of the meninges that leads to erosion of adjacent bone through the pulsations transmitted via the spinal fluid. *A*, Anterior; *P*, posterior.

Fig. 11.12 Solitary Pulmonary Nodule, Enlarging Over Time. Two, close-up images taken one year apart are shown. (A) A small nodular density is present in the left upper lobe (*white circle*) on an image obtained for comparison when image (B) was acquired one year later, by which time the nodule has clearly increased in size and shows an irregular outer margin, both suggestive of malignancy. Biopsy of the lesion demonstrated adenocarcinoma.

Fig. 11.13 Solitary Pulmonary Nodules: CT Patterns. Based on their appearance on CT, small nodules are divided into those with a **solid appearance** (A, *white arrow*) versus those with a **subsolid appearance.** **Subsolid nodules** are further divided into those that are **purely ground-glass nodules** (B, *dotted white arrow*) and those that are **partly solid and partly ground-glass** (C, *white circle*). Note that the vascular markings are still visible in a ground-glass nodule (B, *solid white arrow*). The malignancy rate for subsolid nodules is higher than that of solid nodules and the malignancy rate for partly solid nodules is higher than the rate for pure ground-glass nodules.

- The answer to the question of benign versus malignant will depend on many factors including the availability of **prior imaging studies,** which **can help greatly in establishing stability or growth of a lesion over time** (Fig. 11.12)
- Many nodules are discovered **incidentally** during CT imaging of the lung for an unrelated disease or CT imaging of another body part that contains part of the lungs (e.g., an abdominal CT that includes the lung bases). It is estimated about 1.5 million incidental, solitary pulmonary nodules are found each year in the United States, a number that has been increasing.

- Based on their **appearance on CT,** small nodules have been divided into those with a **solid** appearance versus those with a **subsolid** appearance. The CT appearance of nodules aids in the clinical and radiologic management of their significance and follow-up (Fig. 11.13).
  - **Subsolid nodules** are further divided into those that are **purely ground-glass nodules** and those that are **partly solid and partly ground-glass.**
  - A **ground-glass nodule** is an area of increased attenuation (whiter) on CT in which the vascular and bronchial

markings are **preserved** within the nodule, rather than obliterated by the nodule. Subsolid nodules are important because, when persistent, they may represent **adenocarcinoma** or its precursors (see Fig. 11.13).

- In 2017, an international society of chest radiologists (Fleischner Society) revised a previous set of evidence-based criteria establishing guidelines for the follow-up of **noncalcified nodules** found **incidentally** during **CT** in **adults** over 35 years of age. Their recommendations are shown in a table **included in the appendix of this chapter.**
  - In summary, the new guidelines suggest a less-needed follow-up than previously suggested for many stable, incidental solitary pulmonary nodules. Those that are **solid** and **unchanged** on serial CTs over a **two-year** period, or **subsolid** and **unchanged** over a **five-year** period, are likely benign and **do not need further diagnostic evaluation.**

Signs of a Benign Versus Malignant Solitary Pulmonary Nodule

- **Size of the lesion.** Nodules less than 4 mm rarely show malignant behavior. Masses **larger than 5 cm have a 95% chance of malignancy** (Fig. 11.14).
- **Calcification.** The presence of calcification is usually determined by CT. **Lesions containing central, laminar, or diffuse patterns of calcification are invariably benign** (Fig. 11.15).
- **Margin.** Lobulation, spiculation, and shagginess all suggest malignancy.

Fig. 11.14 Right Upper Lobe Bronchogenic Carcinoma. There is a 3.2 cm spiculated mass in the right upper lobe (*white arrow*). The relatively large size and irregular margins of this mass point toward a malignant process. A percutaneous biopsy revealed an adenocarcinoma of the lung.

Fig. 11.15 Calcified Tuberculous Granulomas and Histoplasmoma. When a pulmonary nodule is heavily calcified, it is almost always benign. (A) Tuberculous granulomas are common sequelae of prior, usually subclinical, tuberculous infection and are usually homogeneously calcified (*black circles*). (B) **Histoplasmomas** (*white arrow*) may contain a central or "target" calcification (*black arrow*) or may have a laminated calcification, which is diagnostic. CT can be used to differentiate between a calcified and a non-calcified pulmonary nodule with greater sensitivity than conventional radiographs.

- **Change in size over time.** Requires a previous study or sufficient confidence so as to obtain a follow-up study that will provide a basis of comparison of size over time.
  - **Malignancies** tend to **increase in size at a rate that is not so brief as to suggest an inflammatory etiology** (changes in weeks) **nor so prolonged as to suggest benignity** (no change over two years) (see Fig. 11.12).
    - **Large cell carcinomas**, as a cell type, **grow the most rapidly.**
    - **Squamous cell carcinomas** and **small cell carcinomas** tend to grow slightly less **rapidly.**
    - **Adenocarcinomas** grow the **most slowly.**

> ## ▶ IMPORTANT POINTS
>
> - **Presence of clinical symptoms.** When clinical signs or symptoms are present (e.g., hemoptysis, weight loss, hoarseness), the chance that a pulmonary nodule is malignant increases. Solitary pulmonary nodules that are surgically removed from those showing **clinical signs or symptoms** and imaging findings that suggest malignancy are **malignant about 50% of the time in men over the age of 50.**

Benign Causes of Solitary Pulmonary Nodules

- **Granulomas.** Tuberculosis and histoplasmosis usually produce calcified nodules less than 1 cm in size, although tuberculomas and histoplasmomas can reach up to 4 cm.
  - **When calcified, they are clearly benign. Tuberculous** granulomas are usually **homogeneously calcified. Histo-** plasmomas may contain a **central** or **"target" calcification** or may have a **laminated calcification,** which is diagnostic.
- **Positron emission tomographic (PET) scans** can also help in differentiating benign from malignant nodules and provide insight into the site of any metastatic disease. Using a glucose analog (**fluorodeoxyglucose or FDG**), the test is based on the enhanced glucose metabolism and uptake of lung cancer cells. Usually, the nodules must be larger than 1 cm in size for accurate characterization as being "PET-avid" (i.e., most likely malignant). (**See online chapter: Nuclear Medicine: Understanding the Principles and Recognizing the Basics**).
- **Hamartomas** are peripherally located lung tumors of **disorganized lung tissue** that characteristically **contain fat and calcification** on CT scan. The **classical calcification** of a hamartoma is called *popcorn calcification* (Fig. 11.16).
- Other, uncommon benign lesions that can produce solitary pulmonary nodules include rheumatoid nodules, fungal diseases, such as nocardiosis; arteriovenous malformations, and granulomatosis with polyangiitis (Wegener granulomatosis).
- Round atelectasis, which may mimic a solitary pulmonary nodule, is discussed in Chapter 7: Recognizing Atelectasis.

BRONCHOGENIC CARCINOMA

- In the United States, **lung cancer is the most common fatal malignancy in men** and the **second most common in women** (next to breast cancer).

Fig. 11.16 Hamartoma of the Lung. Hamartomas classically contain fat and calcification on CT scans. The calcification has been described as **popcorn** in appearance (*white arrow*). The small island of soft tissue in the middle of the right lung (D) is the uppermost part of the right hemidiaphragm. Since you are about halfway through this chapter, now might be a good time to reward yourself with a treat of some real popcorn (if you can).

TABLE 11.4   Carcinoma of the Lung: Cell Types

Cell Type and Clinical Manifestations	Graphic Representation	Cell Type and Clinical Manifestations	Graphic Representation
Squamous Cell Carcinoma • Primarily central in location • Arise in segmental or lobar bronchi • Invariably produce bronchial obstruction leading to obstructive pneumonitis or atelectasis • Tend to grow rapidly		**Small Cell, Including Oat Cell Carcinoma** • Primarily central in location • Many contain neurosecretory granules that lead to an association of small cell carcinoma with paraneoplastic syndromes, such as Cushing syndrome, inappropriate secretion of antidiuretic hormone	
Adenocarcinoma • Primarily peripheral in location • Usually solitary except in the case of diffuse adenocarcinoma, which can present as multiple nodules • Slowest growing		**Large Cell Carcinoma** • Diagnosis of exclusion for lesions that are non-small cell, and not squamous or adenocarcinoma • Larger peripheral lesions • Grow extremely rapidly	

• The **number** of nodules in the lung can help direct the work-up. **Primary lung cancer** usually presents as a **solitary nodule,** whereas **metastatic disease** to the lung from another organ characteristically produces **multiple nodules.**

• Table 11.4 summarizes the classical manifestations and growth tendencies of the four types of bronchogenic carcinoma by cell type.

• **Recognizing a bronchogenic carcinoma**
  • They may be recognized by visualization of the **tumor itself** (i.e., a **nodule/mass in the lung**).
  • They may be suspected by recognizing the **effects of bronchial obstruction** (i.e., **pneumonitis** and/or **atelectasis**).
  • They may be suspected by recognizing the results of either their **direct extension or metastatic spread** to the lung, ribs, or other organs.

Bronchogenic Carcinomas Presenting as a Nodule/Mass in the Lung

• These are most often **adenocarcinomas.**
• The nodule/mass may have **irregular** and **spiculated margins** (see Fig. 11.14).
• The mass **may cavitate**, more often if it is of squamous cell origin (although cavitation also occurs with adenocarcinoma), usually producing a **relatively thick-walled** cavity with a **nodular and irregular inner margin** (Fig. 11.17).

Fig. 11.17 Cavitary Bronchogenic Carcinoma. A large, cavitating neoplasm is seen in the right upper lobe with a thick wall (*double black arrow*), spiculated outer margin (*dotted white arrow*), and a nodular internal margin (*dotted black arrows*). Lung cancers can cavitate due to degeneration of the tumor itself or they can obstruct a bronchus leading to a more distal pneumonia which then cavitates. This was a squamous cell carcinoma.

✳ **IMAGE-GUIDED INTERVENTIONS**

A 68-year-old male with extensive pulmonary disease and smoking history presents for worsening cough with hemoptysis. Chest CT demonstrates a solitary pulmonary nodule in the posterior aspects of the left upper lobe *(arrow)*. How might an image-guided procedure benefit in this case? See the answer in Chapter 29.

Bronchogenic Carcinoma Presenting With Bronchial Obstruction

- **Bronchial obstruction is most often caused by a squamous cell carcinoma.** Endobronchial lesions produce varying degrees of bronchial obstruction that can lead to pneumonitis or atelectasis.
  - **Obstructive pneumonitis and atelectasis** (see Fig. 7.11)
    - It is called *pneumonitis* because the obstructed lung is consolidated, but frequently not infected (though it can be).
    - **Atelectasis** secondary to an endobronchial, obstructing lesion features the usual shifts of the fissures or mobile mediastinal structures **toward** the side of the atelectasis (see Chapter 7) as well as occasional visualization of the obstructing mass itself.

Bronchogenic Carcinoma Presenting With Direct Extension or Metastatic Lesions

- **Rib destruction by direct extension.** *Pancoast tumor* is the eponym for a tumor arising from the superior sulcus of the lung, frequently producing destruction of one or more of the first three ribs on the affected side (Box 11.1).

BOX 11.1 Pancoast Tumor: Apical Lung Cancer (Fig. 11.19)

- Manifests as a soft-tissue mass in the apex of the lung
- Most often squamous cell carcinoma or adenocarcinoma
- Frequently produces adjacent rib destruction
- May invade brachial plexus or cause Horner syndrome on affected side
- On the right side, it may produce superior vena caval obstruction

---

- **Hilar adenopathy.** Usually unilateral on the same side as the tumor (Fig. 11.18).
- **Mediastinal adenopathy.** May be the sole manifestation of a small cell carcinoma, the peripheral lung nodule itself being invisible (see Fig. 11.8).
- **Other nodules in the lung.** One of the manifestations of adenocarcinoma primary to the lung itself may be multiple nodules throughout both lungs and, as such, may mimic metastatic disease.
- **Pleural effusion.** Frequently, there is associated lymphangitic carcinomatosis in the lung when there is a pleural effusion.
- **Metastases to bones.** These tend to be mixed osteolytic and osteoblastic.

Fig. 11.18 Bronchogenic Carcinoma With Hilar and Mediastinal Adenopathy. There is a peripheral lung mass (*solid black arrow*) with evidence of ipsilateral hilar and mediastinal adenopathy (*solid white arrows*) and contralateral mediastinal adenopathy (*dotted white arrow*). Spread to the mediastinal nodes on the side opposite the tumor tends to worsen prognosis for lung cancers. This was an adenocarcinoma of the lung.

Fig. 11.19 Pancoast Tumor, Right Upper Lobe. A large, soft-tissue mass is seen in the apex of the right lung (*white arrow*). It is associated with rib destruction (*black arrow*). On the normal left side, the ribs are intact (*dotted white arrow*). The finding of an apical soft-tissue mass with associated rib destruction is classic for a Pancoast or superior sulcus tumor. The patient had a right-sided constricted pupil (miosis), ptosis, and anhidrosis (Horner syndrome).

TABLE 11.5 Some Common Primary Sites of Metastatic Lung Nodules	
Males	**Females**
Colorectal carcinoma	Breast cancer
Renal cell carcinoma	Colorectal carcinoma
Head and neck tumors	Renal cell carcinoma
Testicular and bladder carcinoma	Cervical or endometrial carcinoma
Malignant melanoma	Malignant melanoma
Sarcomas	Sarcomas

METASTATIC NEOPLASMS IN THE LUNG

Multiple Nodules

- Multiple nodules in the lung are most often metastatic lesions that have traveled through the bloodstream from a distant primary tumor (**hematogenous spread**). Multiple metastatic nodules are **usually of slightly differing sizes,** indicating tumor embolization that occurred at different times.
- They are **frequently sharply marginated,** varying in size from **micronodular** to "cannonball" masses (see Fig. 5.15A).
- For all practical purposes it is **impossible to determine the primary site** by the **appearance of the metastatic nodules** (i.e., all metastatic nodules appear similar).

> ## ⟫ IMPORTANT POINTS
>
> - Tissue sampling, whether by bronchoscopic or percutaneous biopsy, is the best means of determining the organ of origin of the metastatic nodule.

- Table 11.5 summarizes the primary malignancies most likely to metastasize to the lung hematogenously.

Lymphangitic Spread of Carcinoma (Lymphangitic Carcinomatosis)

- In lymphangitic carcinomatosis, the tumor grows in and obstructs lymphatics in the lung, producing a pattern that is **radiologically similar to pulmonary interstitial edema** from heart failure, **including Kerley B lines, thickening of the fissures,** and **pleural effusions.**

> ## ⟫ IMPORANT POINTS
>
> - The findings **may be unilateral or may involve only one lobe,** a pattern that should alert you to suspect the possibility of lymphangitic spread rather than congestive heart failure, which is usually bilateral (Fig. 11.20).

- The **most common primary malignancies to produce lymphangitic carcinomatosis** are those that arise in or around the thorax: **breast, lung, and pancreatic carcinoma.**

PULMONARY THROMBOEMBOLIC DISEASE (PE)

- Over **90% of pulmonary emboli develop from thrombi in the deep veins of the leg,** especially above the level of the popliteal veins. They are usually a **complication of surgery,**

Fig. 11.20 Bronchogenic Carcinoma with Lymphangitic Carcinomatosis. Seen is extensive hilar and mediastinal adenopathy (*solid black arrows*) from a carcinoma of the lung. The interstitial markings are prominent in the right lung compared with the left and there are thickened interlobular septa (Kerley B lines) present (*solid white arrows*) along with a right pleural effusion (*dotted black arrow*). Adenocarcinomas are the most common cause of lymphangitic carcinomatosis. Tumor cells can usually found in the lymphatics and pleural fluid.

Fig. 11.21 Hampton's Hump. A wedge-shaped, peripheral air-space density present (*dotted white arrow*) is associated with filling defects in both the left and right pulmonary arteries (*solid white arrows*). The wedge-shaped infarct is called **Hampton's hump**. Without the associated emboli being present, the peripheral airspace disease could have a differential diagnosis that includes pneumonia, lung contusion or aspiration.

prolonged bed rest, or **cancer.** Because of the **dual** circulation of the lungs (pulmonary and bronchial), **most pulmonary emboli do not result in infarction.**

- Although conventional chest radiographs are frequently abnormal in patients with PE, they mostly demonstrate nonspecific findings such as **subsegmental atelectasis, small pleural effusions,** or **elevation of the hemidiaphragm. Conventional chest radiography** has a **high false–negative rate in detecting PE.**
- Chest radiographs **infrequently** manifest one of the "classical" findings for **pulmonary embolism,** which can include:
  - Wedge-shaped peripheral air-space disease (***Hampton's hump***) (Fig. 11.21).
  - Focally absent or decreased pulmonary vasculature (***Westermark's sign***)
  - **A prominent central pulmonary artery (*Knuckle sign*)**

⟫ IMPORTANT POINTS

- If the chest radiograph is normal, a nuclear medicine ventilation-perfusion scan (V/Q scan) may be diagnostic. If, however, the chest radiograph is abnormal, CT is usually performed.

✴ IMAGE-GUIDED INTERVENTIONS

The contrast-enhanced CT of the chest on a 56-year-old female with chest pain and hemoptysis shows filling defects in both pulmonary arteries *(arrows)*. How might an image-guided procedure benefit in this case? See the answer in Chapter 29.

- **CT pulmonary angiography (CT-PA)** is made possible by the **fast data acquisition** of **spiral CT** scanners (one breath hold) combined with **thin slices** and **rapid bolus intravenous injection of iodinated contrast** that produce maximal opacification of the pulmonary arteries with little or no motion artifact.
- Another benefit of CT-PA studies is the ability to acquire images of the veins of the pelvis and legs by obtaining slightly delayed images following the pulmonary arterial phase of the study. In this way, a **deep venous thrombus** may be detected even if the pulmonary angiogram is nondiagnostic.
- CT-PA has a sensitivity **in excess of 90%** and has replaced the use of ventilation/perfusion (V/Q) scans in patients with **chronic obstructive pulmonary disease** or a **positive chest radiograph** in whom a V/Q scan is known to be less sensitive.
- On CT-PA, acute **pulmonary emboli** appear as **partial or complete filling defects centrally located** within the **contrast-enhanced** lumina of the **pulmonary arteries** (Fig. 11.22).
  - CT-PA has the **additional benefit** of **demonstrating other diseases** that may be present, such as pneumonia, even if the study is negative for pulmonary embolism. CT-PA is also part of the diagnostic imaging examination called the *triple rule-out* in which patients presenting with chest pain can be simultaneously evaluated for **coronary artery disease, aortic dissection**, and **pulmonary embolism**.

CHRONIC OBSTRUCTIVE PULMONARY DISEASE

- Chronic obstructive lung disease (COPD) is defined as a disease of **airflow obstruction caused by chronic bronchitis or emphysema.**
- **Chronic bronchitis** is defined **clinically** by a **productive cough**, whereas **emphysema** is defined **pathologically** by the presence of **permanent and abnormal enlargement and destruction of the air spaces distal to the terminal bronchioles.**
- **Emphysema has three pathologic patterns:**
  - **Centriacinar (centrilobular) emphysema** features focal destruction limited to the respiratory bronchioles and the central portions of the acinus. It is **associated with**

Fig. 11.22 Saddle and Peripheral Pulmonary Emboli. (A) A large pulmonary embolus almost completely fills both the left and right pulmonary arteries *(solid white and black arrows)*. This is called a **saddle embolus** because it straddles several major pulmonary arteries. (B) A small, central filling defect is seen in a more peripheral pulmonary artery *(dotted white arrow)*. This pulmonary artery seems to be floating disconnected in the lung because the plane of this particular image does not display its connection to the pulmonary artery.

Fig. 11.23 Types of Emphysema. (A) *Centriacinar (centrilobular) emphysema* is the most common type. Centrilobular emphysema has a strong association with cigarette smoking. It features focal destruction limited to the respiratory bronchioles and the central portions of the acinus (*white arrows*). It is most severe in the upper lobes. (B) *Panlobular (panacinar) emphysema* involves the entire alveolus distal to the terminal bronchiole; it is most severe in the lower lung zones and generally develops in patients with homozygous alpha 1-antitrypsin deficiency, although it can also be seen in smokers and the elderly. This patient additionally has partial visualization of a nodular liver from cirrhosis (*black arrows*). (C) *Paraseptal emphysema* involves distal airway structures, alveolar ducts, and sacs. It tends to occur around the septae of the lungs or subpleural surfaces.

Fig. 11.24 Emphysema: Conventional Radiography. On conventional radiographs, the imaging findings of chronic obstructive pulmonary disease are hyperinflation, including flattening of the diaphragm, especially on the lateral exposure (*solid white arrow* in B), increase in the size of the retrosternal clear space (*dotted white arrow*), hyperlucency of the lungs with decreased vascular markings and enlargement of the pulmonary arteries secondary to pulmonary arterial hypertension (*solid white arrows* in A).

cigarette smoking and is most severe in the **upper lobes** (Fig. 11.23A).

- **Panacinar emphysema** involves the entire alveolus distal to the terminal bronchiole. It is most severe in the **lower lung zones** and generally develops in patients with homozygous **alpha 1-antitrypsin deficiency** (Fig. 11.23B).

- **Paraseptal emphysema** involves distal airway structures, alveolar ducts, and sacs. Localized to fibrous septa or to the pleura, it can lead to formation of bullae which **may cause pneumothorax.** It is not associated with airflow obstruction (Fig. 11.23C).

- On conventional radiographs, the **most reliable finding of COPD is hyperinflation,** including **flattening of the diaphragm,** especially on the **lateral** exposure (Fig. 11.24). Other findings may include an **increase** in the **retrosternal clear space, hyperlucency** of the lungs with fewer than normal vascular markings visible, and **prominence of the pulmonary arteries** from pulmonary arterial hypertension.

- **With CT, findings of COPD** may include **focal areas of low density** in which the cystic areas lack visible walls except where bounded by interlobular septa. CT is helpful in evaluating the extent of emphysematous disease and in planning for surgical procedures designed to remove bullae to reduce lung volume.

Fig. 11.25 Infected Bulla. (A) In this close-up, there is at least one thin-walled, but air-containing, bulla in the right upper lobe (*solid white arrow*). (B) Several weeks later, the bulla (*dotted white arrow*) now contains both fluid and air (*solid black arrow*). Bullae typically occur at the lung apex and are usually asymptomatic in and of themselves. Patients with infected bullae tend to be less sick than those with a lung abscess, which an infected bulla can mimic.

Fig. 11.26 Bullous Disease: Chest Radiograph and CT. (A) Multiple curvilinear densities are seen in both lungs, representing the walls of bullae (*white arrows*). A paucity of lung markings is seen in the left upper lobe (*white circle*). (B) Multiple, thin-walled bullae are demonstrated by CT (*dotted white arrows*). Characteristically, they contain no blood vessels, but there may be septae that appear to traverse the bulla. Bullae may slowly increase in size and are associated with pneumothorax. If large and compromising the remainder of more normal lung, they can be surgically resected.

BULLAE, CYSTS, AND CAVITIES

- Bullae (singular: bulla), cysts and cavities are all **air-containing lesions in the lung** of differing **size, location,** and **wall composition.**
- Almost any of these lesions can contain **fluid** instead of, or in addition to, air.
- Fluid usually develops as a result of **infection, hemorrhage,** or **liquefaction necrosis.**
- When these lesions are **completely filled with fluid,** they **will appear solid** on conventional radiographs and CT scans, but they will typically demonstrate a **low CT number** that will

differentiate them from a truly solid tumor. When they contain some fluid and some air, they will manifest an **air-fluid level** on a conventional radiograph (exposed with a horizontal x-ray beam) or on CT scans (Fig. 11.25).

Bullae

- Bullae measure **more than 1 cm.** They are usually **associated with emphysema.** They occur in the **lung parenchyma** and have a **very thin wall** (<1 mm) that is frequently **only partially visible** on conventional radiography but well seen on CT. On **conventional radiographs** their **presence is often inferred** by a localized paucity of lung markings (Fig. 11.26).

- They can **grow to fill the entire hemithorax** and compress the lung to such an extent on the affected side that the lung seems to disappear (***vanishing lung syndrome***).
- **Blebs** are **very small** bullae that usually form in the visceral pleura, mostly at the lung **apex**. They may be seen by CT, but are too small to be visible on chest radiographs. They are thought to be associated with spontaneous pneumothoraces.

Cysts

- Lung **cysts** are either **congenital** or **acquired.** They can occur in the **lung parenchyma,** or the **mediastinum.** They

have a **thin wall** that is usually thicker than that of a bulla (**<3 mm**).
- ***Pneumatoceles*** represent acquired **thin-walled cysts** that usually develop after a lung infection caused by such organisms as *Staphylococcus* or *Pneumocystis* (Fig. 11.27).

Cavities

- Cavities can **vary in size** from a few millimeters to many centimeters. They occur in the **lung parenchyma** and usually **result from a process** that produces necrosis of the central portion of the lesion.
- Cavities usually have **the thickest wall** of any of these air-containing lesions **with a wall thickness from 3 mm to several cm** (see Fig. 11.17).
- Differentiation between three of the most frequent causes of cavities (carcinoma, pyogenic abscess, and tuberculosis) is summarized in Table 11.6.

Fig. 11.27 Cysts (Pneumatoceles) in *Pneumocystis* Pneumonia (PCP). Cysts are visible on chest radiographs in 10% of patients with PCP and far more frequently with CT scans (up to 1 of 3 patients). They may occur in the acute or in the postinfective phase of the disease. They have a predilection for the upper lobes and are commonly multiple (*white arrows*). Their etiology is unclear.

TABLE 11.6 Differentiating Three Cavitating Lung Lesions

Lesion	Thickness of the Cavity Wall	Inner Margin of Cavity
Bronchogenic carcinoma (Fig. 11.28A)	Thick[a]	Nodular
Tuberculosis (Fig. 11.28B)	Thin	Smooth
Lung abscess (Fig. 11.28C)	Thick	Smooth

[a]Thick = more than 5 mm; thin = less than 5 mm.

Fig. 11.28 Cavitary Lesions of the Lung. Three of the most common cavitary lesions of the lung can frequently be differentiated from each other by noting the **thickness** of the **wall** of the cavity and the **smoothness** or nodularity of its **inner margin.** (A) Squamous cell bronchogenic carcinoma characteristically produces a cavity with a thick wall (*white arrow*) and a nodular interior margin (*black arrow*). (B) Tuberculosis usually produces a relatively thin-walled, upper lobe cavity with a smooth inner margin (*white arrow*). (C) A staphylococcal lung abscess typically demonstrates a thickened wall (*white arrow*) which, in this case has a small fluid-containing cavity with a smooth inner margin (*black arrow*).

BRONCHIECTASIS

- Bronchiectasis is defined as **localized, irreversible dilatation of part of the bronchial tree.** Although it can be associated with many other diseases, it is **usually caused by necrotizing bacterial infections** such as those of *Staphylococcus* and *Klebsiella* and it usually affects the lower lobes.
- Bronchiectasis may also occur with cystic fibrosis, primary ciliary dyskinesia (*Kartagener syndrome*), allergic bronchopulmonary aspergillosis, and *Swyer-James syndrome* (unilateral hyperlucent lung).
- Clinically, **chronic productive cough** frequently associated with **hemoptysis** are the major symptoms.
- **Conventional radiographs** may demonstrate findings suggestive of the disease, but are **usually not specific.**
  - Findings include parallel-line opacities (*tram-tracks*) from thickened, dilated bronchial walls, **cystic lesions** as large as 2 cm in diameter from cystic bronchiectasis, and **tubular densities** from fluid-filled bronchi (Fig. 11.29).
- **CT is the study of choice for diagnosing bronchiectasis.**
  - The hallmark lesion on CT is the *signet ring sign* in which the **bronchus,** frequently with a thickened wall, **becomes larger than its associated pulmonary artery,** which is the opposite of the normal relationship between the two. The bronchus may also show a failure to taper normally (Fig. 11.30).

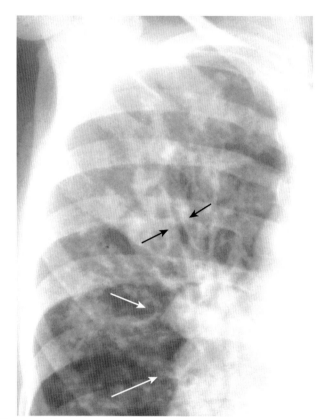

Fig. 11.29 Bronchiectasis in Cystic Fibrosis. Conventional radiographs may demonstrate parallel line opacities called ***tram-tracks*** because of thickened walls of dilated bronchi (*black arrows*). Progressive, bilateral upper lobe bronchiectasis in children is highly suggestive of cystic fibrosis, an autosomal recessive disease secondary to dysfunction of exocrine glands. The hila may be prominent from either hilar adenopathy or pulmonary arterial hypertension (*white arrows*).

Fig. 11.30 Bronchiectasis: CT. (A) The key sign in bronchiectasis is the ***signet ring sign*** in which the bronchus with a thickened wall (*solid white arrow*) becomes larger than its associated pulmonary artery (*dotted white arrow*). (B) The bronchus may also show ***tram-tracking***, thickened walls, and a failure to taper normally (*solid white arrows*). An absence of the normal tapering of the bronchi is one of the most sensitive signs on CT. Cylindrical or tubular bronchiectasis, such as this, is the least severe of several types of bronchiectasis.

🏠 TAKE HOME POINTS

- The mediastinum lies in the central portion of the thorax between the two lungs; it is arbitrarily divided into an anterior, middle, and posterior compartment.
- Masses in the **anterior mediastinum** include substernal thyroid goiters, lymphoma, thymoma, and teratoma.
- The **middle mediastinum** is home primarily to lymphadenopathy from lymphoma and metastatic disease, such as from small cell carcinoma of the lung.
- The **posterior mediastinum** is the location of neurogenic tumors that originate either from the nerve sheath (mostly benign) or tissues other than the sheath (mostly malignant).
- Incidental **solitary pulmonary nodules (SPNs)** less than 4 mm in size are rarely malignant; in those in whom clinical or imaging findings suggest malignancy, 50% over the age of 50 are malignant. The key question is to determine whether a nodule is most likely benign or most likely malignant in any given individual.
- Criteria on which an evaluation of benignity can be made include absolute **size** of the nodule upon discovery, presence of **calcification** within it, the **margin** of the nodule, and **change** in the size of the nodule over time.
- Evidence-based criteria have been developed to help determine the frequency and method of follow-up of the increasing number of solitary pulmonary nodules found **incidentally** on CT scans so as to optimize the role for further diagnostic interventions.
- **Bronchogenic carcinomas** present in one of three ways: visualization of the tumor itself; recognition of the effects of bronchial obstruction, such as pneumonitis and/or atelectasis; or by identification of either their direct extension or metastatic spread to the chest or to distant organs.
- Bronchogenic carcinomas presenting as a solitary nodule/mass in the lung are most often **adenocarcinomas;** adenocarcinomas of the lung may sometimes present with multiple nodules, mimicking metastatic disease.
- Bronchogenic carcinoma presenting with bronchial obstruction is most often caused by **squamous cell carcinoma**, which is the cell type most likely to cavitate.
- **Small cell carcinomas** are highly aggressive, centrally located, peribronchial tumors, the majority of which have already metastasized at the time of initial presentation; they can be associated with paraneoplastic syndromes such as inappropriate secretion of anti-diuretic hormone and Cushing's syndrome.
- Multiple nodules in the lung are most often **metastatic** lesions that have traveled through the bloodstream from a distant primary tumor (**hematogenous spread**); common sites of primaries for such metastases include colorectal, breast, renal cell, head and neck, bladder, uterine and cervical carcinomas, soft-tissue sarcomas, and melanoma.
- In **lymphangitic carcinomatosis,** a tumor grows in and obstructs lymphatics in the lung, producing a pattern that is radiologically similar to pulmonary interstitial edema; primaries that metastasize to the lung in this fashion include breast, lung, and pancreatic cancer.
- Conventional radiography has a high false–negative rate in pulmonary thromboembolic disease because demonstration of "classical" findings such as a Hampton hump, Westermark sign, and knuckle sign is infrequent.
- **CT-pulmonary angiography** is now widely used for the diagnosis of pulmonary embolism producing images of the pulmonary arteries with little or no motion artifact.
- **Chronic obstructive pulmonary disease** consists of emphysema and chronic bronchitis; of the two, chronic bronchitis is a clinical diagnosis, whereas emphysema is defined pathologically and has findings that can be seen on both conventional radiographs and CT scans.
- **Bullae, cysts, and cavities** are all air-containing lesions in the lung that differ in size, location, and wall composition; bullae, cysts, and cavities are seen on CT and may also be visible on conventional radiographs.
- Although **bronchiectasis** may be seen on conventional radiographs, CT is the study of choice; CT demonstrates the **signet-ring sign, tram-tracks,** cystic lesions, or tubular densities.

 More information on recognizing other diseases of the chest is available to registered users online.

Appendix: Fleischner Society Criteria for Follow-Up of Incidental, Non-Calcified Solitary Pulmonary Nodules

	SINGLE SOLID[a] NODULES		
Nodule Size (mm)	<6 mm	6 to 8 mm	>8 mm
Low-risk patients[b]	No routine follow-up	CT at 6–12 months; then consider CT at 18–24 months	Consider CT at 3 months, PET/CT, or tissue sampling
High-risk patients[c]	Optional CT at 12 months	CT at 6–12 months; then CT at 18–24 months	Consider CT at 3 months, PET/CT, or tissue sampling

	SINGLE SUBSOLID[d] NODULES	
Nodule Size (mm)	<6 mm	≥6 mm
Ground-glass[e]	No routine follow-up	CT at 6–12 months to confirm persistence; then CT every 2 years until 5 years
Partly solid	No routine follow-up	CT at 3–6 months to confirm persistence. If unchanged and solid component remains <6 mm, annual CT should be performed for 5 years.

[a]**Solid nodules** are <3 cm well-circumscribed areas of increased attenuation (whiter) on CT that are homogeneous in appearance (see Fig. 11.13A).
[b]**Low-risk patients:** Younger age, minimal or no smoking history, regular margin to nodule, location of nodule in an area **other** than upper lobe.
[c]**High-risk patients:** Older age, heavy smoker, upper lobe location, irregular or spiculated nodule margins.
[d]**Subsolid nodules** are <3 cm well-circumscribed areas of increased attenuation that are either **purely ground-glass** nodules (see Fig. 11.13B) in appearance or **partly ground-glass and partly solid** nodules (see Fig. 11.13C).
[e]**Ground-glass nodules** are <3 cm well-circumscribed areas of greater attenuation on CT in which the bronchial and vascular markings are preserved rather than obliterated (see Fig. 11.13B).
CT, Computed tomography; PET, positron emission tomography.
From MacMahon H, Naidich DP, Goo JM, et al: Guidelines for Management of Incidental Pulmonary Nodules Detected on CT Images: From the Fleischner Society 2017. Radiology 2017;284:228–243.

12

Recognizing Adult Heart Disease

This chapter will discuss how to assess heart size, then describe the normal and abnormal contours of the heart on the frontal radiograph, and, finally, illustrate some imaging findings in common cardiac diseases.

RECOGNIZING AN ENLARGED CARDIAC SILHOUETTE

- The cardiac silhouette ("heart shadow") can appear enlarged on conventional radiographs for three main reasons (arranged in the order in which they will be discussed, not by frequency of occurrence):
    - **Pericardial effusion** that mimics the appearance of cardiomegaly on conventional radiographs
    - **Extracardiac** factors that produce apparent cardiac enlargement
    - And most importantly, true cardiac enlargement (**cardiomegaly**)

Pericardial Effusion

- Normally, there are 15 to 50 mL of fluid in the pericardial space between the parietal and visceral pericardial layers. Abnormal accumulations of fluid begin in the **dependent portions of the pericardial space** that in the supine position, is **posterior to the left ventricle** (Fig. 12.1A)**.** As the pericardial effusion increases in size, it tends to accumulate more **along the right heart border** until it fills the pericardial space and **encircles the heart** (Fig. 12.1B).
- Computed tomography (CT) scans can demonstrate small pericardial effusions, although pericardial ultrasonography is usually the imaging study of first choice. Conventional radiographs are poor at defining a pericardial effusion.
- Some of the causes of pericardial effusions are outlined in Box 12.1.

BOX 12.1   Causes of Pericardial Effusion

- Congestive heart failure
- Infection (TB, viral)
- Metastatic malignancy (lung and breast, especially)
- Uremic pericarditis
- Collagen-vascular disease (lupus)
- Trauma
- Postpericardiotomy syndrome

Fig. 12.1 Pericardial Effusions, Small and Large. (A) There is fluid in the pericardial space posterior to the heart in this unenhanced CT of the lower chest (*white arrow*). (B) In another patient, after intravenous contrast opacifies the heart, a larger pericardial effusion surrounds the heart (*dotted white arrows*). Conventional chest radiographs may show an enlarged cardiac silhouette, but cannot differentiate the soft-tissue density of the heart from the fluid density of the effusion.

Fig. 12.2 Cardiomegaly on a Portable Radiograph. (A) If the heart is about 50% of the cardiothoracic ratio (ratio of length of the *solid black arrows* to *dotted black arrows*), then the heart is not enlarged. (B) If the heart (*dotted black arrow*) is near or touching the lateral chest wall (*solid black arrow*), then the heart is enlarged.

TABLE 12.1 **Extracardiac Causes of Apparent Cardiomegaly**	
Cause	**Reason for Enlarged Appearance**
AP portable supine chest is the most common cause	Magnification due to AP projection
Suboptimal inspiration	In expiration, the diaphragm moves upward and compresses the heart, making the heart appear larger than it would be in full inspiration.
	If there are eight to nine posterior ribs visible on the frontal chest radiograph, then the inspiration is adequate (see Fig. 2.4).
Obesity, pregnancy, ascites	These conditions prevent an adequate inspiration.
Pectus excavatum deformity, a congenital deformity of the lowermost section of the sternum, causes it to bow inward and compress the heart	The heart is compressed between the sternum and the spine.
Rotation	Especially when it occurs to the patient's left, rotation may make the heart appear larger (see Fig. 2.8).
Pericardial effusion	Other imaging modalities (most commonly ultrasound), CT or electrocardiographic findings will help to identify pericardial fluid.

AP, Anteroposterior; *CT,* computed tomography.

Extracardiac Causes of Apparent Cardiac Enlargement

> **❗ DIAGNOSTIC PITFALLS**
>
> - Sometimes, there is an **extracardiac** cause of *apparent* cardiac enlargement on conventional radiography that may cause the cardiothoracic ratio to appear greater than 50% (see Fig. 2.9), **whereas the heart itself may actually be normal in size**.

- The extracardiac causes of apparent cardiomegaly are outlined in Table 12.1. **Magnification** of the heart produced by projection, usually on an anteroposterior (AP), supine, **portable chest examination,** is the most common cause of apparent cardiomegaly (see Fig. 2.9).

TABLE 12.2 **Recognizing Cardiomegaly on an AP Chest Radiograph**	
Appearance of Heart on AP Study	**Likely "Actual" Heart Size**
Borderline enlarged	Normal size
Significantly enlarged	Enlarged
Touching, or almost touching, the left lateral chest wall	Definitely enlarged

Identifying Cardiac Enlargement on an AP Chest Radiograph

- So, is it possible to estimate the size of the heart on a portable chest radiograph? The answer is "yes." A good rule of thumb: If the heart appears enlarged on a well-inspired, portable chest radiograph, it probably is enlarged (see Table 12.2 and Fig. 12.2).

Fig. 12.3 Normal and Enlarged Appearance of the Cardiac Silhouette in the Lateral Projection. (A) In most normal patients, the posterior border of the heart (*black arrow*) does not overlap the thoracic spine (*white arrow*). (B) In this patient with cardiomegaly, the posterior border of the heart (*black arrow*) overlaps the anterior border of the thoracic spine (*white arrow*). The lateral projection can be used as a helpful confirmatory sign of enlargement of the cardiac silhouette.

Recognizing Cardiomegaly on the Lateral Chest Radiograph

- Generally speaking, evaluation of cardiac size using conventional radiography is best made on the frontal chest radiograph. To evaluate for the presence of enlargement of the cardiac silhouette in the lateral projection, **look at the space posterior to the heart and anterior to the spine at the level of the diaphragm.** In a normal person, the **cardiac silhouette will usually not extend posteriorly and project over the spine** (Fig. 12.3A).
- As the **heart enlarges,** whether that enlargement is caused by cardiomegaly or pericardial effusion, the **posterior border of the heart may extend to, or overlap, the anterior border of the thoracic spine.** This can be useful as a confirmatory sign of an enlarged cardiac silhouette (Fig. 12.3B).

RECOGNIZING COMMON CARDIAC DISEASES

- In this section, several diseases will be discussed in more detail. Most of them produce abnormalities in size and contour of the heart or great vessels. For a **systematic approach** to recognizing the cardiac contour abnormalities on chest radiographs in adults, see **"The ABCs of Heart Disease"** available online to registered users. The diseases to be discussed here are:
  - Congestive heart failure and pulmonary edema
    - Cardiogenic versus noncardiogenic pulmonary edema
  - Hypertensive cardiovascular disease
  - Mitral stenosis
  - Pulmonary arterial hypertension
  - Aortic stenosis
  - Cardiomyopathy
  - Thoracic aortic aneurysm and aortic dissection
  - Coronary artery disease

Congestive Heart Failure

- The incidence of congestive heart failure (CHF) has grown rapidly over the last two decades so that CHF is **the most common diagnosis in hospitalized patients over the age of 65.**
- **Causes of congestive heart failure**
  - In the United States, the **two most common causes of CHF are coronary artery disease and hypertension.**
  - Other causes of CHF:
    - **Cardiomyopathy,** such as from longstanding alcohol abuse
    - **Cardiac valvular lesions,** such as aortic stenosis and mitral stenosis
    - **Arrhythmias**
    - **Hyperthyroidism**
    - **Severe anemia**
    - **Left-to-right shunts**
- Typically, **congestive heart failure** presents with **one of two radiographic patterns: pulmonary interstitial edema** or **pulmonary alveolar edema.** Not every feature of each pattern is always present and there is often an overlap between the two patterns.

Pulmonary Interstitial Edema

> **IMPORTANT POINTS**
>
> - The **four key radiographic signs of pulmonary interstitial edema** are:
>   - **Thickening of the interlobular septa**
>   - **Peribronchial cuffing**
>   - **Fluid in the fissures**
>   - **Pleural effusions**

Thickening of the Interlobular Septa: The Kerley B Line

- The interlobular septae are not detectable on a normal chest radiograph, but can become visible if they accumulate excessive fluid, usually at a pulmonary (venous) capillary wedge pressure of about **15 mm Hg.** The thickened septae are called **septal lines** or **Kerley B lines** (named after Peter James Kerley, an Irish neurologist and radiologist).
- **Recognizing Kerley B lines**
  - Kerley B lines actually do exist. They will be visible on a frontal radiograph usually **at the lung bases,** at or **near the costophrenic angles.**
  - They are **very short** (1 to 2 cm long), **very thin** (≈1 mm) and **horizontal in orientation,** which means they are **perpendicular to the pleural surface.**
  - They **usually extend to and abut the pleural surface** (Fig. 12.4).
  - After repeated episodes of pulmonary interstitial edema, the **septal lines may fibrose** and, therefore, **remain, even after all other signs of pulmonary interstitial edema clear.** These are called **chronic Kerley B lines** and they may be present even if the patient is not clinically in congestive failure.

- **Kerley A Lines**
  - Kerley named other lines seen in congestive heart failure besides the "B" line.
  - **Kerley A** lines appear when connective tissue around the bronchovascular sheaths in the lung distends with fluid. **Kerley A lines extend from the hila for several centimeters,** but **do not reach the periphery of the lung** as do Kerley B lines (Fig. 12.5).
  - Once he started, Kerley apparently had trouble stopping and he also described "C" lines, but there is some doubt that they exist as separate entities.

Peribronchial Cuffing

- In adults, bronchi may **normally** be visible on-end (*en face*) in the region of the hila, but their walls are usually too thin and they are **not visible** more peripherally in the lung.
- When fluid accumulates in the interstitial tissue around and in the wall of a bronchus, such as in congestive heart failure, the **bronchial wall becomes thicker and may appear as a ring-like density that can be seen on-end** in radiographs.

Fig. 12.4 Kerley B Lines. There are numerous, thin, horizontal white lines seen at the lung base abutting the pleural surface (*white oval*). Interlobular septae are not visible on a normal chest radiograph.

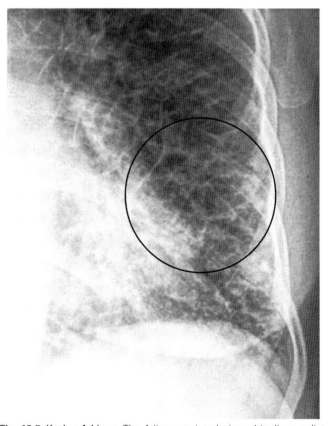

Fig. 12.5 Kerley A Lines. The A lines are interlacing white lines radiating from the hila, but not reaching the chest wall (*circle*). They are longer than Kerley B lines. A network of Kerley lines is produced in the lungs of patients with congestive heart failure producing the "prominence of the pulmonary interstitial markings" described in that disease.

Fig. 12.6 Peribronchial Cuffing. When fluid accumulates in the interstitial tissue around and in the wall of a bronchus as it does in CHF, the normally invisible bronchial wall becomes thicker and can appear as ring-like densities when seen on end (*white arrows and circle*). Peribronchial cuffing may not always produce perfectly round circles.

Fig. 12.8 Pleural Effusions in Congestive Heart Failure (CHF). There are bilateral pleural effusions (*solid white arrows*). It is common for the right pleural effusion in CHF to be slightly larger than the left. It is uncommon in CHF to have a large left pleural effusion alone, a finding that might prompt investigation of another cause for the effusion, such as a malignancy or tuberculosis. This patient had congestive heart failure.

Fig. 12.7 Normal Fissures and Fluid in the Fissures. (A) The major (*solid white arrow*) and minor fissures (*dashed white arrow*) may normally be barely visible as very thin, smooth, white lines. (B) When fluid collects in the major (*solid black arrow*) and minor (*dashed black arrow*) fissures, they become thicker and more irregular in their appearance. When the patient's heart failure clears, the fissures will return to normal appearance, but after repeated and prolonged bouts of failure, fibrosis may result in permanent thickening of the fissures.

- When seen on-end, *peribronchial cuffing* appears as numerous, small, ring-like shadows that look like little *doughnuts* (Fig. 12.6).

Fluid in the Fissures

- The major (or oblique) and minor (or horizontal) **fissures may be visible normally,** but are almost never thicker than a line you could draw with the **point of a sharpened pencil** (Fig. 12.7A).
- **Fluid can collect between the two layers of visceral pleura that form the fissures or in the subpleural space** between the visceral pleura and the lung parenchyma. This **fluid** distends the fissure and makes it **thicker,** more **irregular in contour,** and therefore **more visible** than normal (Fig. 12.7B).

Pleural Effusion

- As a result of either increased production or decreased absorption of pleural fluid, fluid in excess of the normal 2 to 5 mL can collect in the pleural space, typically at a pulmonary capillary wedge pressure of about **20 mm Hg.**
- **Pleural effusions accompanying congestive heart failure are usually bilateral,** but can be asymmetric (Fig. 12.8).
  - When **unilateral,** they are **almost always right-sided.**

Fig. 12.9 Congestive Heart Failure: CT. This is an axial CT scan of the chest following intravenous injection of contrast. Note that the right side of the heart is opacified, but the contrast has not yet passed through the lungs a sufficient number of times to fully opacify the left side of the heart. Bilateral pleural effusions are present and they layer posteriorly because the patient is being scanned supine (*solid black arrows*). Fluid has insinuated itself into the fissure (*dotted black arrow*). The thickened interlobular septae (*solid white arrows*) are Kerley B lines. *LV*, Left ventricle; *RV*, right ventricle.

 IMPORTANT POINTS

- About 15% the time, the effusion can be unilateral and on the left, but if you see a unilateral left pleural effusion, you should think of causes other than CHF, such as metastases, tuberculosis, or pulmonary thromboembolic disease.

- At times, pleural fluid accumulates in the form of a **laminar effusion** in which the fluid assumes a **thin, band-like density along the lateral chest wall, beginning near the costophrenic sulcus,** but often preserving the sulcus itself (see Fig. 8.15).
- For more about pleural effusions, see **Chapter 8: Recognizing a Pleural Effusion.**
- All of these findings can be seen on CT as well as on conventional radiographs (Fig. 12.9).
- The key findings of **pulmonary interstitial edema** are summarized in Box 12.2.

Pulmonary Alveolar Edema
- When the **pulmonary venous pressure is sufficiently elevated (≈25 mm Hg), fluid spills out of the interstitial tissues of the lung into the airspaces.** This results in *pulmonary alveolar edema* (most often shortened to *pulmonary edema* without including "alveolar").

 IMPORTANT POINTS

- The **radiographic findings** of **pulmonary alveolar edema are:**
  - **Fluffy, indistinct patchy airspace densities that are frequently centrally located.** The outer third of the lung may be spared and the lower lung zones are more affected than the upper. This produces the ***bat-wing, angel-wing,* or *butterfly*** configuration of pulmonary edema (Fig. 12.10).
  - **Pleural effusions** and **fluid in the fissures** are commonly found in pulmonary alveolar edema on a cardiogenic basis.

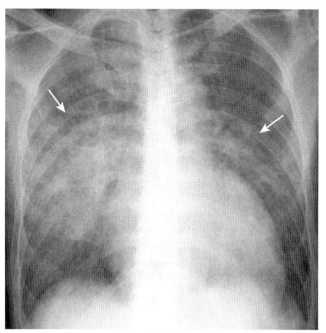

Fig. 12.10 Bat-Wing Pattern of Pulmonary Edema. Central airspace disease that spares the lung periphery is called the **bat-wing (angel-wing)** or **butterfly** pattern (*solid white arrows*) and, although it may not be the most common manifestation of pulmonary edema, it is suggestive of that disease versus other airspace diseases, such as pneumonia. The bat-wing pattern is seen in rapidly developing cardiac failure, such as massive myocardial infarction and papillary muscle rupture. The patient had suffered an acute myocardial infarction.

BOX 12.2 Four Key Findings in Pulmonary Interstitial Edema

- Thickening of the interlobular septa—**Kerley B lines**—and fluid in the central connective tissue of the lungs—**Kerley A lines**
- ***Peribronchial cuffing:*** fluid-thickened bronchial walls visualized on-end
- ***Fluid in the fissures:*** opacification and thickening of the interlobar fissures
- ***Pleural effusion:*** usually bilateral but, when unilateral, usually right-sided

BOX 12.3 Key Findings in Pulmonary Alveolar Edema

- Fluffy, indistinct patchy airspace densities
- ***Bat-wing*** or ***butterfly*** configuration frequently sparing the outer third of lungs
- Pleural effusions are usually present when the edema is cardiogenic in origin

- The key findings in pulmonary alveolar edema are summarized in Box 12.3.
- **What happened to cardiomegaly and cephalization?**
  - Although most patients with CHF have an enlarged heart, most patients with an enlarged heart are not in congestive heart failure. In any individual, **cardiomegaly itself is not a particularly sensitive indicator for the presence or absence of congestive heart failure.**

Fig. 12.11 Rapidly Clearing Pulmonary Edema. (A) This patient demonstrates bilateral, perihilar airspace disease suggestive of pulmonary edema. (B) Four days later, the lungs are clear. Acute respiratory distress syndrome (ARDS) is not likely to clear this quickly, nor are patients who have coexisting diseases such as renal or hepatic failure or superimposed pneumonia.

- **Cephalization,** defined as redistribution of flow in the lungs such that the upper lobe pulmonary vasculature becomes larger than the lower lobe vessels**, is difficult to identify for most beginners** and is meaningful only if you are certain the patient was **upright** at the time of the chest exposure. Because many or most patients suspected of having CHF are imaged supine, the sign is not very reliable.
- **How pulmonary edema resolves**
  - Pulmonary edema generally is both **abrupt in onset** and **quick to clear**–typically in a matter of a few hours to a few days (Fig. 12.11).
  - Resolution frequently begins peripherally and moves centrally. Radiologic resolution may lag behind clinical improvement, especially if the patient has large pleural effusions that may last long after other radiographic signs have cleared.

Noncardiogenic Pulmonary Edema: General Considerations

- Although congestive heart failure accounts for most cases of pulmonary edema (*i.e., cardiogenic pulmonary edema*), there are other, **noncardiogenic causes of pulmonary edema.**
- Among the causes of noncardiogenic pulmonary edema is a diverse group of diseases including:
  - **Increased capillary permeability,** which includes all of the various causes of *acute (adult) respiratory distress syndrome* or *ARDS,* such as:
    - Sepsis
    - Uremia
    - Disseminated intravascular coagulopathy
    - Smoke inhalation
    - Near-drowning
  - **Volume overload**

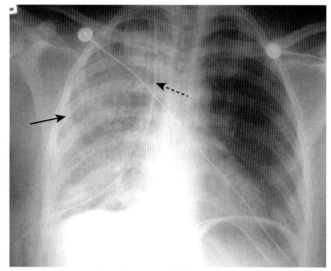

Fig. 12.12 Reexpansion Pulmonary Edema. Unilateral airspace disease affects the entire right lung (*solid black arrow*). In addition, a chest tube (*dotted black arrow*) is seen on the same side. Reexpansion pulmonary edema results from the overly rapid expansion of a lung that has typically been chronically collapsed by pneumothorax or a large pleural effusion (as had been the case in this patient). Its exact cause is not known. Other causes of unilateral pulmonary edema can include either an abnormality on the same side as the pulmonary edema (e.g., prolonged positioning with the affected side dependent) or an abnormality on the opposite side (e.g., a large pulmonary embolus occluding flow to the opposite lung).

- **Lymphangitic spread of malignancy**
- Other causes of noncardiogenic pulmonary edema may include:
  - **High-altitude pulmonary edema**
  - **Neurogenic pulmonary edema**
  - **Re-expansion pulmonary edema** (Fig. 12.12)
  - **Heroin or other drug overdoses (e.g., crack cocaine)**

Fig. 12.13 Noncardiogenic Pulmonary Edema. Although this airspace disease has a perihilar distribution similar to cardiogenic pulmonary edema (*white arrows*), there is no pleural fluid, fluid in the fissures, or cardiomegaly. The patient had just used inhaled crack cocaine. The lungs are the principal organs affected by crack cocaine use. Onset of pulmonary edema usually occurs with inhalation of a large dose. Black sputum is characteristic of crack cocaine smoking, from the carbonaceous residue that occurs from the process used to produce the inhaled product.

Noncardiogenic Pulmonary Edema: Imaging Findings

- **Acute respiratory distress syndrome (ARDS) represents one form of noncardiogenic pulmonary edema.**
  - Characteristically, **patients with ARDS are radiographically normal for 24 to 36 hours** after the initial insult. Then, pulmonary abnormalities become evident in the form of **pulmonary interstitial edema, patchy airspace disease,** or in the typical pattern of bilateral **pulmonary alveolar edema.**
  - Clinically, the **patient demonstrates severe hypoxia, cyanosis, tachypnea, and dyspnea.**
  - Typically, the findings of ARDS stabilize after 5 to 7 days and begin improving in about 2 weeks. Complete clearing, when it occurs, may take months.
  - In the later stages of ARDS, a **reticular interstitial lung pattern may develop,** although the majority of patients who survive tend to have little impairment of lung function.

Differentiating Cardiac From Noncardiac Pulmonary Edema

> ### ⏩ IMPORTANT POINTS
>
> - The **patterns of cardiac (cardiogenic) and noncardiac (noncardiogenic) pulmonary edema overlap considerably** and the patient's **history and clinical picture are keys** to establishing the most likely cause of pulmonary edema.

- In general, **noncardiogenic pulmonary edema** is:
  - **Less likely** to demonstrate **pleural effusions** and **Kerley B lines than cardiogenic pulmonary edema.**
  - **More likely** to demonstrate **a normal pulmonary capillary wedge pressure (PCWP)** of less than 12 mm Hg **than cardiogenic pulmonary edema.**

TABLE 12.3 Cardiogenic Versus Noncardiogenic Pulmonary Edema

Imaging Finding	Cardiogenic	Noncardiogenic
Pleural effusions	Common	Infrequent
Kerley B lines	Common	Infrequent
Heart size	Frequently enlarged	May be normal
Pulmonary capillary wedge pressure	Elevated	Normal

- **More likely** to be associated with a **normal-sized** heart (Fig. 12.13).
- **More likely** to demonstrate airspace disease that is more **patchy** and **peripheral** than that in cardiogenic pulmonary edema, but this is highly variable.
- The key differences between cardiogenic and noncardiogenic pulmonary edema are summarized in Table 12.3.

Hypertensive Cardiovascular Disease

- Chronic elevation of systemic blood pressure leads to left ventricular hypertrophy in about 20% of patients and more than twice as often if the patient is obese. Most of the time (90%), the hypertension is *essential* hypertension with no identifiable cause. Heart failure, coronary artery disease, and cardiac arrhythmias are common complications of hypertension.
- Systemic hypertension can lead to left ventricular hypertrophy. Left ventricular hypertrophy occurs at the expense of the lumen, the wall becoming thicker while the lumen becomes smaller. Therefore, **the heart is usually normal or slightly increased in size** early in the disease, especially on conventional radiographs. It is not until the muscle begins

Fig. 12.14 Hypertensive Cardiovascular Disease. Systemic hypertension can lead to hypertrophic cardiomyopathy. (A) The aorta itself is *uncoiled* (*solid white arrows*) from increased systemic blood pressure (see also Fig. 4.3). The left ventricle (*dotted white arrow*) appears only slightly enlarged, but a contrast-enhanced CT scan through the heart (B) demonstrates marked concentric hypertrophy of the left ventricular wall (*white and black arrows*) that has occurred at the expense of the lumen (LV).

to decompensate that the heart increases dramatically in size (Fig. 12.14).

- **The aorta**, under increased systemic pressure, pivots outward around the aortic valve and the aortic hiatus in the diaphragm and **gradually uncoils**, becoming more prominent in **both** its **ascending** and **descending** portions (see Fig. 4.03).

- Prolonged systemic hypertension may eventually lead to congestive heart failure.

Mitral Stenosis

- In developed nations, the incidence of mitral stenosis from rheumatic heart disease has declined markedly, but it is still seen in the elderly and in younger individuals from developing countries. The **most common symptoms** are from **left heart failure:** dyspnea on exertion, orthopnea, and paroxysmal nocturnal dyspnea.

- Mitral stenosis leads to obstruction to the outflow of blood from the left atrium and usually becomes symptomatic when the **valve area falls below one-third** of its normal size. As the left atrial pressure builds, the left atrium enlarges and the increased pulmonary venous pressure (*i.e., pulmonary venous hypertension*) is reflected retrograde into the pulmonary circulation (Fig. 12.15).

- Upper lobe vessels become as large as, or more prominent than, lower lobe vessels (*cephalization*). Pulmonary venous hypertension eventually leads to congestive heart failure. With prolonged elevation of pulmonary venous pressure, there may be physical changes in the pulmonary vasculature leading to escalating *pulmonary vascular resistance* requiring ever-increasing levels of pulmonary arterial pressure.

- Eventually there is *pulmonary arterial hypertension* and right-sided heart failure (Fig. 12.16).

Fig. 12.15 Mitral Stenosis. This is a contrast-enhanced axial CT image through the heart. The left atrium (LA) is markedly enlarged in this patient because of the obstruction of outflow from the left atrium by the stenotic mitral valve. Eventually, the increase in left atrial pressure is transmitted backward through the pulmonary venous and then pulmonary arterial circulations. *Ao,* Aorta; *RA,* right atrium.

Pulmonary Arterial Hypertension

- Normal mean pulmonary artery pressure is about 15 mm Hg. Pulmonary arterial hypertension may be **idiopathic (primary)** or **secondary** to another disease, usually emphysema. Mitral stenosis is another cause of secondary pulmonary arterial hypertension.

- With **primary** pulmonary hypertension, the leading cause of death is **progressive right heart failure.** Secondary pulmonary hypertension shares comorbidities with the diseases that cause it, such as emphysema, recurrent thromboembolic disease, mitral stenosis, and CHF.

- The **imaging hallmark of pulmonary arterial hypertension** is a discrepancy in size between the central pulmonary vasculature (i.e., the main, right, and left pulmonary arteries are **large**) and the peripheral pulmonary vasculature. This discrepancy has been called *pruning.*

- On CT scans, the **main pulmonary artery is normally about the same diameter as the ascending aorta,** but in **pulmonary arterial hypertension** the main pulmonary artery itself is usually **3 cm or larger** in size (Fig. 12.17).

Aortic Stenosis

- The classic triad of clinical symptoms in aortic stenosis is composed of **chest pain,** symptoms related to **heart failure,** and **syncope.**
- Aortic stenosis may be secondary to a **congenital bicuspid aortic valve,** from **degeneration of a tricuspid valve** or, less frequently now, **rheumatic heart disease.**

- Because there is obstruction to left ventricular outflow from aortic stenosis and the ventricles respond to obstruction by undergoing hypertrophy of their walls, the heart is usually normal in size **early** in the course of the disease.
- The **ascending aorta** may be unusually prominent because of *poststenotic dilatation,* a hallmark of a significantly stenotic lesion in any major artery in which, because of **eddy currents** and **turbulent flow,** there is increased intraluminal pressure for several centimeters **distal** to a partially obstructing lesion (Fig. 12.18A).

Fig. 12.16 Chronic Mitral Stenosis With Tricuspid Regurgitation. The left atrium and left atrial appendage are enlarged (*white arrow*). Pulmonary venous hypertension has produced a redistribution of flow in the lungs *(cephalization)* so that the upper lobe vessels have become more prominent than the lower lobe vessels (*white circle*). Because of increased pulmonary vascular resistance and subsequent pulmonary arterial hypertension, the right heart has developed tricuspid regurgitation with marked enlargement of the right atrium (*black arrow*).

Fig. 12.17 Pulmonary Arterial Hypertension. Normally, the main pulmonary artery (MPA) is about the same diameter as the ascending aorta (A). In this patient, with pulmonary arterial hypertension, the MPA is much larger than the aorta. There is also a rapid attenuation in the size of the pulmonary arteries (*white arrows*) called *pruning,* another feature of pulmonary arterial hypertension. This patient had a history of chronic pulmonary thromboembolic disease.

Fig. 12.18 Aortic Stenosis. (A) Poststenotic dilatation is isolated to the ascending aorta (*solid white arrow*). The ascending aorta should normally not project farther to the right than the right heart border (*black arrow*). Notice that the heart is not enlarged overall and the descending aorta (*dotted white arrow*) is normal in appearance. (B) This unenhanced axial CT scan of the heart shows dense calcification of the aortic valve (*black arrow*) and a markedly thickened left ventricular wall (*double white arrows*) from hypertrophy. *LV,* Left ventricular lumen.

- **Calcification** of the aortic valve, which is easily seen on CT, has been shown to be predictive of the increased likelihood of aortic stenosis and mortality from cardiovascular disease (Fig. 12.18B).
- Eventually, when the heart begins to decompensate it will become **enlarged** and congestive heart failure may ensue.

Cardiomyopathy
Dilated Cardiomyopathy

- Dilated cardiomyopathy is, by definition, a condition in which there is **increased systolic and diastolic volume of the ventricles** associated with a **decreased (<40%) ejection fraction.** It is the **most common** form of **cardiomyopathy** (90%).
- It can be **idiopathic (primary)** or **associated with known diseases,** such as cardiac ischemia, diabetes, and alcoholism.
- **Decreased contractility** and **ventricular dilatation** are **hallmarks,** so it is usually characterized by an **enlarged heart,** frequently associated with the imaging signs of **congestive heart failure** (Fig. 12.19).
- The diagnosis can usually be made by echocardiography following the initial chest radiograph, in concert with the clinical findings.
- **Magnetic resonance imaging (MRI)** can provide the most accurate and reproducible findings for this disease. Using electrocardiographic (ECG)-gated, cine-magnetic resonance angiography (MRA), **cardiac ejection fraction** and **cardiac dimensions** can be accurately assessed.
- **Radionuclide ventriculography** using small quantities of intravenously injected radioisotope can also determine **ejection fraction** and can be useful in differentiating between **ischemic** and **nonischemic causes of cardiomyopathy.**

Hypertrophic Cardiomyopathy

- **Hypertrophic cardiomyopathy** is an abnormality (divided into primary [genetic] and secondary forms). It causes **asymmetric** or **concentric thickening of the myocardium,** sometimes with obstruction to left ventricular outflow caused by **systolic anterior motion** of the anterior **mitral valve leaflet** (in the primary form).
  - **Systolic anterior motion (SAM)** of the mitral valve refers to a **paradoxical motion** of the anterior (and sometimes posterior) mitral valve leaflet **toward the left ventricular outflow tract** during systole.
  - It **may lead to sudden cardiac death** and has been implicated as the cause of death in several high-profile athletes.
- The secondary form (the most common manifestation of hypertrophic cardiomyopathy) is caused by **hypertensive cardiovascular disease,** which produces **concentric** and **diffuse** hypertrophy of the left ventricle not usually associated with left ventricular outflow tract obstruction (see Fig. 12.14).
- The primary form may be diagnosed with echocardiography or ECG-gated MRI of the heart in which the **asymmetric hypertrophy of the ventricular septum (ASH)** may be demonstrated.

Restrictive Cardiomyopathy

- Restrictive cardiomyopathy is a **rare form** of cardiomyopathy characterized by **high diastolic filling pressures of the ventricles** in association with relatively well-preserved systolic function. It is usually secondary to an **infiltrative process** in the myocardium. Such diseases include **amyloid, autoimmune disease, and prior chest radiation.** The predominant presenting symptoms are related to **congestive heart failure.**

Fig. 12.19 Dilated Alcoholic Cardiomyopathy. Cardiomyopathies comprise a diverse group of diseases that affect the heart muscle. In this patient with dilated cardiomyopathy, the cardiac silhouette is markedly enlarged, primarily as a result of biventricular enlargement. The patient had a long history of alcohol abuse. Dilated cardiomyopathy is frequently associated with congestive heart failure.

- Although clinically similar to **constrictive pericarditis,** the key difference is that the **pericardium is normal in restrictive cardiomyopathy,** whereas it is **thickened in constrictive pericarditis.** The importance in differentiating the two is that constrictive pericarditis, unlike restrictive cardiomyopathy, is surgically curable.
- In restrictive cardiomyopathy, the **heart is usually not enlarged.** There are pulmonary changes of **congestive heart failure.**
- MRI can demonstrate the thickness of the pericardium and, if the pericardium is normal in size (<4 mm), constrictive pericarditis can effectively be excluded. If there is pericardial calcification, better seen on CT, restrictive cardiomyopathy can be excluded (Fig. 12.20).

Aortic Aneurysms: General Considerations

- Aneurysms are **defined as enlargement of a vessel greater than 50% of its original size. Atherosclerosis is the most common cause** of a descending thoracic aortic aneurysm. The majority of patients with aortic aneurysms are also hypertensive.
- Most patients with aneurysms are **asymptomatic** and the **aneurysm is discovered serendipitously.** When an aneurysm of the descending thoracic aorta expands, it may cause pain that classically, but not always, radiates to the back.

- As measured on CT or MRI scans, the **ascending aorta is usually less than 3.5 cm** in diameter and the **descending aorta is less than 3 cm.**
- An **aneurysm** of the thoracic aorta is usually defined as a **persistent enlargement greater than 4 cm.**
- In general, **aneurysms of 5 to 6 cm are at risk to rupture** and will require surgical intervention. The **rate of growth** of an aneurysm is also important in determining the need for surgical intervention and repair. Annual aneurysm growth rates should be less than 1 cm/year or elective resection may be considered.

Recognizing a Thoracic Aortic Aneurysm

- The **appearance** of a thoracic aortic aneurysm on chest radiographs **will depend,** in part, **from which portion of the thoracic aorta it arises.** Aneurysms of the **ascending aorta** may extend **anteriorly and to the right.** Aneurysms of the **aortic arch** produce a **middle mediastinal mass.** Aneurysms of the **descending aorta** project **posteriorly, laterally,** and to the **left** (Fig. 12.21).
- **Contrast-enhanced CT** is the modality **most often used** to diagnose a thoracic aortic aneurysm; MRI is also excellent at demonstrating aneurysms, but is usually less available and more expensive.
- Aneurysms can appear as **fusiform (long)** or **saccular (globular)** in shape.
- Their anatomy will be **more readily delineated on CT studies** using iodinated contrast material injected intravenously as a bolus, but they may be visible on noncontrast (unenhanced)

Fig. 12.20 Constrictive Pericarditis. There is extensive pericardial calcification (*white arrows*), most likely postinflammatory in etiology in this patient. Although **restrictive cardiomyopathy** and **constrictive pericarditis** can have identical clinical findings, the presence of pericardial calcifications **excludes** restrictive cardiomyopathy. If indicated, pericardiectomy holds the potential for cure for constrictive pericarditis.

Fig. 12.21 Aortic Aneurysm. The entire thoracic aorta is enlarged in this 67-year-old man. The ascending aorta is abnormally prominent (*solid white arrow*). The descending thoracic aorta should normally parallel and almost disappear with the thoracic spine; as it becomes larger, it swings farther away from the spine, as in this case (*dotted white arrows*).

Fig. 12.22 Aortic Aneurysm: Conventional Chest Radiograph and CT. (A) Close-up view of a frontal radiograph of the chest demonstrates a large mediastinal soft-tissue mass (*solid white arrow*). This soft-tissue density represents a large aneurysm of the proximal descending aorta seen also on the CT scan (B). The aneurysm measured 6.7 cm, which placed it at significant risk for rupture. Calcification in the wall of an aneurysm is common (*dotted white arrow*). Contrast material mixes with blood flowing in the lumen of the aorta (*solid white arrow*), but the flowing blood is separated from the intimal calcification by a considerable amount of noncontrast-containing thrombus adherent to the wall (*black arrow*).

studies as well. Often, both unenhanced and contrast-enhanced CT studies are obtained to fully evaluate the aneurysm and its contained clot.

- Frequently **calcification is seen in the intima,** which may be **separated** from the **contrast-filled lumen by varying amounts of clot** (Fig. 12.22).

Thoracic Aortic Dissection

- **Aortic dissections most often originate in the ascending aorta (Stanford type A)** or may involve only the **descending aorta (Stanford type B).**
- They result from a tear that allows blood to dissect in the wall for varying lengths of the aorta, usually along the media.
- In general, **patients with aortic dissection have been hypertensive and may have an underlying condition that can predispose to dissection,** such as cystic medial degeneration, atherosclerosis, Marfan syndrome, Ehlers-Danlos syndrome, trauma, syphilis, or crack cocaine abuse.
- In many patients, **abrupt onset of ripping or tearing chest pain,** which is **maximal at its time of onset,** is the characteristic history.
- **Conventional radiographs** are **not significantly sensitive to be diagnostically reliable,** but they **may point to the diagnosis** when several imaging findings occur together, especially in the proper clinical setting. The findings are:
    - "Widening of the mediastinum" is a **poor means of establishing the diagnosis** because (1) it is commonly over-interpreted on portable supine radiographs, whereas, (2) it occurs in only about 1 in 4 cases of aortic dissection.
    - **Left pleural effusion** (which **frequently represents a transudate** caused by pleural irritation, although transient hemorrhage from the aorta can also produce a hemothorax) (Fig. 12.23).
    - **Left apical pleural cap** of fluid or blood
    - **Loss of the normal shadow of the aortic knob**

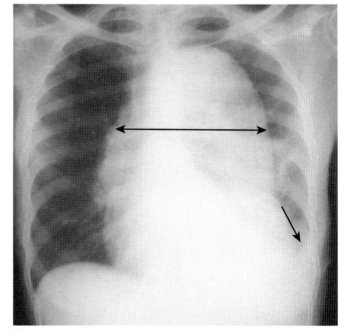

Fig. 12.23 Aortic Dissection. This 60-year-old patient has two signs suggestive of an aortic dissection on the chest radiograph: an indisputable widening of the mediastinum (*double black arrow*) and a left pleural effusion (*solid black arrow*). He also had ripping chest pain. That combination should alert you to the presence of an aortic dissection. The diagnosis was confirmed by CT examination.

- **Increased deviation of the trachea or esophagus to the right**
- Various studies have shown MRI and contrast-enhanced CT to be equally as sensitive and specific for aortic dissection, so the imaging modality used will depend in part on the patient's hemodynamic stability and the availability of resources. Transesophageal ultrasound is also used to establish the diagnosis.

Fig. 12.24 Aortic Dissections: Types A and B. (A) An intimal flap is seen to traverse both the ascending (*solid black arrow*) and descending aorta (*dotted black arrow*). This is a Stanford type A dissection because of its involvement of the ascending aorta. (B) In another patient, there is a normal-appearing ascending aorta (*dotted white arrow*) and an intimal flap noted by the black line traversing the descending aorta (*solid black arrow*). An **intimal flap** is the characteristic lesion of an aortic dissection. The smaller lumen is usually the **true** (original) lumen and the larger, **false** lumen, is actually a channel that has been produced by blood dissecting through the media.

> ## ❯❯ IMPORTANT POINTS
>
> - On both **MRI and CT**, the **diagnosis of an aortic dissection rests on identification** of the **intimal flap** that separates the **true (original)** from the **false lumen** (canal created by the dissection) (Fig. 12.24**).**

- In general, **type A (ascending aortic) dissections are treated surgically,** whereas **type B (descending aortic dissections) are treated medically.**

Coronary Artery Disease

- Coronary artery disease (CAD) is the **leading cause of death worldwide.**
- The coronary artery lumen becomes narrowed by varying amounts of atheromatous plaque. Calcium deposits in the muscular layers of the artery's walls. Vulnerable plaque may rupture, there may be vasospasm or there may be emboli that produce enough stenosis to lead to *ischemia* and possibly *infarction* of cardiac muscle (Fig. 12.25).
- MRI, CT, and nuclear medicine studies can be used in the evaluation of CAD. MRI can demonstrate **postinfarct scar formation** and **myocardial contractility.** Ventricular **function** can be quantitatively assessed.
- Cardiac CT is used for imaging of the coronary arteries. It has a **very high negative predictive value**: a negative test virtually rules out CAD. One of the major drawbacks in the use of cardiac CT angiography has been the relatively high x-ray dose delivered, but changes in equipment and new algorithms are reducing this dose considerably. Cardiac CT angiography requires injection of iodinated contrast material (eVideo 12.1).

Fig. 12.25 Cardiac CT: Coronary Artery Stenosis and Calcification. Contrast fills the lumen of the left anterior descending coronary artery except where atheromatous plaque (*solid white arrows*) narrows the lumen by about 70%, a significant stenosis. Rupture of this soft plaque, hemorrhage or clot formation can further narrow or completely occlude the lumen. Calcified plaque is also present (*dotted white arrows*).

- CT may also be used in asymptomatic patients for **calcium scoring** in which the calcium found in the coronary arteries is used as a **marker** for coronary artery disease. The amount of calcium detected on a cardiac CT scan, and calculated by computer, can be a helpful **prognostic** tool. The findings on cardiac CT are expressed as a **calcium score**, the higher the score the more extensive the evidence for CAD and the higher the potential mortality from a cardiovascular event. Calcium scoring is performed without intravenous contrast (see Fig. 4.11).

- CT can also demonstrate complications of myocardial infarction, such as ventricular aneurysms and intracardiac clots.
- **Single photon emission computed tomography (SPECT)** is an imaging technique that blends the intravascular injection of a **radioactive isotope** with acquisition of images using a rotating nuclear gamma camera capable of 3D localization

of disease. Stress and resting myocardial perfusion images using SPECT imaging can demonstrate areas of **ischemia**, especially compared with the same study done at rest. Nuclear medicine studies can also estimate left ventricular function. **(Registered users can learn more in the bonus online chapter entitled Nuclear Medicine: Understanding the Principles and Recognizing the Basics.)**

- For detecting coronary artery stenosis, coronary angiography remains the gold standard (see eVideo 4.1).

TAKE HOME POINTS

- In adults, a quick assessment of heart size can be made using the **_cardiothoracic ratio,_** which is the ratio of the widest transverse diameter of the heart compared with the widest internal diameter of the rib cage. In normal adults, the cardiothoracic ratio is usually less than 50%.
- **Extracardiac causes** can make the heart appear to be enlarged, even if it is actually normal, including anteroposterior (AP) portable studies, factors that inhibit a deep inspiration, abnormalities of the bony thorax, and the presence of a pericardial effusion.
- The heart will appear slightly **larger on an AP projection** than a PA projection of the chest because the heart is closer to the imaging surface on a PA exposure.
- On the lateral projection, the heart usually does not extend posteriorly to overlap the spine unless it is enlarged or there is a pericardial effusion.
- Two major patterns of congestive heart failure are pulmonary interstitial and pulmonary alveolar edema.
- The four key findings of **pulmonary interstitial edema** are thickening of the interlobular septa, peribronchial cuffing, fluid in the fissures, and pleural effusions.
- The key findings in **pulmonary alveolar edema** are fluffy, indistinct, patchy airspace densities; bat-wing or butterfly pattern of disease that frequently spares the outer third of lungs; pleural effusions, especially with cardiogenic pulmonary edema.
- Causes of pulmonary edema can be divided into two major categories: cardiogenic and noncardiogenic causes.
- **Cardiogenic pulmonary edema** is more likely to have pleural effusions and Kerley B lines, cardiomegaly, and an elevated pulmonary capillary wedge pressure than noncardiogenic pulmonary edema.
- The **noncardiogenic causes of pulmonary edema** are a diverse group of diseases that include uremia, disseminated intravascular coagulopathy, smoke

inhalation, near-drowning, volume overload, and lymphangitic spread of malignancy.

- **Acute respiratory distress syndrome** (ARDS) can be considered a subset of noncardiogenic pulmonary edema in which the clinical picture is one of severe hypoxia, cyanosis, tachypnea, and dyspnea.
- Essential **hypertension** is a common disease that can lead to congestive heart failure and coronary artery disease, as well as to secondary hypertrophic cardiomyopathy.
- **Mitral stenosis** has become less common with antibiotic treatment of rheumatic fever, but can lead to left, and then right, heart failure through chronic elevation of the pulmonary venous and arterial pressures with increased pulmonary vascular resistance.
- **Pulmonary arterial hypertension** may either be idiopathic (primary) or secondary to emphysema or recurrent thromboembolic disease. It produces **_pruning_** of the pulmonary vasculature and might be suspected when the main pulmonary artery achieves a diameter of 3 cm or more on CT or MRI.
- **Aortic stenosis** in the elderly is most often secondary to degeneration of a tricuspid aortic valve and can lead to angina, syncope, and/or congestive heart failure. The ascending aorta may be prominent from _poststenotic dilatation._
- **Cardiomyopathies** are divided into dilated, hypertrophic, and restrictive forms. Restrictive cardiomyopathy must be differentiated from constrictive pericarditis with which it shares its clinical findings.
- **Aortic aneurysms** can be saccular, fusiform, or can dissect. Most thoracic aortic dissections begin in the ascending aorta (Stanford Type A) and are treated surgically.
- **Coronary artery disease** is the leading cause of death worldwide and it, or its sequelae, can be imaged using a variety of techniques including CT, MRI, and SPECT.

 More information on recognizing adult heart disease is available to registered users online.

13

Recognizing the Normal Abdomen and Pelvis: Conventional Radiographs

- Although imaging of the abdomen is now largely performed utilizing computed tomography (CT), ultrasound, (US), or magnetic resonance imaging (MRI), many patients still have "plain films" of the abdomen as a **first step** before other imaging studies are performed or as a method of **following up** on findings demonstrated by other modalities. The principles that guide the interpretation of conventional radiographs also apply to the modalities of CT, MRI, and US.
- To recognize *abnormal* findings on conventional radiographs of the abdomen, you must first familiarize yourself with the appearance of *normal*.

RECOGNIZING THE NORMAL ABDOMEN: WHAT TO LOOK FOR

> **IMPORTANT POINTS**
>
> - **First,** look at the **overall gas pattern** (Box 13.1).
>   - You are looking for the **overall** pattern, so do not spend too much time trying to identify every bubble of bowel gas you see.
> - **Second,** check to see if there is **extraluminal air.**
> - **Third,** look for abnormal **abdominal calcifications.**
> - **Fourth,** look for any **soft-tissue masses.**

Recognizing the Normal Abdomen: Normal Bowel Gas Pattern

- Virtually all gas in the bowel comes from swallowed air. Only a fraction comes from the bacterial fermentation of food. For the purposes of this chapter, the terms "gas" and "air" are used interchangeably to refer to the contents of the bowel.
- Loops of bowel that contain a sufficient amount of air to fill the lumen completely are said to be **distended.** **Distension** of bowel is **normal.**
- Loops of bowel that are filled beyond their normal size are said to be **dilated.** **Dilatation** of the bowel is **abnormal.**
- **Stomach**
  - There is almost **always air in the stomach,** unless:
    - The patient has recently vomited, or
    - There is a nasogastric tube in the stomach and the tube is attached to suction.

> **BOX 13.1 Recognizing the Normal Abdomen: What to Look For**
>
> - Gas pattern
> - Extraluminal air
> - Calcifications
> - Soft-tissues masses

Fig. 13.1 Normal Supine Abdomen. This is the "scout" film of the abdomen, the supine view that gives you a general idea of the bowel gas pattern, allows you to search for abnormal calcifications and detect organomegaly. Usually air is seen in the stomach (*solid black arrow*), in about two or three loops of nondilated small bowel (*solid white arrow*) and in the rectosigmoid (*dotted black arrow*). Depending on the amount of fat around the visceral structures, their outlines may be partially visible on conventional radiographs such as the psoas muscles on this image (*dotted white arrows*).

- **Small Bowel**
  - There is usually a small amount of **air in about two or three loops of non-dilated small bowel** (Fig. 13.1).
  - The **normal diameter of small bowel is less than 2.5 cm,** which is about 1 inch or the diameter of one United States quarter.

- **Large Bowel**
  - There is **almost always air in the rectum or sigmoid.** There may be **varying amounts of gas** in the remainder of the **colon** (Fig. 13.2).
  - Use this rule to decide if the **large bowel** is dilated or not:
    - **The large bowel can normally distend to about the same size as it does on a barium enema examination.** To give you an idea of how large that is, look at Fig. 13.3.
    - Stool is recognizable by the **multiple, small bubbles of gas** present within a semisolid appearing soft-tissue mass. Recognizing the appearance of stool will help in localizing the large bowel (Fig. 13.4).

Fig. 13.2 Normal Prone Abdomen. In the prone position, the ascending and descending colon (*solid white arrows*) as well as the rectosigmoid, all posterior structures, are the highest parts of the large bowel and thus most likely to fill with air. There is air in the "S-"shaped rectosigmoid (*solid black arrow*).

Fig. 13.3 Normal Colonic Distension. To illustrate the size the normal colon may appear on a plain film, the normal diameter of the colon is shown on this barium enema (*white arrows*). Beyond this the colon would be considered dilated. This patient has had a ***double-contrast barium enema*** examination in which both air and barium were instilled as contrast agents. The combination allows for excellent visualization of the mucosal surface of the colon.

> **▶▶ IMPORTANT POINTS**
>
> - Individuals who swallow large quantities of air may develop ***aerophagia,*** characterized by numerous polygonal-shaped, air-containing loops of bowel, none of which is dilated (Fig. 13.5).

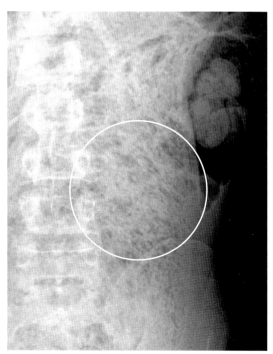

Fig. 13.4 Appearance of Stool. Stool contains numerous small bubbles of gas within a soft-tissue density (*white circle*). Stool marks the location of the large bowel and can help in identification of individual loops of bowel on conventional radiographs. This patient had a markedly dilated sigmoid colon from chronic constipation.

Fig. 13.5 Aerophagia. Virtually all bowel gas comes from swallowed air. Swallowing large quantities of air may produce a picture called ***aerophagia,*** characterized by numerous irregularly shaped, air-containing loops of bowel (*white circle*). The bowel loops are distended and overlapping but not dilated.

Recognizing the Normal Abdomen: Normal Fluid Levels

- **Stomach**
  - There is almost always **air and fluid** in the stomach so there is **almost always an air-fluid level in the stomach** on either an upright abdomen, a study done with the patient in the decubitus position or an upright chest radiograph.
    - **To see an air-fluid level, the x-ray beam must be directed horizontally** – parallel to the floor (**see Terminology online**).
- **Small Bowel**
  - **Two or three air-fluid levels** in small bowel may be seen normally on an upright or decubitus view of the abdomen.
- **Large Bowel**
  - The large bowel functions, in part, to remove fluid so **there are usually no** or **very few air-fluid levels** in the colon (Fig. 13.6).

⟫ IMPORTANT POINTS

- There may be many air-fluid levels present in the colon if the patient has had a recent enema or if the patient is taking medication with a strong anticholinergic, antiperistaltic effect.

- The normal distribution of bowel gas and fluid is summarized in Table 13.1.

Differentiating Large from Small Bowel

- **Recognizing large bowel**
  - **Large bowel is peripherally placed** around the perimeter of the abdominal cavity, except for the right upper quadrant, which is occupied by the liver (Fig. 13.7).
  - **Haustral markings usually do not extend completely across the large bowel** from one wall to the other. If they should connect one wall with another, **haustral markings are spaced more widely apart** than the valvulae conniventes of the small bowel (Fig. 13.8).

TABLE 13.1 Normal Distribution of Gas and Fluid in the Abdomen

Organ	Normally Contains Gas	Normally has Air/Fluid Levels
Stomach	Yes	Yes
Small bowel	Yes, 2–3 loops	Yes
Large bowel	Yes, especially rectosigmoid	No

Fig. 13.6 Normal Air-Fluid Levels, Upright Abdomen. The two things to look for on an upright view of the abdomen are **air-fluid levels** and **free intraperitoneal air**. Normally, there is an air-fluid level in the stomach (*solid black arrow*). There may be short, air-fluid levels in a few nondilated loops of small bowel (*black circle*). There are usually very few or no air-fluid levels in the colon. Free air, were it present, would be visible just below the right hemidiaphragm (*dotted black arrow*) and would be easier to recognize on the right than the left.

Fig. 13.7 Location of Large Bowel. Large bowel usually occupies the periphery of the abdomen. The small bowel is located more centrally. Here, large bowel (*black arrows*) contains a normal amount of air. The liver (L) occupies the right upper quadrant and normally displaces all bowel from this area.

- **Recognizing small bowel**
  - **Small bowel is centrally placed** in the abdomen. **Valvulae markings typically extend across the lumen** of small bowel from one wall to the other. The **valvulae are spaced much closer together** than the haustra of the large bowel (Fig. 13.9).
    - Small bowel can achieve a maximally dilated diameter of about 5 cm. Large bowel can dilate to many times that size.

ACUTE ABDOMINAL SERIES: THE VIEWS AND WHAT THEY SHOW

- Almost every Department of Radiology has a series of radiographic images (a protocol) that is routinely obtained in patients who have acute abdominal pain. These series are sometimes called "obstructions series," "complete abdominal series," "acute abdominal series," or something similar. For the purposes of this book, we will call such series "**acute abdominal series.**"
- **Acute abdominal series: what it may contain**
  - **Supine view** of the abdomen
    - This view is almost always obtained.
  - **Prone or lateral rectum view**
    - The inclusion of either of these views is the most variable in different hospitals' acute abdominal series.
  - **Upright or left-side down (left lateral) decubitus view**
    - One or the other is almost always included.

- **Chest: upright or supine view**
  - Inclusion of a chest radiograph depends upon hospital practices.
- Table 13.2 summarizes **what to look for on each of the views** of an acute abdominal series.

Acute Abdominal Series: Supine View ("Scout Film")

- **What is it good for?**
  - **Overall appearance of the gas pattern**
    - The **overall appearance of the bowel gas pattern,** including how much air and fluid there is and its most likely location, is **more important** than identifying every small bubble of air on the radiograph.

TABLE 13.2 Acute Abdominal Series: The Views and What to Look For

View	Look For
Supine abdomen	Overall bowel gas pattern, calcifications, masses
Prone abdomen	Gas in the rectosigmoid
Upright abdomen	Free air, air-fluid levels in the bowel
Upright chest	Free air, pneumonia, pleural effusions

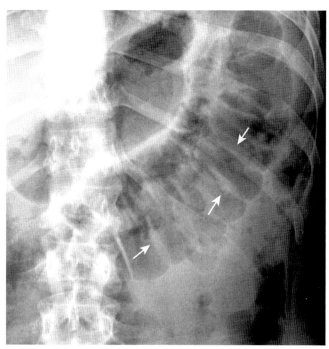

Fig. 13.8 Normal Large Bowel Haustral Markings. Most haustral markings in the colon do not traverse the entire lumen and therefore do not extend from one wall to the opposite wall (*white arrows*). This is unlike the appearance of the **valvulae conniventes** in the small bowel that do appear to traverse the entire lumen. The haustral markings are also spaced more widely apart than the valvulae of the small bowel (see Fig. 13.9).

Fig. 13.9 Small Bowel Valvulae. Markings representing the **valvulae conniventes** usually traverse the full width of the lumen of the small bowel, from one wall to the other. In addition, the valvulae are spaced closer together than the haustra of the large bowel, even when the small bowel is dilated, as it is here. The white arrows point to two valvulae that traverse the entire lumen in this close-up of dilated small bowel.

- Identifying the **presence or absence of calcifications**
- Identifying the **presence of soft-tissue masses** (see Fig. 13.1)
- **How it is obtained**
  - Patients lie on their back on the x-ray table or stretcher and the x-ray beam is directed vertically downward (Fig. 13.10).
- **Substitute view**
- No other view really substitutes for a supine view of the abdomen. Virtually all patients, regardless of their condition, can tolerate this part of the examination.

Acute Abdominal Series: Prone View

- **What is it good for?**
  - **Identifying gas in the rectum and/or sigmoid**
    - Because the rectum and sigmoid are the **highest points of the large bowel** with the person lying prone on the x-ray table, air will rise into the rectosigmoid.
      - By the way, almost no air is introduced into the rectosigmoid during the course of a routine rectal examination.
  - **Identifying gas in ascending and descending colon**
    - Because these two parts of the large bowel, besides the rectosigmoid, are posteriorly positioned, air will also collect in them when the patient is lying prone (see Fig. 13.2).
- **How it is obtained**
  - Patients lie on their abdomen on the x-ray table or stretcher and the x-ray beam is directed vertically downward (Fig. 13.11).
- **Substitute view**
  - Frequently, patients are **unable to lie prone** because of their physical condition (e.g., recent surgery, severe abdominal pain).
- These patients can turn on their **left side** and have a **lateral view of the rectum** exposed with a **vertical beam** to substitute for the prone radiograph (Fig. 13.12). The lateral view of the rectum will usually demonstrate the presence or absence of air in the rectum and/or sigmoid (Fig. 13.13).

Fig. 13.11 Positioning for Prone View of the Abdomen. The patient lies on their abdomen on the x-ray table or stretcher and the x-ray beam is directed vertically downward. Once again, the camera icon represents the x-ray tube, positioned about 40 inches above the cassette, represented by the gray rectangle under the patient.

Fig. 13.12 Positioning for the Lateral Rectum View. Patients who cannot lie prone can usually turn on their left side to have a lateral view of the rectum exposed with a vertical beam. This can substitute for a prone view of the abdomen.

Fig. 13.10 Positioning for Supine View of the Abdomen. The patient lies on their back on the x-ray table or stretcher. The x-ray beam is directed vertically downward. The camera icon represents the x-ray tube, which would actually be positioned about 40 inches above the **cassette**, represented by the gray rectangle under the table.

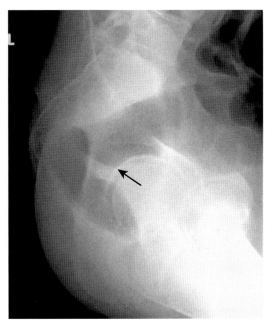

Fig. 13.13 Normal Lateral View of the Rectum. The lateral view of the rectum will usually demonstrate the presence of air in the rectum and/or sigmoid (*black arrow*). This, as we shall see in Chapter 15, can be helpful in suggesting mechanical obstruction of the bowel, at times.

Acute Abdominal Series: Upright View of Abdomen

- **What is it good for?**
  - Seeing **free air in the peritoneal cavity** (i.e., extraluminal air)
  - Seeing **air-fluid levels within the bowel lumen** (see Fig. 13.6)
- **How it is obtained**
  - The patient stands or sits up and the exposure is made with the **x-ray beam directed horizontally**, parallel to the plane of the floor (Fig. 13.14).
- **Substitute view**
  - Frequently, patients with the signs and symptoms of an acute abdomen cannot tolerate standing or sitting up for an upright view of their abdomen.

- In such cases, a **left lateral decubitus view** of the abdomen can be substituted for the upright radiograph. For a left lateral decubitus view, the **patient lies on their left side on the x-ray table.** This is done so that any **"free air"** will **distribute itself at the highest part of the abdominal cavity** on the patient's **right** side (Fig. 13.15).
  - **Free air should be easily visible** over the **outside edge of the liver** where there is normally no bowel gas present (Fig. 13.16).
    - If a right lateral decubitus view were obtained, any free air, if present, would rise to the left side of the abdomen. The left side of the abdomen is normally the location of the stomach bubble as well as gas in the splenic flexure of the colon, either of which could be mistaken for free air.
  - **To see** the **free air, the x-ray beam must be directed horizontally**, parallel to the floor, when a decubitus view is obtained.

Fig. 13.14 Positioning of Patient for an Upright View of the Abdomen. The patient stands or sits upright and the x-ray beam is directed horizontally, parallel to the plane of the floor for this view. The x-ray tube represented by the camera icon is again positioned about 40 inches from the cassette, represented by the gray rectangle behind the patient.

Fig. 13.15 Positioning of the Patient for a Left Lateral Decubitus View of the Abdomen. Patients who cannot tolerate an upright view of their abdomen usually have a left lateral decubitus view as a substitute. The patient lies on their left side on the examining table, the x-ray tube is usually positioned anteriorly (*camera icon*) and the cassette (*gray rectangle*) is placed in back of the patient. The x-ray beam is directed horizontally, parallel to the floor at a distance of about 40 inches from the patient.

Fig. 13.16 Normal Left Lateral Decubitus View of the Abdomen and Free Air. With the patient lying on the examining table left side down, an exposure is made with a horizontal x-ray beam (parallel to the floor), so that any "free air" will distribute itself at the highest part of the abdominal cavity, above the liver on the patient's right side. (A) There is no free air in this patient (*white arrows*). (B) In another patient with a perforated ulcer, free air (letter A) is visible as a black crescent over the outside edge of the liver along with an air-fluid level from free fluid in the peritoneal cavity (*black arrows*). F, Direction of patients' feet; H, direction of patients' head.

- Box 13.2 summarizes the ingredients that must be present in order to visualize air-fluid levels in the abdomen.

Acute Abdominal Series: Upright View of Chest

- **What is it good for?**
  - Seeing **free air beneath the diaphragm**
  - Finding **pneumonia at the lung bases,** which might mimic the symptoms of an acute abdomen
  - Finding **pleural effusions,** which could be secondary to an intraabdominal process and help identify its presence
    - **Pancreatitis,** for example, **may be associated with a left pleural effusion.**
    - Some **ovarian tumors** may occasionally be associated with **right-sided or bilateral pleural effusions.**
    - An abscess beneath the right hemidiaphragm (**subphrenic abscess) may be associated with a right pleural effusion.**

BOX 13.2 To See an Air-fluid Level on Conventional Radiographs, You Must Have...

- Air
- Fluid
- A horizontal x-ray beam (parallel to the plane of the floor)
- Air-fluid interfaces cannot be visualized on conventional radiographs taken with a vertical x-ray beam (e.g., supine studies).

- See Chapter 8 for more on the laterality of pleural effusions.
- **How it is obtained**
  - The **patient stands or sits up** and an exposure of the thorax is made using a **horizontal x-ray beam** (Fig. 13.17)**.**
- **Substitute view for an upright chest x-ray**
  - Frequently, patients with the signs and symptoms of an acute abdomen cannot tolerate standing for an upright view of their chest. In those cases, **a supine view of the chest may be obtained** with the patient lying on the stretcher or x-ray table.
  - In a supine view, the x-ray beam is directed **vertically downward** and **free air, especially small amounts, may not be visible.**

RECOGNIZING THE NORMAL ABDOMEN: EXTRALUMINAL AIR

- Extraluminal air is discussed in **Chapter 16: Recognizing Extraluminal Air in the Abdomen.**

RECOGNIZING THE NORMAL ABDOMEN: CALCIFICATIONS

- Abdominal calcifications are discussed in **Chapter 17: Recognizing Abnormal Calcifications and Their Causes.**

Fig. 13.17 Positioning of Patient for an Upright Chest Radiograph. The patient sits upright or stands with the anterior chest wall closest to the cassette. The x-ray beam passes horizontally. Any free air in the abdomen will rise to a position under the diaphragm and be visible.

! DIAGNOSTIC PITFALLS

- Two common calcifications should not be confused with pathologic calcifications of the abdomen.
  - **Phleboliths** are small, rounded calcifications that represent calcified venous thrombi that occur with increasing age, most often in the pelvic veins of women. They classically have a **lucent center** that helps to differentiate them from ureteral calculi with which phleboliths can be confused (Fig. 13.18).
  - **Calcification of the rib cartilages** occurs with advancing age and, although not a true abdominal calcification, can sometimes be confused for renal or biliary calculi when these rib calcifications overlie the kidney or region of the gallbladder. Calcified cartilage tends to have an **amorphous, speckled appearance** and the calcified cartilage will occur in an arc corresponding to that of the anterior rib cartilage as it sweeps back toward articulation with the sternum (Fig. 13.19).

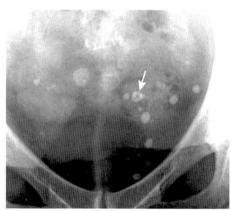

Fig. 13.18 Phleboliths. Phleboliths are calcifications most often found in the pelvis in women with increasing age. Unlike ureteral calculi, they classically have a lucent center (*white arrow*). They are almost always incidental and nonpathologic, but they can prove challenging diagnostically because their location and appearance can be similar to ureteral calculi.

Fig. 13.19 Calcified Rib Cartilages. Calcification of the rib cartilages (*white circle*) appears to be a physiologic process that is more common in females and rare under the age of 35. It has been postulated that it may be a response to strains imposed by muscular activity. A difference between males and females in the pattern of rib cartilage calcification has been used by forensic pathologists to help identify gender in postmortem examinations.

RECOGNIZING THE NORMAL ABDOMEN: ORGANOMEGALY

- **Conventional radiographic evaluation of soft-tissue structures in the abdomen** (e.g., the liver, spleen, kidneys, gallbladder, urinary bladder, or soft-tissue masses such as tumors or abscesses) **is limited** because these structures are **soft-tissue densities** and they are **surrounded by other soft tissues or fluid** of similar density. Only a **difference in density** between two adjacent structures **will render their outlines visible** on conventional radiographs.
- Still, conventional radiographs are easy to obtain and frequently the first study ordered in a patient with abdominal symptoms.

▶▶ IMPORTANT POINTS

- There are **two fundamental ways of recognizing the presence** and **estimating the size of soft-tissue masses or organs** on conventional radiographs of the abdomen:
  - The first is by **direct visualization of the edges of structure** that can occur only if it is surrounded by something of a different density other than soft tissue, such as **fat or free air**.
  - The second is to recognize **indirect evidence of the mass** or enlarged visceral organ by **recognizing pathologic displacement of air-filled loops of bowel**.

Liver

- **Normal**
  - The liver normally displaces all bowel gas from the right upper quadrant.
  - Occasionally, a **tongue-like projection of the right lobe** of the liver may extend to the iliac crest, **especially in females.** This is called a **_Riedel lobe_** and is normal (Fig. 13.20).

Fig. 13.20 Riedel Lobe of the Liver. A normal anatomic variant, particularly found in females, is this tongue-like, inferior projection of the right lobe of the liver (*black arrows*). It can mimic a palpable liver mass.

- **Enlarged liver**
  - **An enlarged liver might be suggested** from conventional radiographs if there is displacement of all bowel from the right upper quadrant **down to the iliac crest** and **across the midline** (Fig. 13.21). **Conventional radiographs are poor for estimating the size of the liver.** Imaging evaluation of liver size is best made using CT, MRI, or US.

Spleen

- **Normal**
  - The adult **spleen is about 12 cm in length and usually does not project below the 12th posterior rib.** As a general rule, the spleen is about as large as the left kidney.
- **Enlarged spleen**
  - As an aid in identifying splenomegaly, keep in mind that the normal position of the **stomach bubble** (i.e., air in the gastric fundus) **is nestled beneath the highest part of the left hemidiaphragm** about midway between the abdominal wall and the spine (see Fig. 13.1).
  - If the spleen projects well **below the 12th posterior rib** and/or **displaces the stomach bubble** toward or across the midline, the spleen is probably enlarged. (Fig. 13.22).

Kidneys

- **Normal**
  - Portions of the kidney outlines may be visible on conventional radiographs if an adequate amount of perirenal fat is present.

- The **kidney length is approximately the height of four lumbar vertebral bodies** or about **10 to 14 cm in size in an adult.**
- The liver depresses the right kidney so that the **right kidney is usually lower in the abdomen than the left kidney** (Fig. 13.23).

Fig. 13.22 Splenomegaly. The spleen is about 12 cm in length and usually does not project below the 12th posterior rib. If the spleen (*white arrows*) projects well below the 12th posterior rib (*black arrow*) and/or displaces the normally left-sided stomach bubble toward or across the midline, the spleen is probably enlarged, as it is in this patient with leukemia.

Fig. 13.23 Position of the Kidneys. This is one image from an *intravenous urogram* (aka, *intravenous pyelogram, IVP*) in which the patient receives an intravenous injection of iodinated contrast which is then excreted by the kidneys. Both kidney outlines (*solid white arrows*), ureters (*solid black arrows*), and urinary bladder (B) can be seen. Other images of the kidneys, including oblique views, were often obtained to visualize the entire contour of the kidney. IVPs have largely been replaced by computed tomography (CT) scans in the form of CT urograms. The liver (L) normally depresses the right kidney more inferiorly than the left kidney.

Fig. 13.21 Hepatomegaly. Although conventional radiographs are notoriously poor for evaluating liver size, sometimes the liver can become so enlarged it will be obvious even on plain films. If the liver displaces all bowel loops from the right upper quadrant (*white arrow*) down to the iliac crest and across the midline (*black arrows*), then hepatomegaly is suggested, such as in this patient with cirrhosis.

- The left **kidney is roughly the same length as the spleen.**
- **Enlarged kidney**
  - Usually only extremely enlarged kidneys or very large renal masses will be recognizable on conventional radiographs by displacement of bowel gas (Fig. 13.24).

Urinary Bladder

- **Normal**
  - The bladder frequently is surrounded by **enough extravesical fat that at least the dome is visible** in most

individuals. It appears as the top of an oval structure with its long axis parallel to the long axis of the pelvis and the **base of the bladder just above the top of the symphysis pubis.**

- The urinary bladder is about the size of a small cantaloupe when distended and about the size of a lemon when contracted (Fig. 13.25).
- **Enlarged urinary bladder**
  - Bladder enlargement is usually recognized by displacement of bowel upward and out of the pelvis by a mass of

Fig. 13.24 Enlarged Kidney. Soft-tissue masses or organomegaly can be diagnosed from a conventional radiograph either by visualizing the **edge of the mass** if fat or air is surrounding it or by **displacement of bowel.** (A) On the conventional radiograph, there is a soft-tissue mass in the left upper quadrant (*white arrows*) that is displacing bowel to the right (*black arrow*). (B) A coronal reformatted CT scan of the same patient demonstrates a large renal cyst (*white arrows*) arising from the compressed left kidney (*black arrow*), displacing it and the adjacent bowel. The spleen (S) is also being compressed by the cyst.

Fig. 13.25 Normal Urinary Bladder. Close-up of the pelvis demonstrates the outline of the urinary bladder made visible by perivesical fat (*white arrows*). In males, the sigmoid colon usually occupies the space just above the bladder (*black arrow*), whereas in females, the soft tissue above the bladder may be either the uterus or sigmoid colon.

soft-tissue density. Bladder outlet obstruction is much more common in men from enlargement of the prostate, so that a pelvic soft-tissue mass is more likely to be a dilated bladder in a male than a female (Fig. 13.26A).

Uterus

- **Normal**
  - The uterus usually sits atop the dome of the bladder. Frequently a lucency is produced by fat between the top of the bladder and the bottom the uterus. The **normal uterus is about 8 cm by 4 cm by 6 cm.**

- **Enlarged uterus**
  - **Ultrasound** is the **best** tool for **evaluating the size of the uterus and ovaries.**
  - **Occasionally uterine enlargement,** when marked, **may be visible** on **conventional radiographs.** (Fig. 13.26B).

Psoas Muscles

- One or both psoas muscles may be visible if adequate extraperitoneal fat surrounds them. Inability to visualize one or both psoas muscles is not a reliable indicator of retroperitoneal disease (see Fig. 13.1).

Fig. 13.26 Distended Urinary Bladder and Enlarged Uterus. (A) The distended bladder (letter *B*) is visualized as a soft-tissue mass that ascends from the pelvis into the lower abdomen displacing the bowel into the mid-abdomen (*black arrows*). This was a 72-year-old man with bladder outlet obstruction from benign prostatic hypertrophy. (B) In a different patient, the uterus (letter *U*) is slightly enlarged. It can be distinguished from the bladder because there is a fat plane (*white arrows*) between it and the urinary bladder (letter *B*) below it.

🏠 TAKE HOME POINTS

- Evaluation of the abdomen should focus on four main areas: the gas pattern, free air, soft-tissue masses or organomegaly, and abnormal calcifications.
- Normally air is present in the stomach and colon, especially the rectosigmoid, whereas a small amount of air (two to three loops) may normally be seen in small bowel.
- Normally an air-fluid level is seen in the stomach; there may be two to three air-fluid levels in nondilated small bowel, but usually no air-fluid level is visible in the colon.
- An **acute abdominal series** may consist of: supine abdomen, prone abdomen (or its substitute, which is a lateral rectum view), upright abdomen (or its substitute, which is a left lateral decubitus view), and an upright chest (or its substitute, which is a supine chest).

- The **supine view** of the abdomen is the general scout view for the bowel gas pattern and is useful for identifying calcifications and for detecting organomegaly or soft-tissue masses.
- The **prone view** allows air, if present, to be seen in the rectosigmoid, which is important in the identification of mechanical obstruction of the bowel.
- The **upright abdomen** may demonstrate air-fluid levels in the bowel or free intraperitoneal air.
- The **upright chest radiograph** may demonstrate free air beneath the diaphragm, pleural effusion (which may provide a clue as to the presence and the nature of intraabdominal pathology) or pneumonia (which can mimic an acute abdomen).
- CT, US, and MRI have essentially replaced conventional radiography in the assessment of organomegaly or abdominal soft-tissue masses.

🛜 More information on the appearance of the normal abdomen on conventional radiographs is available to registered users online.

14

Recognizing the Normal Abdomen and Pelvis on Computed Tomography

INTRODUCTION TO ABDOMINAL AND PELVIC CT

- It is estimated that around 80 million computed tomography (CT) scans of all kinds are performed in the United States each year. Almost 10% of all visits to the emergency department are for abdominal pain of a nontraumatic nature. Many of those patients undergo a CT scan of the abdomen and pelvis performed to detect or clarify their clinical findings. Since the advent of CT, exploratory surgery has become rare and the need for emergency surgery has dramatically decreased.
- As with all imaging studies, one of the guiding principles in CT scanning of the abdomen and pelvis is to maximize the differences in density between tissues to best demonstrate their unique anatomy. Toward that end, CT studies make extensive use of **intravenous** and **oral contrast** agents.

INTRAVENOUS CONTRAST IN CT SCANNING

- CT scans **can be performed with and/or without the intravenous administration of iodinated contrast** material but, **in general, they yield more diagnostic information** that is more easily detectable **when intravenous contrast can be used.**
- CT scans done with **intravenous contrast** are called *contrast-enhanced* or simply *enhanced*. Typically, the radiologist will choose the scanning parameters to optimize the CT study for the patient's particular clinical issues. For example, different rates of contrast administration and timing of the scan will allow diagnostic enhancement of hepatic vessels versus the liver parenchyma.
- Although it might sound like a great idea to give everyone contrast, keep in mind that **iodinated contrast** can have **adverse effects** and produce **serious reactions** in **susceptible individuals** (Box 14.1).

ORAL CONTRAST IN CT SCANNING

- For abdominal and pelvic CT imaging, **oral contrast** may also be administered to define the bowel, although its use has diminished as the quality of CT images has improved. Oral contrast is usually **not employed in chest CT scanning** unless there is a particular question concerning the esophagus.
- Orally administered contrast, frequently given in doses divided over time to allow earlier contrast to reach the colon while

---

BOX 14.1 Contrast Reactions

- Intravenous contrast materials available today are **nonionic, low-osmolar solutions containing a high concentration of iodine** which circulate through the bloodstream, opacify those tissues and organs with high blood flow, are absorbed by x-rays (and therefore appear "whiter" on images), and are finally excreted in the urine by the kidneys.
- In some patients (e.g., those with diabetes, dehydration, or multiple myeloma) who have compromised renal function evidenced by creatinine greater than 1.5 mg/dL, iodinated contrast can produce a nephrotoxic effect resulting in **acute tubular necrosis.** Although usually reversible, in a small number of patients with underlying renal insufficiency, renal dysfunction may permanently worsen. This effect is contrast dose-related.
- Iodinated contrast agents can sometimes produce **mild side-effects** including a feeling of warmth, nausea and vomiting and local irritation at the site of injection, itching and hives; these side-effects usually require no treatment. Occasional idiosyncratic, allergic-like reactions may also include itching, hives, and laryngeal irritation.
- Asthmatics and those with a history of severe allergies or prior reactions to intravenous contrast have a higher likelihood of contrast reactions (but still very low overall) and may benefit from steroids, diphenhydramine (Benadryl), and cimetidine (e.g., Tagamet) administered prior to and/or after injection. Prior shellfish allergy bears absolutely NO relationship to iodinated contrast reactions.
- In about 0.01 to 0.04% of all patients, **severe and idiosyncratic reactions** to contrast can occur that can produce intense bronchospasm, laryngeal edema, circulatory collapse and, very rarely, death (1 in 200,000 to 300,000).
- In patients with a history of intravenous contrast reactions, oral contrast can be safely administered without the need for premedication.

---

later contrast opacifies the stomach, is utilized for many abdominal CT scans except those performed for **trauma,** the **stone search study,** and studies specifically directed toward evaluating vascular structures such as the **aorta.**

- One of two different types of oral contrast may be used. The most widely used is a dilute solution of **barium sulfate,** the same contrast agent employed in upper gastrointestinal studies and barium enemas. If there is concern for bowel perforation and the possibility that contrast may exit from the lumen of the bowel, an iodine-based, water-soluble contrast is sometimes used (e.g., **Gastrografin**). Contrast may also be introduced rectally to opacify the distal colon more quickly than it would take for orally administered contrast to reach the large bowel or through a Foley catheter to quickly opacify the urinary bladder.

- You will probably not be required to make the decision of when or if to use contrast as **the radiologist will usually tailor the examination to best answer the clinical question being asked.** That means it is **always important** to provide as much clinical information as possible when requesting a study.

- Table 14.1 summarizes, in general, **when intravenous and oral contrast are utilized** for particular problems.
- Table 14.2 outlines some of the common **patient preparations** that are generally suggested for a variety of imaging studies. Preparation instructions may vary depending on the facility and individual patient needs. In general, a patient

TABLE 14.1 CT Scans: When Contrast is Used

IV Contrast Used	IV Contrast Usually Not Used
Chest	
CT-Pulmonary angiogram (CT-PA) for pulmonary embolism	Evaluation of diffuse infiltrative lung diseases using HRCT
Evaluation of the mediastinum or hila for mass or adenopathy	Confirmation of the presence of a nodule suspected from conventional radiographs
Detect aortic aneurysm or dissection	Detect pneumothorax/pneumomediastinum
Evaluation of blunt or penetrating trauma	Calcium scoring for the coronary arteries
Characterization of pleural disease (metastases, empyema)	Known allergies to contrast or renal failure
CT densitometry of pulmonary masses	
Evaluation of the coronary arteries	
IV Contrast Used	**IV Contrast Usually Not Used**
Abdomen and Pelvis	
Evaluate for the presence of and/or to characterize a mass and to stage or follow-up malignancies	CT colonography, unless staging a suspected cancer detected by colonoscopy
Trauma	Search for a ureteral calculus
Abdominal pain (e.g., appendicitis)	
Detect aortic aneurysm or dissection	
WHEN ORAL CONTRAST IS USED	
Most cases of nontraumatic abdominal pain	
Inflammatory bowel disease	
Abdominal or pelvic abscess	
Locate the site of bowel perforation, including fistulae	

HRCT, High-resolution computed tomography; *IV*, intravenous.

TABLE 14.2 Preparations for Imaging Studies

Study	Before the Order is Placed	Before the Start of the Study	After the Study is Done
CT			
Head CT with or without contrast	Solicit history of previous contrast reaction	Serum creatinine may be needed before contrast injections	Nothing
Body CT without contrast	Nothing	No preparation needed	Nothing
Body CT with oral **contrast** and/ or IV contrast	Solicit history of previous contrast reaction	Serum creatinine may be needed before contrast injections; oral contrast is given just before study	Nothing
US			
Upper abdomen, general survey study: aorta, gall bladder, inferior vena cava, liver, pancreas, renal stenosis, retroperitoneal, spleen	Nothing	Nothing to eat or drink for several hours prior to examination	Nothing
Renal or kidney	Nothing	Patient may be asked to drink a prescribed amount of water to distend bladder 1 to 2 hours before procedure; patient should not empty bladder	Nothing

Continued

TABLE 14.2 Preparations for Imaging Studies—cont'd

Study	Before the Order is Placed	Before the Start of the Study	After the Study is Done
Male or female pelvis or lower abdomen; obstetric/gynecologic US	Nothing	Patient may be asked to drink a prescribed amount of water to distend bladder 1 to 2 hours before procedure; patient should not empty bladder	Nothing
Renal transplant; thyroid, and vascular studies	Nothing	No preparation needed	Nothing
MRI **Without contrast**	Solicit history of working with metal, grinding, welding or possible metal in eyes; patient may need an orbital x-ray; solicit history of pacemaker, aneurysm clips, neural stimulators, IUD, permanent makeup, cochlear implants, artificial heart valves, pregnancy, metallic fragments; claustrophobia	No preparation needed	Nothing
With contrast	Solicit history of working with metal, grinding, welding or possible metal in eyes; patient may need an orbital x-ray; solicit history of pacemaker, aneurysm clips, neural stimulators, IUD, permanent makeup; cochlear implants, artificial heart valves, pregnancy, metallic fragments; claustrophobia	Serum creatinine may be needed before contrast injections or in patients with renal insufficiency	Nothing
Barium Study **Esophagram** or video fluoroscopic swallowing examination	Nothing	No preparation needed	Nothing
Upper gastrointestinal series/ small bowel series	Nothing	Nothing to eat or drink for several hours prior to study	Nothing
Barium enema; virtual colonography	Nothing	Bowel preparation to cleanse colon before study may consist of oral laxatives, suppositories, fluids	Mild laxative if desired
Mammography **Mammogram**	Nothing	Patient should not use any deodorant, perfume, powder, ointment, or any other skin products on chest, breast, or under arms on the day of appointment	Nothing
Nuclear Medicine **Thyroid** uptake and scan	No intravenous, iodinated contrast studies within previous 4 to 8 weeks	Stop thyroid medications or foods high in iodine content	Nothing
Bone density	Is the patient pregnant?	No contrast or barium studies for 48 hours prior to the procedure. No food restriction	Nothing
Bone scan	Is the patient pregnant?	No food restriction	Nothing
Cardiac treadmill and pharmacologic stress test	Is the patient pregnant?	Nothing to eat or drink for several hours prior to the examination. No caffeine several hours prior to the examination	Nothing

is permitted to take medications with a small sip of water, even when instructions are nothing to eat or drink before the study.

ABDOMINAL CT: GENERAL CONSIDERATIONS

- Conventional radiography, ultrasonography (US), CT, and magnetic resonance imaging (MRI) are all utilized in the imaging evaluation of abdominal abnormalities.
- Each has advantages and disadvantages inherent to its own particular technology and the choice of modality is frequently based on the patient's clinical condition (Table 14.3).
- Although advances in CT imaging have resulted in better diagnostic studies, they may have come with an unintended consequence: potentially higher **radiation dose.** The radiation dose delivered by CT studies is dependent on many factors, including the type of equipment, the energy of the x-rays used to produce the images, and the size of the patient. Dose-reducing measures are being employed, including the use of optimized CT settings, reduction in the x-ray energy used, limiting the number of repeat scans, and assuring—through appropriate consultation—that the **benefits** derived from obtaining the study **outweigh** any potential **risks** of the radiation exposure.

▶▶ IMPORTANT POINTS

- **History and physical examination continue to be an essential part of evaluating abdominal abnormalities** not only to suggest an etiology but also in helping to determine which, if any, imaging studies will provide the best yield in establishing the correct diagnosis.

ABDOMINAL CT: BY ORGAN

Liver

- By convention, **CT scans**, like most other radiologic studies, **are viewed** with the **patient's right on your left and the patient's left on your right.** If the patient is scanned in the supine position, as most usually are, the **top** of each image is **anterior** and the **bottom** of each image is **posterior.**
- The liver receives its blood **supply** from both **hepatic arteries** and **portal veins** and **drains** to the inferior vena cava via the **hepatic veins.** The normal parenchyma is supplied 80% by the portal vein and 20% by the hepatic artery, so it will enhance mostly in the portal venous phase.
- For practical purposes, the **vascular distribution of the liver defines its anatomy** because the vascular anatomy is what directs the surgical approach to liver lesions.
- The liver is divided into **right, left, and caudate lobes** by its vessels.
  - The **right lobe** is subdivided into **two segments:** the **anterior** and **posterior.** The **left** lobe is subdivided into **two segments:** the **medial** and **lateral.**
  - A prominent, fat-filled fissure that contains the **falciform ligament** and **ligamentum teres** (formerly the umbilical

TABLE 14.3 Imaging of the Abdomen and Pelvis Modalities Compared

Uses	Advantages	Disadvantages
CONVENTIONAL RADIOGRAPHY		
Primarily used for screening in cases of abdominal pain	Readily available Relatively low cost Can be portable Patients tolerate procedure well	Has lower sensitivity Uses ionizing radiation
ULTRASONOGRAPHY (US)		
Primary imaging mode for gallbladder and biliary tree Screening for aortic aneurysm Identification of vascular abnormalities and flow Detection of ascites Primary imaging mode for the female pelvis	Readily available Relatively low cost Uses no ionizing radiation Patients tolerate procedure well Can be portable (point-of-care studies)	Operator dependent More difficult to interpret
COMPUTED TOMOGRAPHY		
Diagnostic modality of choice for most abdominal abnormalities, including trauma	Usually available Lower cost than MRI High spatial-resolution and image reconstruction Evaluates multiple organ systems simultaneously	Higher cost than US Uses ionizing radiation Inability to use intravenous contrast in renal insufficiency Possibility of contrast reactions Patient weight and size may affect scanning
MAGNETIC RESONANCE IMAGING (MRI)		
Problem-solving for difficult diagnoses Extension of known disease into surrounding soft tissues (staging) Vascular anatomy	High soft-tissue contrast No ionizing radiation No iodinated contrast Image reconstruction in any plane	Usually highest cost of imaging modalities Limited availability Longer scan times Claustrophobia; patient weight and size may preclude study Monitoring issues in acutely ill patients Incompatible with certain medical devices or foreign bodies in patient

vein) separates the **medial and lateral segments** of the **left lobe** of the liver (Fig. 14.1).

- The outer surface of the liver is normally smooth. The normal liver usually appears homogeneous in density on CT, and its attenuation should always be **denser than or equal to the density of the spleen on noncontrast scans.**

- The adult liver usually measures **15 cm or less on coronal scans at its maximum height**. Care must be taken not to measure the length at the site of a Riedel lobe of the liver, a normal inferior projection from the right lobe seen mainly in females (**see Fig. 13.20**). The liver's greatest **transverse measurement is 20 to 26 cm.**

- The diaphragmatic surface of the liver is affixed by connective tissue to a triangular section of the undersurface of the diaphragm, termed the *bare area*. This will have importance later in differentiating ascites from pleural effusion (Chapter 18) (Fig. 14.2).

- **Liver volume** can be calculated using CT (as well as US and MRI). The volume of the liver will vary by gender and by patient weight. The adult liver volume is about 1500 cm³. Liver volume determinations may be used for liver resection, transplantation, and in evaluating the progression of various diseases, such as alcohol-related liver disease.

Spleen

- On early contrast-enhanced scans, the spleen may be inhomogeneous in its attenuation, a finding that should disappear over the course of the next several minutes.

- The **normal** adult spleen may have **lobulations,** not to be confused with lacerations. The splenic artery and vein enter and exit at the hilum of the spleen.

- The spleen is usually **about 12 cm long, does not project** substantially below the margin of the **12th rib,** and is about the **same size as the left kidney.**

Pancreas

- The pancreas is a retroperitoneal organ oriented obliquely so that the entire organ is not seen on any one axial image of the upper abdomen.
  - The **tail** is usually **most superior,** lying in the hilum of the spleen.
  - Proceeding inferiorly, the **body of the pancreas** crosses the midline and rests anterior to the **superior mesenteric artery.** The **head of the pancreas** is nestled in the duodenal loop (Fig. 14.3). The **uncinate process,** a part

Fig. 14.1 Normal Liver Anatomy. The ligamentum teres (*dotted black arrow*) divides the left lobe of the liver into a medial (M) and lateral segment (L) with the larger right lobe (R) lying more posterior. The portal vein (PV) lies just posterior to the hepatic artery (*solid black arrow*). The splenic artery (*solid white arrow*) follows the path of the pancreas (P) toward the spleen (S). The inferior vena cava (IVC) lies to the right of the aorta (A).

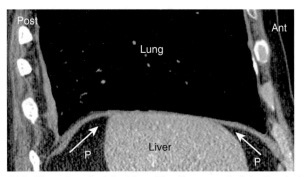

Fig. 14.2 "Bare Area" of the Liver. The "bare area" of the liver (*white arrows*) has no peritoneal covering, but is affixed directly to the undersurface of the diaphragm. As such, it will be impossible for ascitic fluid in the peritoneal cavity (P) to insert itself between the liver and the lung, which will be important for differentiating pleural effusion from ascites on CT (see Chapter 18). *Ant,* Anterior; *Post,* Posterior.

Fig. 14.3 Normal Pancreas. (A) Body of pancreas (*thick white arrow*) and splenic artery (*thin white arrow*). Additionally well seen are both adrenal glands (*dotted white arrows*) and gallbladder (*black arrow*). (B) Normal head of pancreas (*solid white arrow*). Because of its oblique orientation, the entire pancreas is not visualized on a single axial image of the abdomen. The tail is most superior and the body and then head are usually seen on successively more inferior slices.

of the head, curves around the **superior mesenteric vein.**

- The **splenic vein** courses along the posterior border of the pancreas to the **superior mesenteric vein** and the **splenic artery** runs along the superior border of the pancreas from the **celiac axis** to the spleen. The main pancreatic duct empties into the duodenum as the **Duct of Wirsung** and sometimes through an **accessory Duct of Santorini.** The pancreatic duct may be visible and measures 3 to 4 mm in diameter.
- The **head** of the pancreas measures **3 cm** in maximum dimension, the **body 2.5 cm,** and the **tail 2 cm.** The gland is about **12 to 15 cm in length.** As a person ages, the gland may undergo fatty infiltration giving it a "feathery" appearance.

Kidneys

- The kidneys are retroperitoneal organs, encircled by varying amounts of fat and enclosed within a fibrous capsule.
- They are surrounded by the *perirenal space* that, in turn, is delimited by the **anterior and posterior renal fasciae.** Certain fascial attachments, muscles, and other organs define a series of spaces that produce predictable patterns of abnormality when those spaces are filled with fluid, pus, blood, or air.
- In adults, the **left kidney** is **minimally larger** than the **right,** each kidney being about **11 cm** in size or about the **same size** as the **spleen.**
- The **right renal artery** passes **posterior** to the inferior vena cava (IVC). The **renal veins** lie **anterior to the arteries;** the longer left renal vein passes anterior to the aorta before draining into the IVC (Fig. 14.4).
- The **renal hilum** contains the renal pelvis and the renal artery and vein. The upper poles of the kidneys are more posterior than the lower poles and are tilted medially toward the spine.

- Dedicated renal CT scans frequently utilize a precontrast view of the kidneys followed by a series of images obtained at timed intervals after the injection of intravenous contrast (**multiphasic study**) (Fig. 14.5).
- So long as they are functioning properly, the **kidneys are the major route** for excretion of **iodinated contrast** material. They should therefore **enhance** whenever intravenous contrast is administered. Over time, the urine will become more opacified, increasing significantly from its normal water density, a process sometimes requiring delayed imaging of the urinary tract.
- If the kidneys are not functioning properly, contrast is excreted though alternative pathways (e.g., bile, bowel), a process called *vicarious excretion* of contrast.

Fig. 14.4 Normal Kidneys. The kidneys (K) lie in the renal fossae bilaterally. The normal renal sinus, containing fat, occupies the central portion of the kidneys (*dotted black arrows*). The right renal artery (*solid black arrow*) runs posterior to the inferior vena cava (IVC). The left renal vein (*dotted white arrow*) here lies anterior to the left renal artery (*solid white arrow*). *A,* Abdominal aorta.

Fig. 14.5 Multiphasic CT, Normal Left Kidney. (A) The **corticomedullary phase** occurs about 30 to 70 seconds after the start of intravenous contrast injection and shows the corticomedullary junction between the outer, brighter cortex (*solid white arrow*) and the inner, less dense medulla (*solid black arrow*). This phase can provide information about the renal vasculature and renal perfusion. (B) The **nephrographic phase** occurs about 80 to 100 seconds after injection and demonstrates homogeneous opacification of the kidney (*dotted black arrows*). It is useful in evaluating the renal parenchyma, especially for renal neoplasms, as well as scarring and inflammatory disease. (C) The **excretory phase** is obtained about 5 to 10 minutes postinjection and may show urothelial abnormalities, such as tumors, papillary necrosis, and ureteral stricture. The intrarenal collecting system (*dotted white arrows*) and ureter (*solid white arrow*) are now opacified.

Small and Large Bowel

- **Opacification** and **distension** of the bowel lumen are helpful for proper evaluation of the bowel wall regardless of the modality used to evaluate it. Wall thickness may seem artificially increased if the bowel is collapsed.
- The **small bowel** is usually **2.5 cm** or less in **diameter** with a **wall thickness** usually less than **3 mm**. Adjacent loops of small bowel are usually in contact with each other, depending in part on the amount of intraperitoneal fat present.
- The **colonic wall** is usually **less than 3 mm** thick with the colon **distended** and **less than 5 mm** with the colon **collapsed.** The **cecum** is recognizable by the presence of the terminal ileum. The positions of the transverse and sigmoid segments of the colon are variable, depending on their degree of redundancy (Fig. 14.6).

Fig. 14.6 Normal Small Bowel. Contrast fills a nondilated lumen (<2.5 cm). The small bowel wall is so thin that it is normally almost invisible (*white arrows*). The terminal ileum can be recognized by the fat-containing "lips" of the ileocecal valve (*black arrows*) outlined with orally administered contrast in the lumen.

Urinary Bladder

- The bladder is an **extraperitoneal organ,** the extraperitoneal space being continuous with the retroperitoneum. The **dome of the bladder** is covered by the **inferior reflection of the peritoneum.**
- The bladder's location in **males** is superior to the prostate gland and anterior to the rectum. In **females,** the bladder is anterior to the vagina and anteroinferior to the uterus. The ureters enter the posterolateral aspect of the bladder at the trigone.
- The **bladder wall measures 5 mm or less with the bladder distended.**
- The bladder is **best evaluated when distended** with either urine or urine-containing contrast, but the **bladder wall is usually visible** whether or not intravenous contrast has been administered (Fig. 14.7).

Fig. 14.7 Normal Bladder. The urinary bladder (B) contains unopacified urine in this early image of a contrast-enhanced CT scan of the pelvis. The bladder wall (*solid white arrows*) is thin and of equal thickness around the circumference of the bladder. The rectum lies posterior to the bladder (*dotted white arrow*).

🏠 TAKE HOME POINTS

- Computed tomography studies make extensive use of intravenous and oral contrast agents to maximize the differences in density between structures so as to best demonstrate their anatomy.
- In general, intravenous, contrast-enhanced CT scans yield more diagnostic information, which is more easily recognizable when intravenous contrast can be used.
- Iodinated contrast agents may occasionally produce **side-effects,** such as warmth or nausea and vomiting; rarely idiosyncratic **allergic-like reactions** occur, leading to more severe symptoms and death.
- Oral and/or rectal contrast may be used to define the bowel and help in differentiating bowel from adjacent lymph nodes or pathologic, fluid-containing lesions.
- In a number of clinical settings, either iodinated and/or oral contrast improve the diagnostic accuracy of CT scanning and imaging studies are usually tailored by the radiologist based on the clinical problem.

- It is essential to provide an **appropriate history** to help in determining which, if any, imaging study (studies) will provide the best yield in establishing the correct diagnosis.
- Advances in CT imaging have resulted in better diagnostic studies, but they may carry the potential for a **higher radiation dose.** Dose-reducing measures are being employed, including the use of optimized CT settings, reduction in the x-ray energy used, limiting the number of repeat scans, and assuring that the benefits derived from obtaining a study outweigh any potential risks of the radiation exposure.
- Some of the common patient preparations that are used for a variety of imaging studies are outlined.
- The normal CT appearances of the liver, spleen, pancreas, kidneys, bowel, and bladder are described.

More information on recognizing the normal abdomen and pelvis on CT is available to registered users online.

15

Recognizing Bowel Obstruction and Ileus

- In Chapters 13 and 14, we discussed how to recognize the normal intestinal gas pattern on conventional radiographs and computed tomography (CT). In this chapter, you will learn how to recognize and categorize the four most common abnormal bowel gas patterns and their causes. These patterns of abnormal bowel gas will appear the same whether imaged initially by conventional radiography or by CT scanning. CT is superior in revealing the location, degree, and cause of an obstruction and in demonstrating any signs of reduced bowel viability.
- Abnormalities of bowel function are suggested by the history and clinical findings.
- The key questions in assessing the bowel gas pattern on imaging studies are:
  - Are there **dilated loops of small and/or large bowel?**
  - On CT, is there a **transition point?**
  - On plain films, is there **air in the rectum or sigmoid?**

ABNORMAL GAS PATTERNS

- Abnormal intestinal gas patterns can be divided into two main categories, each of which can be subdivided into two subcategories (Box 15.1).
- **Functional ileus** is one main category in which it is presumed that **one or more loops of bowel lose their ability to propagate the peristaltic waves of the bowel,** usually because of some **local irritation or inflammation,** and hence cause a **functional type of "obstruction"** proximal to the affected loop(s).
- There are **two kinds** of **functional ileus.**
  - **Localized ileus affects only one or two loops** of (usually small) bowel *(also called sentinel loops).*
  - **Generalized adynamic ileus** affects **all loops of large and small bowel,** and frequently the stomach.

- **Mechanical obstruction** is the other main category of abnormal bowel gas pattern.
  With mechanical obstruction, a **physical, organic, obstructing lesion prevents the passage of intestinal content** past the point of either the small or large bowel blockage.
- There are **two kinds** of **mechanical obstruction.**
  - **Small bowel obstruction** (frequently abbreviated SBO)
  - **Large bowel obstruction** (frequently abbreviated LBO)

LAWS OF THE GUT

▶▶ IMPORTANT POINTS

- The bowel reacts to a mechanical obstruction in more or less predictable ways.
- After the obstruction occurs, **peristalsis continues** (except in the loops of bowel involved in a functional ileus) in an attempt to propel intestinal contents through the bowel.
- Loops **proximal** to the **obstruction** soon become **dilated with swallowed air and/or secreted fluid.**
  - This can occur within a few hours of a complete small bowel obstruction.
- Loops **distal** to an **obstruction** will eventually become **decompressed or airless,** as their contents are evacuated.
- In a mechanical obstruction, **the loop(s) that will become the most dilated** will either be the **loop of bowel with the largest resting diameter before the onset of the obstruction** (e.g., the **cecum** in the large bowel), or the **loop(s) of bowel just proximal to the obstruction.** The **transition point,** the **site** of obstruction and the location where the bowel changes in caliber from dilated to collapsed, will frequently be visible on CT.

- Most patients with a mechanical obstruction will present with some form of **abdominal pain**, **abdominal distension,** and **constipation.** Patients may present with **vomiting early** in the course of a **proximal small bowel obstruction** and **later** in the course of the illness if it is **a distal small bowel obstruction.**
- **Prolonged obstruction** with persistently elevated intraluminal pressures can lead to vascular compromise, **necrosis,** and **perforation** in the affected loop of bowel. At this point, bowel sounds may become **hypoactive** or **absent.**

BOX 15.1 Abnormal Bowel Gas Patterns

Functional Ileus
- Localized ileus (sentinel loops)
- Generalized adynamic ileus

Mechanical Obstruction
- Small bowel obstruction (SBO)
- Large bowel obstruction (LBO)

- We'll look at each of the four abnormal bowel gas patterns in detail (Table 15.1).
- For each of the four abnormal gas patterns, we will examine their **pathophysiology, causes, key imaging features,** and **diagnostic pitfalls.**

FUNCTIONAL ILEUS: LOCALIZED—SENTINEL LOOPS

- **Pathophysiology**
  - **Focal irritation** of a loop or loops of bowel **occurs most often from inflammation of an adjacent visceral organ** (e.g., pancreatitis may affect bowel loops in the left upper quadrant, diverticulitis in the left lower quadrant).
  - The **loop(s) affected** are almost always loops of **small bowel** and, because they **herald the presence of underlying pathology,** they are called *sentinel loops.*
  - The **irritation causes these loops to lose their normal function and become aperistaltic,** which in turn leads to **dilatation** of these loops.
  - Because a **functional ileus does not produce the degree of obstruction that a mechanical obstruction does,** some gas continues to pass through the defunctionalized bowel past the point of the localized ileus.
  - **Air** usually reaches and **is visible in the rectum or sigmoid** on conventional radiographs.
- **Causes of a localized ileus**
  - The **dilated loops of bowel tend to occur** in the **same anatomic area** as the **inflammatory or irritative process** of the adjacent abdominal organ, although this may not always be the case.
  - On conventional radiographs, the exact cause of the functional ileus can only be inferred by the location of the ileus. On CT scans of the abdomen, however, the **cause** of the localized ileus is frequently visible.

- Table 15.2 summarizes **sites of a localized ileus** and their **most common cause.**
- **Key imaging features of a localized ileus**
  - On conventional radiographs, there are **one or two** *persistently dilated* loops of small bowel.
    - *Persistently* means that these **same loops remain dilated** on **multiple views** of the abdomen (supine, prone, upright abdomen) or on **serial studies** done over the course of time.
    - *Dilated* means the small bowel loops are **persistently larger than 2.5 cm.** Small bowel loops involved in a **functional ileus** usually **do not dilate as greatly as** those that are **mechanically obstructed.**
  - Infrequently, the sentinel loop may be **large bowel,** rather than small bowel. This can especially occur in the **cecum,** with diseases such as appendicitis.
  - **Air-fluid levels are frequently** seen in **sentinel loops.**
  - There is usually **gas in the rectum or sigmoid** in a localized ileus (Fig. 15.1).

TABLE 15.2 Causes of a Localized Ileus

Site of Dilated Loops	Cause(s)
Right upper quadrant (RUQ)	Cholecystitis
Left upper quadrant (LUQ)	Pancreatitis
Right lower quadrant (RLQ)	Appendicitis
Left lower quadrant (LLQ)	Diverticulitis
Mid-abdomen	Ulcer or kidney/ureteral calculus

TABLE 15.1 Abnormal Gas Patterns: Summary

	Air in Rectum or Sigmoid	Air in Small Bowel	Air in Large Bowel
Normal	Yes	Yes, 1–2 loops	Rectum and/or sigmoid
Localized ileus	Yes	2–3 distended loops	Rectum and/or sigmoid
Generalized ileus	Yes	Multiple distended loops	Yes, distended
Small bowel obstruction (SBO)	No	Multiple dilated loops	No
Large bowel obstruction (LBO)	No	None, unless ileocecal valve incompetent	Yes, dilated

Fig. 15.1 Sentinel Loops From Pancreatitis. A single, persistently dilated loop of small bowel is seen in the left upper quadrant on both the supine (A) (*solid white arrow*) and prone (B) (*dotted white arrow*) radiographs of the abdomen representing a sentinel loop or **localized ileus.** A localized ileus is called a **sentinel loop** because it often signals the presence of an adjacent irritative or inflammatory process. This patient had acute pancreatitis.

⚠ DIAGNOSTIC PITFALLS

- **Differentiating a localized ileus from an early SBO**
  - A **localized ileus may resemble an** *early* **mechanical SBO** (i.e., there may be a few dilated loops of small bowel with air in the colon in both). *Early* means the **patient has had symptoms for a day or two.** Patients who have had obstructive symptoms for a week or more usually no longer demonstrate imaging findings of an "early" obstruction.
  - **Solution.** A combination of the clinical and laboratory findings and CT scanning of the abdomen that demonstrates the underlying pathology should differentiate localized ileus from small bowel obstruction (Fig. 15.2).

Fig. 15.2 Pancreatitis Producing Focal Bowel Dilatation. Although the cause of a sentinel loop can usually only be inferred from conventional radiographs, CT scans can depict the underlying abnormality producing the bowel irritation. In this contrast-enhanced, axial CT scan of the upper abdomen with oral contrast, the pancreas is inflamed, enlarged, and edematous (*white arrows*) and there is haziness of the peripancreatic fat. The inflammation can affect peristalsis in adjacent loops of small bowel (SB) and lead to dilatation of the loops.

FUNCTIONAL ILEUS: GENERALIZED ADYNAMIC ILEUS

- **Pathophysiology**
  - In a generalized adynamic ileus, the **entire bowel is aperistaltic or hypoperistaltic.** Swallowed **air dilates and fluid fills most loops of both small and large bowel.**
  - A **generalized adynamic ileus is almost always the result of abdominal or pelvic surgery** in which the bowel is manipulated during the surgery.
- **Causes of a generalized adynamic ileus** are summarized in Table 15.3.
- **Key imaging features of a generalized adynamic ileus**
  - The **entire bowel is usually air-containing and dilated,** both large and small bowel. The stomach may be dilated as well.
  - The absence of peristalsis and the continued production of intestinal secretions usually produce **many long air-fluid levels in the bowel.**
  - Because this is not a mechanical obstruction, there usually is **gas in the rectum or sigmoid. No transition point** is identified on CT of the abdomen.
  - **Bowel sounds are frequently absent or hypoactive** (Fig. 15.3).
- **Differentiating other causes of dilated bowel**
  - Patients do not present to the emergency department with a generalized adynamic ileus unless they are one or two days

TABLE 15.3 Causes of a Generalized Adynamic Ileus

Cause	Remarks
Postoperative	Usually abdominal surgery
Electrolyte imbalance	Especially diabetics in ketoacidosis

Fig. 15.3 Generalized Adynamic Ileus, Supine (A) and Upright Abdomen (B). There are dilated loops of large (*solid white arrows*) and small bowel (*dotted white arrow*) with gas down to and including the rectum (*solid black arrows*). The patient had absent bowel sounds and had undergone colon surgery the day before.

postoperative (abdominal or gynecologic surgery) or they have a severe electrolyte imbalance (e.g., hypokalemia).
- Many patients who have either **intestinal pseudo-obstruction** (see the end of this chapter) **or aerophagia** may be mistakenly thought to have a generalized ileus on abdominal radiographs.

MECHANICAL OBSTRUCTION: SMALL BOWEL OBSTRUCTION

- **Pathophysiology**
  - A lesion, either inside or outside of the small bowel, obstructs the lumen.

» IMPORTANT POINTS

- Over time, **from the point of obstruction backward,** the **small bowel dilates** from continuously swallowed air and from intestinal fluid that is still produced by the stomach, pancreatic, biliary systems, and small bowel.
- **Peristalsis continues and may increase** in an effort to overcome the obstruction.
  - This can lead to **high-pitched, hyperactive bowel sounds.**
- As time passes, the peristaltic waves **empty the small bowel along with the colon** of their contents **from the point of obstruction *forward*.**

- If the obstruction is **complete** and if enough time has elapsed since the onset of symptoms, **there is usually no air in the rectum or sigmoid.**
- **Causes of a mechanical small bowel obstruction** are summarized in Table 15.4.

TABLE 15.4 Causes of a Mechanical Small Bowel Obstruction

Cause	Remarks
Postsurgical adhesions	Most common cause of a small bowel obstruction; most frequent following appendectomy, colorectal surgery, and pelvic surgery; **transition point** on small bowel CT without other identifying cause
Malignancy	Primary malignancies of the small bowel are rare; secondary tumors, such as gastric and colonic carcinomas and ovarian cancers, may compromise the lumen of small bowel.
Hernia	An inguinal hernia may be visible on conventional radiographs if air-containing loops of bowel are seen over the obturator foramen; easily seen on CT (see Fig. 15.4).
Gallstone ileus	May be visible on conventional radiographs or CT if air is seen in the biliary tree and (rarely) a gallstone in RLQ **(see Chapter 16)**
Intussusception	Ileocolic intussusception, the most common form, produces SBO.
Inflammatory bowel disease	Thickening of the bowel wall may occur with compromise of the lumen in patients with Crohn disease; this is most likely to occur in the terminal ileum.

Fig. 15.4 Small Bowel Obstruction From Inguinal Hernia. (A) The scout image from a CT scan of the abdomen reveals dilated loops of small bowel (*solid black arrow*) caused by a left inguinal hernia (*white circle*). Loops of bowel should normally not be present in the scrotum. (B) Coronal-reformatted CT scan on another patient shows multiple fluid-filled and dilated loops of small bowel (*solid white arrows*) from an inguinal hernia (*white circle*) containing another dilated loop of small bowel (*dotted white arrow*).

- **Key imaging features of mechanical small bowel obstruction**
  - On conventional radiographs, **there are multiple dilated loops** (>2.5 cm) **of small bowel** proximal to the point of the obstruction.
    - As they begin to dilate, **small bowel loops** *stack-up* **on one another forming a** *step-ladder* **appearance**, usually beginning in the left upper quadrant and proceeding, depending on how distal the small bowel obstruction is, to the right lower quadrant (Fig. 15.5).
    - Generally speaking, **the more proximal the small bowel obstruction** (e.g., proximal jejunum), **the fewer the dilated loops** there will be; the **more distal the obstruction** (e.g., at the ileocecal valve), the **greater the number of dilated small bowel loops.**
  - On upright or decubitus radiographs, there will usually be **numerous air-fluid levels in the small bowel** proximal to the obstruction.
  - If enough time has elapsed to decompress and empty the bowel distal to the point of obstruction, **there will be little or no gas in the colon, especially the rectum.**

>> **IMPORTANT POINTS**

- In a mechanical small bowel obstruction there should always be a **disproportionate dilatation of small bowel compared with the collapsed large bowel** (Fig. 15.6).

- **The CT findings of a small bowel obstruction:**
  - **Fluid-filled and dilated loops of small bowel** (>2.5 cm in diameter) proximal to the point of obstruction.

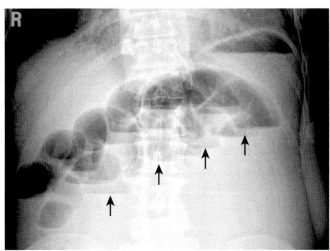

Fig. 15.5 "Step-Ladder" Appearance of Obstructed Small Bowel. This sign may be seen on upright, abdominal views of patients with a mechanical small bowel obstruction (SBO) caused by the arrangement of fluid-filled and dilated small bowel loops in a step-wise configuration following the locations of the jejunum in the left upper quadrant to the ileum in the right lower quadrant (*black arrows*). This was a distal SBO caused by a carcinoma of the colon that obstructed the ileocecal valve.

Fig. 15.6 Mechanical Small Bowel Obstruction. Although a small amount of air is seen in the right colon (*white arrow*), the **overall** bowel gas pattern is one of disproportionate dilation of multiple loops of small bowel (*black arrows*), which is consistent with a mechanical small bowel obstruction. The obstruction was secondary to adhesions.

! DIAGNOSTIC PITFALLS

- Differentiating a partial SBO from a functional (localized) adynamic ileus
  - An **intermittent,** (also known as a **partial** or **incomplete**) **mechanical small bowel obstruction** is one that **allows some gas to pass the point of obstruction**, at least at times, and can lead to a confusing picture because gas may pass into the colon long after the large bowel would be expected to be devoid of such gas. **Partial or incomplete small bowel obstruction** occurs **more often in patients** in whom **adhesions** are the etiology (Fig. 15.7).
  - CT with or without oral contrast should be able to demonstrate a partial small bowel obstruction or identify the abnormality producing sentinel loops (Fig. 15.8).

» IMPORTANT POINTS

- **CT is the most sensitive study** for diagnosing the site and cause of a mechanical small bowel obstruction.
  - CT scans for bowel obstruction can be performed with or without oral contrast, utilizing the fluid already present in the bowel as contrast. Orally administered contrast (either barium or iodinated contrast) may help in **identifying dilated loops** of bowel and in finding the **transition point** between the **proximal dilated** bowel and the **distal collapsed** bowel, but the oral contrast could also obscure important findings displayed by the use of intravenous contrast.
- **Intravenous contrast** is used to detect **complications** of bowel obstruction, such as **ischemia** and **strangulation**.

- Identification of a **transition point**, which is where the **bowel changes caliber** from **dilated to normal** indicating the site of the obstruction. In the absence of identifying a mass or other obstructive cause at the transition point, the cause is almost certainly adhesions (Fig. 15.9).

Fig. 15.8 Partial Small Bowel Obstruction. Coronal-reformatted CT scan with oral contrast shows dilated and contrast-containing loops of small bowel (*solid white arrows*). Although air is seen in the collapsed colon (*dotted white arrows*), the disproportionate dilatation of small bowel identifies this as a small bowel obstruction.

Fig. 15.9 Small Bowel Obstruction Caused by a Spigelian Hernia. A Spigelian hernia is one that occurs at the lateral edge of the rectus abdominis muscle at the semilunar line. This patient has a **transition point** (*solid white arrow*) as the small bowel enters the hernia (*dotted white arrow*). More proximally, there are multiple dilated loops of small bowel (*solid black arrows*) indicating obstruction. The colon lies beyond the point of obstruction and is collapsed (*dotted black arrow*).

Fig. 15.7 Partial Small Bowel Obstruction, Supine (A) and Upright (B). The important observation is that even though there is air in the large bowel (*solid black arrows*), the small bowel is disproportionately dilated in both views (*dotted white arrows*) compared with the large bowel, a finding suggestive of small bowel obstruction. Small bowel obstructions are more common in patients with adhesions from previous surgery, which the surgical clips (*white circles*) indicate happened in this patient.

- **Collapsed small bowel and/or colon distal to the point of obstruction** (Fig. 15.10)
- **Small-bowel feces sign.** Proximal to the transition point of a small bowel obstruction, intestinal debris and fluid may accumulate producing the appearance of fecal material in the small bowel. This is a sign of SBO (Fig. 15.11).

- **Closed-loop obstruction** occurs when **two points** of the **same loop** of bowel are **obstructed** at a **single location.** The closed loop usually remains dilated and may form a U- or C-shaped structure. Most closed-loop obstructions are caused by adhesions. In the small bowel, a closed-loop obstruction carries a higher risk of strangulation of the

Fig. 15.10 Small Bowel Obstruction: CT With Oral and Intravenous Contrast. There are multiple fluid- and contrast-filled, dilated loops of small bowel (*solid black arrows*) and a collapsed colon (*solid white arrows*), indicating a small bowel obstruction. Bowel wall enhancement or lack thereof may be obscured by oral contrast, a drawback to the use of oral contrast. Incidentally noted is a right renal cyst (*dotted black arrow*).

Fig. 15.11 Small Bowel Feces Sign. Air is mixed with debris and old oral contrast in a dilated loop of small bowel (*solid white arrows*). There are proximal fluid-containing, dilated loops of small bowel (*dotted white arrows*). The patient had a CT scan with oral contrast several days earlier for abdominal pain and returned for this noncontrast scan when symptoms persisted. Intestinal debris and fluid may accumulate in the loop found just proximal to a small bowel obstruction and present with this finding, which resembles fecal material in the colon.

bowel. In the large bowel, a closed-loop obstruction is called a *volvulus* (Fig. 15.12).

- **Strangulation.** Vascular compromise can be identified by circumferential thickening of the wall of the bowel with (frequently) absence of normal wall enhancement following intravenous contrast administration. There may be associated edema of the mesentery and ascites (Fig. 15.13).

Fig. 15.12 Closed-Loop Obstruction, CT Lower Abdomen. A loop of small bowel (CL) is obstructed twice at the same point of a twist (*solid white arrow*) producing a closed loop. No oral contrast enters the closed-loop, but is present in a more proximal loop of small bowel (*dotted white arrow*). Closed-loop obstructions are important because of their higher incidence of bowel necrosis from strangulation of the bowel.

Fig. 15.13 Bowel Necrosis: Contrast-Enhanced CT. A dilated loop of small bowel demonstrates faint, but normal enhancement of the wall (*white arrow*) on this coronal reformat of a contrast-enhanced CT, whereas more distal, dilated loops of small bowel show no wall enhancement (*black circle*). The lack of enhancement is an indication of vascular compromise of the distal loops with bowel necrosis.

MECHANICAL OBSTRUCTION: LARGE BOWEL OBSTRUCTION (LBO)

- **Pathophysiology**
  - A lesion, either inside or outside the colon, causes obstruction to the lumen.
  - Over time, from the point of obstruction *backward*, the **large bowel dilates** and the **cecum frequently attains the greatest diameter** even if the obstruction is as far away as the sigmoid colon.
  - The large bowel normally functions to reabsorb water, so there are **usually few or no air-fluid levels** in the obstructed colon.
  - As time passes, continuing peristaltic waves from the point of obstruction *forward* **empty the colon distal to the obstruction.**
  - **Usually little or no air is seen in the rectum in a mechanical large bowel obstruction.**
- **Causes of a mechanical large bowel obstruction** are summarized in Table 15.5
- **Key imaging features of a mechanical large bowel obstruction**
  - The **colon is dilated to the point of obstruction.**
    - Because there are a limited number of large bowel loops, they tend not to overlap (as do the loops of small bowel) so **it is sometimes possible to identify the site of obstruction** as the **last air-containing** segment of the colon (Fig. 15.14).
    - Regardless of the point of obstruction, the **cecum is often the most dilated** part of the colon. **When the cecum reaches a diameter above 12 to 15 cm, there is danger of cecal rupture.**
  - The **small bowel is not dilated** (unless the ileocecal valve becomes *incompetent* (see below) (Fig. 15.15).
  - Because it is distal to the point of obstruction, **the rectum usually contains little or no air.**
  - Because the large bowel functions to reabsorb water, **usually no (or very few) air-fluid levels are seen in the large bowel.**

TABLE 15.5	Causes of a Mechanical Large Bowel Obstruction	
Cause	**Remarks**
Tumor (carcinoma)	Most common cause of LBO; more frequently obstructs when it involves the left colon
Hernia	May be visible on conventional radiographs if air is seen over the obturator foramen
Volvulus	Either the sigmoid (more commonly) or cecum may twist on its axis and obstruct the colon and/or small bowel (Box 15.2)
Diverticulitis	Uncommon cause of colonic obstruction
Intussusception	Colocolic intussusception usually occurs because of a tumor acting as a lead point

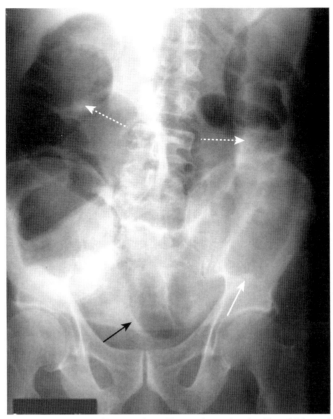

Fig. 15.14 Mechanical Large Bowel Obstruction. The entire colon is dilated (*dotted white arrows*) to a cut-off point in the distal descending colon (*solid white arrow*), the site of this patient's obstructing carcinoma of the colon. Some gas has passed backward through an incompetent ileocecal valve and outlines a dilated ileum (*solid black arrow*). Notice that the large bowel is disproportionately dilated compared with the small bowel, consistent with a large bowel obstruction.

Fig. 15.15 Large Bowel Obstruction: CT. Two CT images from the same patient demonstrate (A) dilated and fluid-filled loops of large bowel (*white arrows*). The orally administered contrast had not yet reached the large bowel at the time of this study, but does fill loops of small bowel. A large soft-tissue mass in the sigmoid (*dotted white arrow*) represents the patient's obstructing carcinoma of the sigmoid colon (B).

> ! **DIAGNOSTIC PITFALLS**

- **A large bowel obstruction can mimic a small bowel obstruction** if the intracolonic pressure rises high enough that the **ileocecal valve opens** (such a valve is called *incompetent*) and **gas from the dilated large bowel decompresses backward into the small bowel**, much like the air escaping from a balloon (Fig. 15.16).

- **Oral contrast containing barium is usually not administered to a patient with a suspected large bowel obstruction** because water will be absorbed from the barium when it reaches the obstructed colon, increasing the viscosity of the barium and possibly leading to impaction.
- **Recognizing a large bowel obstruction on CT**
  - CT is obtained to identify the cause of the obstruction, assess for free intraperitoneal air, and to identify associated lesions, such as metastases to the liver or lymph nodes if the obstruction is produced by a malignancy.
  - The large bowel is **dilated** to the **point of obstruction** (the **transition point**), then **normal** in caliber **distal** to the obstructing lesion.
  - The point of obstruction, frequently a carcinoma, can usually be located on CT as a **soft-tissue mass.** Hernias containing large bowel are also easy to identify on CT (Fig. 15.17).

VOLVULUS OF THE COLON

- Volvulus of the colon is a particular kind of large bowel obstruction that produces a striking and characteristic picture that is summarized in Box 15.2.

> **BOX 15.2 Volvulus: A Cause of Mechanical Large Bowel Obstruction**
>
> - Either the cecum or the sigmoid colon can twist upon itself producing a mechanical obstruction known as a *volvulus.*
> - Sigmoid volvulus is more common and tends to occur in older men.
> - The volvulated sigmoid assumes a massive size rising up from the pelvis with the wall between the twisted loops of sigmoid forming a line that points from the left lower to the right upper quadrant.
> - The appearance of the dilated sigmoid has been likened to a *coffee-bean* (Fig. 15.18).
> - When the **cecum** volvulates, it usually moves across the midline into the **left upper quadrant** producing loops of bowel forming a line that characteristically points from the right lower to the left upper quadrant.
> - Endoscopic decompression is the usual treatment for a sigmoid volvulus. Sigmoid colectomy may be used to reduce or prevent recurrent volvulus.

INTESTINAL PSEUDOOBSTRUCTION (OGILVIE SYNDROME)

- **Ogilvie syndrome (acute intestinal pseudoobstruction)** may occur in elderly individuals who are usually already hospitalized or at chronic bed rest.
  - Drugs with **anticholinergic effects, like antidepressants, phenothiazines, anti-Parkinsonian agents, and narcotics,** may cause or exacerbate the condition.

- The syndrome is characterized by a **loss of peristalsis,** resulting in sometimes **massive dilatation of the right colon or the entire colon resembling a large bowel obstruction** (Fig. 15.19).
  - Unlike a mechanical obstruction, **no obstructing lesion can be demonstrated** on CT or with barium enema. Unlike a generalized adynamic ileus, **patients have more marked abdominal distension** and bowel sounds may be **normal or hyperactive** in almost half of patients with Ogilvie syndrome.

> ⏩ **IMPORTANT POINTS**
>
> - The supine abdominal radiograph shows **marked bowel dilatation, almost always confined to the colon.**

- Management is **pharmacologic stimulation of colonic contractions,** usually with drugs such as neostigmine.

Fig. 15.16 Large Bowel Obstruction Masquerading as a Small Bowel Obstruction. There are air-filled and dilated loops of small bowel (*solid white arrows*) in this patient who actually had a mechanical large bowel obstruction from a carcinoma of the mid-descending colon. The pressure in the colon was sufficient to open the ileocecal valve, which then allowed much of the gas in the colon to decompress backward into the small bowel. The ascending and descending colon are dilated and still contain air (*dotted white arrows*), a clue that this is really a distal large bowel obstruction. Abdominal CT can resolve the question of whether the large or small bowel is obstructed.

Fig. 15.17 Large Bowel Obstruction From Carcinoma of the Colon. This coronal reformatted CT scan of the abdomen and pelvis shows a dilated cecum containing stool (*dotted white arrow*) and dilated large bowel **(LB)** to the level of the distal descending colon where a large soft-tissue mass is identified (*solid white arrow*). This mass was surgically removed; it was an adenocarcinoma of the colon.

Fig. 15.18 Sigmoid Volvulus, Supine Abdomen. A massively dilated sigmoid colon (*white arrows*) is twisted upon itself at some point in the pelvis. The dilated sigmoid has a **coffee-bean** shape (*white line*). Because the point of obstruction is in the distal colon, there is air and stool in the more proximal portion of the colon (*dotted white arrow*). Volvulus can produce massively dilated loops of sigmoid colon.

Fig. 15.19 Ogilvie Syndrome. This syndrome, which most often occurs in elderly and bedridden patients who are already severely ill, results in acute, massive dilatation of the colon, particularly the right colon and cecum, without mechanical obstruction. It can result in perforation and peritonitis and has a high overall mortality. Treatment may include a nasogastric tube, colonoscopic decompression, or pharmacologic stimulation of the bowel.

TAKE HOME POINTS

- Abnormal bowel gas patterns can be divided into two main groups: **functional ileus** and **mechanical obstruction.**
- There are two varieties of functional ileus: **localized** ileus (sentinel loops) and **generalized** adynamic ileus. There are two varieties of mechanical obstruction: **small bowel obstruction (SBO)** and **large bowel obstruction (LBO).**
- In **mechanical obstruction,** the gut reacts in predictable ways: loops proximal to the obstruction become dilated, peristalsis attempts to propel intestinal contents through the bowel and loops distal to the obstruction eventually are evacuated; the loop(s) that become the most dilated will either be the loop of bowel with the largest resting diameter or the loop(s) of bowel just proximal to the obstruction.
- The key findings of a **localized ileus** are two to three dilated loops of small bowel (**sentinel loops**) with air in the rectosigmoid and an underlying irritative process that frequently is adjacent to the dilated loops.
- Some causes of **sentinel loops** include pancreatitis (LUQ), cholecystitis (RUQ), diverticulitis (LLQ), and appendicitis (RLQ). All can be readily identified using ultrasound or CT.
- The key findings in a **generalized adynamic ileus** are dilated loops of large and small bowel with gas in the rectosigmoid and long, air-fluid levels. Postoperative patients develop generalized adynamic ileus.

- The key imaging findings in a **mechanical small bowel obstruction** are disproportionately dilated and fluid-filled loops of small bowel with little or no gas in the rectosigmoid. CT is best at identifying the cause and site of obstruction, or its complications.
- The most common cause of an SBO is **adhesions;** other causes include hernias, intussusception, gallstone ileus, malignancy, and inflammatory bowel disease, such as Crohn disease
- A **closed-loop obstruction** is one in which two points of the bowel are obstructed in the same location producing the "closed loop." In the small bowel, a closed-loop obstruction carries a higher risk of strangulation of the bowel. In the large bowel, a closed-loop obstruction is called a volvulus.
- The key imaging findings in **mechanical LBO** include dilatation of the colon to the point of the obstruction and absence of gas in the rectum with no dilatation of the small bowel as long as the ileocecal valve remains competent. CT will often demonstrate the cause of the obstruction.
- Causes of mechanical LBO include malignancy, hernia, diverticulitis, and intussusception.
- **Ogilvie syndrome** is characterized by a loss of peristalsis, resulting in sometimes massive dilatation of the entire colon resembling a large bowel obstruction, but without a demonstrable point of obstruction; it can sometimes be confused for a generalized adynamic ileus.

 More information on recognizing bowel obstruction and ileus is available to registered users online.

16

Recognizing Extraluminal Gas in the Abdomen

- Recognition of extraluminal gas is an important finding that can have an immediate effect on the course of treatment. Air is normally not present in the peritoneal or extraperitoneal spaces, bowel wall, or biliary system. **Air outside of the bowel lumen** is called *extraluminal air.* For the purposes of this text, the terms "air" and "gas" are used interchangeably.
- **The four most common locations of extraluminal air are:**
  - **Intraperitoneal (pneumoperitoneum)** (frequently called *free air*)
  - **Retroperitoneal air**
  - **Air in the bowel wall (pneumatosis intestinalis)**
  - **Air in the biliary system (pneumobilia)**

SIGNS OF FREE INTRAPERITONEAL AIR

> ### IMPORTANT POINTS
> - The **three major radiographic signs of free intraperitoneal air** are arranged below in the order in which they are most commonly seen:
>   - **Air beneath the diaphragm**
>   - **Visualization of both sides of the bowel wall**
>   - **Visualization of the falciform ligament**

Air Beneath the Diaphragm
- Free air will generally rise to the highest part of the abdomen. In the upright position, **free air** will usually reveal itself **under the diaphragm** as a **crescentic lucency** that parallels the undersurface of the diaphragm (Fig. 16.1).

Fig. 16.1 Free Air Beneath the Diaphragm. Thin crescents of air seen beneath both the right (*solid white arrow*) and left (*dotted white arrow*) hemidiaphragms represent free intraperitoneal air. The patient had undergone abdominal surgery 3 days earlier. Free air can remain for up to 7 days after surgery in an adult, but serial studies should demonstrate a progressively decreasing amount of air.

- The **size of the crescent** will be **roughly proportional to the amount of free air.** The smaller the amount of free air, the thinner the crescent; the larger the amount of free air, the larger the crescent (Fig. 16.2).
- **Although free air is best demonstrated on CT scans of the abdomen** because of its greater sensitivity in detecting very small amounts of free air (Fig. 16.3), most surveys of the

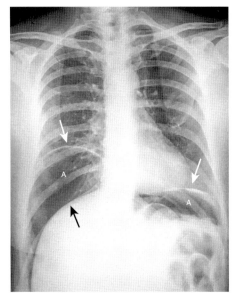

Fig. 16.2 Large Amount of Free Air. Upright view of the chest demonstrates a large amount of free air (A) beneath each hemidiaphragm (*white arrows*). The top of the liver (*black arrow*) is made visible by the air above it. The patient had a perforated gastric ulcer.

Fig. 16.3 Small Amount of Free Air, CT. Axial CT scan of the upper abdomen performed with the patient supine shows a very small collection of free air beneath the anterior abdominal wall (*solid white arrows*). Characteristically, free air has no surrounding bowel wall, as does air within bowel loops (*dotted white arrows*). This amount of free air was not visible on conventional radiographs.

abdomen begin with conventional radiographs. Conventional radiographs **serve as an important screening tool** on which many previously unsuspected cases of free air are discovered

>> **IMPORTANT POINTS**

- On conventional radiographs, **free air is best demonstrated with the x-ray beam directed parallel to the floor** (i.e., a horizontal beam) (see Figs. 13.14 and 13.15). **Small amounts of free air will not be visible on** radiographs in which the x-ray beam is directed vertically downward, such as a supine or prone views.

- Free air is **easier to recognize under the right hemidiaphragm** because that is normally the location of the liver, which is soft-tissue density. Free air is **more difficult to recognize under the left hemidiaphragm** because air-containing structures, such as the fundus of the **stomach** and the splenic flexure of the **colon**, already reside in that location, and they may mimic free air (Fig. 16.4).
- If the patient is unable to stand or sit upright, then a view of the abdomen with the patient lying on their left side (meaning the right side is pointing up) taken with a horizontal x-ray beam may show free air rising above the right edge of the liver (see Fig. 13.15). This is called a **left lateral decubitus view** of the abdomen (Fig. 16.5).

Fig. 16.4 Normal Left Hemidiaphragm (A) and Free Air Under Hemidiaphragm (B). (A) It is more difficult to detect free air in the left upper quadrant than the right because of the normal presence of air-containing structures such as the stomach (S) and splenic flexure (SF). (B) In another patient, there is a crescent of free air (*white arrows*) below the left hemidiaphragm and above the splenic flexure (SF).

Foot   Head

Fig. 16.5 Left Lateral Decubitus View: Free Air. Close-up of the right upper quadrant in a patient lying on their left side in the left lateral decubitus position shows a crescent of air (*dotted white arrows*) above the outer edge of the liver (*black arrow*), beneath the right hemidiaphragm (*solid white arrow*). The head/foot orientation of the patient is indicated.

> **! DIAGNOSTIC PITFALLS**
>
> - **Chilaiditi sign**
>   - Occasionally, normal colon may be interposed between the dome of the liver and the right hemidiaphragm and, unless a **careful search** is made **for the presence of haustral folds** characteristic of the colon, it may be mistaken for free air (Fig. 16.6). This normal interposition of the colon between the liver and right hemidiaphragm is called the **Chilaiditi sign (pronounced kyla-ditty).** If in doubt, obtain a left lateral decubitus view of the abdomen or, if necessary, a CT scan of the abdomen.

Visualization of Both Sides of the Bowel Wall

- In the **normal** abdominal radiograph, we visualize only the air **inside** the lumen of the bowel, **not the wall of the bowel itself.** This is because the wall is soft-tissue density and is normally surrounded by tissue of the same density.
- Introduction of **air into the peritoneal cavity enables us to visualize the wall of the bowel itself** because the wall is now surrounded on both inside and outside by air.

- The **ability to see both sides of the bowel wall is a sign of free intraperitoneal air** called the **Rigler sign** (Fig. 16.7).
- The Rigler sign can be seen on supine, upright, or prone films of the abdomen so long as there is a relatively large amount of free air present.

> **! DIAGNOSTIC PITFALLS**
>
> - When **dilated loops** of small bowel **overlap**, they may occasionally produce the mistaken impression that you are seeing both sides of the bowel wall (Fig. 16.8). If in doubt, confirm the presence of free air with an upright view, left lateral decubitus view, or CT scan of the abdomen.

Fig. 16.7 Rigler Sign. When a significant amount of air fills the peritoneal cavity, both sides of the bowel wall will be outlined by air, making the bowel walls visible as discrete lines (*solid white arrows*). This is known as the **Rigler sign** and indicates the presence of a pneumoperitoneum. Note that with free air the bowel wall is still visible in locations the loops of bowel **do not overlap** (*dotted white arrows*) (see Fig. 16.8). This patient was immediately postoperative abdominal surgery.

Fig. 16.6 Chilaiditi Sign. Close-up of the right hemidiaphragm on a conventional chest radiograph (A) and an axial CT scan at the level of the diaphragm (B) both demonstrate air beneath the diaphragm that could be confused for free air (*dotted black arrows in both photos*). Careful evaluation of this air demonstrates it contains several haustral folds (*solid black arrows* in [A] and *solid white arrows* in [B]) that indicate this is a loop of colon interposed between the liver and the diaphragm rather than free air.

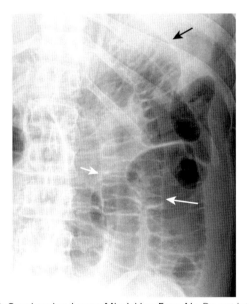

Fig. 16.8 Overlapping Loops Mimicking Free Air. Do not let overlapping loops of dilated small bowel (*white arrows*) fool you into thinking you are seeing both sides of the bowel wall because of free air. Notice that where the loops do not overlap, both sides of the bowel wall are not seen (*black arrow*). This has been called a **Pseudo-Rigler sign**.

Fig. 16.9 Falciform Ligament Sign. (A) Free intraperitoneal air surrounds the normally invisible falciform ligament on the anterior edge of the liver causing that thin, soft-tissue structure to become visible (*solid white arrows*) just to the right of the upper lumbar spine. Notice also that both sides of the stomach wall are visible (Rigler sign) (*dotted white arrow*) and there is increased lucency to the entire right upper quadrant (*solid black arrow*) in this patient with a large pneumoperitoneum from a perforated gastric ulcer. (B) On CT, the falciform ligament (*white arrow*) is outlined by free air (FA) on either side of it, anterior to the liver (L).

TABLE 16.1	Three Signs of Free Air
Sign	**Remarks**
Air beneath diaphragm	Requires patient to be in the upright or left lateral decubitus position and a horizontal x-ray beam, unless free air is massive in amount
Visualization of both sides of the bowel wall	Usually requires large amount of free air; will be visible in any position
Visualization of the falciform ligament	Usually requires large amounts of free air; best seen when patient is supine

Visualization of the Falciform Ligament

- The **falciform ligament** courses over the **free edge of the liver anteriorly** just to the **right of the upper lumbar spine**. It contains a remnant of the obliterated umbilical vein. **It is normally invisible**, composed of soft tissue and surrounded by tissue of similar density.
- When a (usually) large amount of free air is present and the **patient is in the supine position, free air** may rise over the anterior surface of the liver, **surrounding the falciform ligament** and **rendering it visible.** Visualization of the falciform ligament is aptly called the **falciform ligament sign** (Fig. 16.9).
- The linear appearance of the falciform ligament combined with the oval-shaped collection of free air that distends the abdomen has been likened to the appearance of a football with its laces and is is called the *football sign* (Fig. 16.10).
- Table 16.1 summarizes the **three major signs of free air** on conventional radiographs.

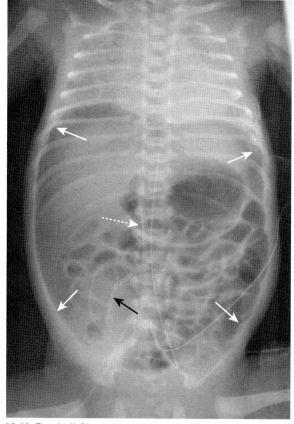

Fig. 16.10 Football Sign. A large amount of free air fills and distends the entire abdominal cavity (*solid white arrows*) with visibility of the falciform ligament (*dotted white arrow*) and both sides of bowel wall (*black arrow*) in this infant with pneumoperitoneum from necrotizing enterocolitis. The combination of the oval-shaped abdomen and the line of "laces" made by the falciform ligament led to this being named the **football sign.** This infant also has hyaline membrane disease of the lungs and two umbilical catheters in place.

Causes of Free Air

- The **most common cause of free intraperitoneal air is rupture of an air-containing loop of bowel,** either stomach, small or large bowel.

> ## ⏩ IMPORTANT POINTS
>
> - **Perforated peptic ulcer** is the most common cause of a perforated stomach or duodenum and is still the most common cause of free air.

- **Trauma,** whether accidental or iatrogenic, can also produce free air. **Free air following penetrating trauma** usually **implies a perforation of the bowel,** not free air generated simply by penetration of the abdominal wall itself.
- **For several days following abdominal surgery (≈5 to 7 days).** Whether the surgery had been performed on the bowel or not, **it is normal to see free air** on postoperative studies. The **amount** of free air following surgery **should diminish with each successive study.** A complication of the surgery or of the original disease should be considered **if free air persists for longer than a week** or if the amount **increases** on successive studies.
- **Perforated diverticulitis and perforated appendicitis** usually produce walled-off abscess collections around the site of the perforation and **rarely lead to significant amounts of free air.**
- **Perforation of a carcinoma,** usually of the colon, is unusual, but can also lead to free air.

SIGNS OF EXTRAPERITONEAL AIR (RETROPERITONEAL AIR)

- Unlike the collections of free intraperitoneal air that outline loops of bowel and usually move freely in the abdomen, **extraperitoneal air can be recognized** by:
    - **Streaky, linear appearance outlining extraperitoneal structures**
    - **Mottled, blotchy appearance** (anterior pararenal space, especially)
    - **Relatively fixed position, moving little** if at all **with changes in patient positioning**
- Extraperitoneal air may outline extraperitoneal structures such as:
    - **Psoas muscles**
    - **Kidneys, ureters, or urinary bladder**
    - **Aorta or inferior vena cava** (Fig. 16.11)
    - Inferior border of the diaphragm by collecting in the **subphrenic tissues**
- **Extraperitoneal air may extend through a diaphragmatic hiatus into the mediastinum** (and produce ***pneumomediastinum***) or **may extend to the peritoneal cavity**

Fig. 16.11 Extraperitoneal Air Seen on CT. Air is seen in the retroperitoneum (*solid black arrow*) on this axial CT scan of the upper abdomen. Air outlines the inferior vena cava (*solid white arrow*) and the aorta (*dotted white arrow*). Unlike free air, extraperitoneal air is streaky, relatively fixed in position, and outlines extraperitoneal structures.

TABLE 16.2   Signs of Extraperitoneal Air
• Streaky, linear collections of air that outline extraperitoneal structures
• Mottled, blotchy collections of air that remain in a fixed position

through openings in the peritoneum (and produce ***pneumoperitoneum***).
- Table 16.2 summarizes the signs of extraperitoneal air

Causes of Extraperitoneal Air

- **Extraperitoneal air is most frequently the result of bowel perforation** secondary to either:
    - **Inflammatory disease (e.g., ruptured appendix),** or
    - **Ulcerative disease (e.g., Crohn disease** of the ileum or colon)
- **Other causes of extraperitoneal air** include:
    - **Blunt or penetrating trauma**
    - **Iatrogenic manipulation** (e.g., perforation of the bowel during **sigmoidoscopy**)
    - **Foreign body** (e.g., perforation of extraperitoneal ascending colon by an ingested foreign body)
- **Gas-producing infection** originating in extraperitoneal organs (e.g., **perforated diverticulitis**)

SIGNS OF AIR IN THE BOWEL WALL

- Air in the bowel wall is called **pneumatosis intestinalis.**
- Air in the bowel wall is **most easily recognized** on abdominal radiographs **when it is seen in profile** producing a **linear**

radiolucency (black line) whose contour exactly parallels the bowel lumen (Fig. 16.12).

- **Air** in the bowel wall **seen *en face*** is **more difficult to recognize,** but frequently has a **mottled appearance that resembles gas mixed with fecal material** (Fig. 16.13).
  - Clues to help differentiate pneumatosis from fecal material include:
    - **Presence of such mottled gas in an area of the abdomen unlikely to contain colon**
    - **Lack of change** in the appearance of the mottled gas pattern over several images in **different positions**
- Table 16.3 summarizes the signs of air in the bowel wall.

TABLE 16.3 Signs of Air in the Bowel Wall

Sign	Remarks
Linear radiolucency paralleling the contour of air in the adjacent bowel lumen	Appearance when seen in profile
Mottled appearance that resembles air mixed with fecal material	Appearance when seen *en face*; may occur in an area of the abdomen not expected for colon; does not change over time
Globular, cyst-like collections of air that parallel the contour of the bowel	Unusual, benign condition affecting the colon, most often left colon

Fig. 16.12 Pneumatosis Seen in Profile. Close-up of the right lower quadrant in an infant demonstrates a thin curvilinear lucency that parallels the lumen of the adjacent bowel (*white arrows*), an appearance characteristic of gas in the bowel wall seen in profile. In infants, the most common cause for this finding is ***necrotizing enterocolitis,*** a disease found mostly in premature infants in which the terminal ileum is most affected **(see Chapter 28)**. Pneumatosis intestinalis is pathognomonic for necrotizing enterocolitis in infants.

Causes and Significance of Air in the Bowel Wall

- Pneumatosis intestinalis can be divided into two major categories.
  - A rare, **primary form called *pneumatosis cystoides intestinalis*** that usually **affects the left colon** producing **cyst-like collections of air in the submucosa or serosa** (Fig. 16.14).

Fig. 16.13 Pneumatosis Seen *En Face*. Close-up of the right lower quadrant in another infant shows multiple faint, mottled lucencies in the right lower quadrant, which is the appearance of pneumatosis intestinalis when seen *en face* (*white circle*). The density has the same appearance as air mixed with stool. This infant also had necrotizing enterocolitis.

Fig. 16.14 Pneumatosis Cystoides Intestinalis. Axial CT scan of the upper abdomen windowed for lung technique shows a cluster of air-containing cysts (*solid white arrows*) associated with the left colon, characteristic of ***pneumatosis cystoides intestinalis,*** a rare condition of unknown etiology. The cysts are usually subserosal or submucosal in location and the patient is often asymptomatic.

- A **more common, secondary form** that can occur in:
  - **Chronic obstructive pulmonary disease,** presumably secondary to air from ruptured blebs dissecting through the mediastinum to the abdomen
  - Diseases in which there is **necrosis of the bowel** wall such as:
    - **Necrotizing enterocolitis** in infants (see Figs. 16.12 and 16.13).
    - **Ischemic bowel disease** in adults (Fig. 16.15)
  - **Obstructing lesions of the bowel,** which raise intraluminal pressure such as:
    - **Hirschsprung disease or pyloric stenosis** in children
    - **Obstructing carcinomas** in adults

> ## ▶▶ IMPORTANT POINTS
>
> - **Pneumatosis intestinalis associated with** diseases that produce **necrosis of bowel** is usually **a more ominous prognostic sign** than pneumatosis associated with **obstructing lesions of the bowel** or chronic obstructive pulmonary disease.

- **Complications of pneumatosis intestinalis** can include:
  - **Rupture into the peritoneal cavity** leading to intraperitoneal free air **(pneumoperitoneum)**
  - Dissection of air into the portal venous system (Fig. 16.16)

SIGNS OF AIR IN THE BILIARY SYSTEM

- Air in the biliary system presents as **one or two tube-like, branching lucencies in the right upper quadrant overlying the central portion of the liver that conform to the location and appearance of the major bile ducts** (i.e., the common duct, cystic duct and/or the hepatic ducts) (Fig. 16.17).
- Table 16.4 summarizes the signs of **air in the biliary system.**

Fig. 16.16 Portal Venous Gas. (A) Numerous small black branching structures are visible over the periphery of the liver (*white circle*). This is air in the portal venous system, a finding most often associated with necrotizing enterocolitis in infants, but which can also be seen in adults, usually with bowel necrosis. Unlike air in the biliary system, this air is peripheral rather than central and has numerous branches rather than the few tubular structures seen with pneumobilia. (B) Close-up of axial CT scan through the liver shows air in the portal venous system (*white arrows*) in a patient with mesenteric vascular disease.

Fig. 16.17 Air in the Biliary Tree (Pneumobilia). Frontal view of the upper abdomen from an upper gastrointestinal series demonstrates several air-containing tubular structures over the central portion of the liver consistent with air in the biliary system (*white circle*). Also seen is barium that has entered the gallbladder from the bowel (*white arrow*). This patient had a history of a prior sphincterotomy for gallstones so that reflux of air and barium into the biliary system would be expected.

Fig. 16.15 Necrosis of Bowel from Mesenteric Ischemia. Axial CT image of the pelvis demonstrates multiple loops of bowel with curvilinear collections of air throughout their walls consistent with pneumatosis (*white arrows*). The patient had widespread ischemia of bowel from mesenteric vascular disease. Pneumatosis that results from bowel necrosis is an ominous sign.

TABLE 16.4   **Signs of Air in the Biliary Tract**
• Tube-like, branching lucencies in the right upper quadrant overlying the liver
• Tubular structures are central in location and few in number compared with portal venous gas, which is peripheral in location and fills innumerable vessels
• Air may be seen in the lumen of the gallbladder

Causes of Air in the Biliary System

- Gas in the biliary system **may be a "normal" finding** if the sphincter of Oddi, which guards the entrance of the common bile duct as it enters the duodenum, is open (said to be "incompetent").
- Prior **sphincterotomy,** such as might be done to allow gallstones to exit from the ductal system into the bowel
- **Prior surgery** that results in the **reimplantation of the common bile duct** into another part of the bowel (i.e., choledochoenterostomy) is frequently accompanied by the persistent presence of gas in the biliary ductal system.

- Pathologic conditions that can produce pneumobilia include **uncommon causes,** such as:
  - **Gallstone ileus,** in which a **gallstone erodes through the wall of the gallbladder** into the **duodenum** (usually) producing a **fistula between the bowel and the biliary system.** The **gallstone impacts in the small bowel,** most often in the narrower terminal ileum, and produces a mechanical obstruction (which has historically been called an "ileus" even though it is a mechanical obstruction) (Fig. 16.18).
  - **Gas-forming pyogenic cholangitis,** particularly from *Escherichia coli*

Fig. 16.18 Gallstone Ileus. The three key findings of gallstone ileus are present on this study. (A) Axial CT scan of the upper abdomen shows **air in the lumen of the gallbladder** (*black arrow*) and dilated small bowel (*white arrow*), which is consistent with a mechanical **small bowel obstruction.** (B) At a lower level, another axial CT scan of the abdomen shows a **large calcified gallstone** inside the small bowel (*dotted white arrow*) and additional proximal, dilated loops of small bowel (*solid white arrow*).

🏠 TAKE HOME POINTS

- Gas in the abdomen outside of the normal confines of the bowel is called **extraluminal air.**
- The four most common locations for extraluminal air are intraperitoneal (**pneumoperitoneum,** frequently called **free air**), retroperitoneal air, air in the bowel wall (pneumatosis), and air in the biliary system (pneumobilia).
- The three key signs of free air are air beneath the diaphragm, visualization of both sides of the bowel wall (**Rigler sign**), and visualization of the falciform ligament.
- The most common causes of free air are perforated peptic ulcer, trauma whether accidental or iatrogenic, perforated diverticulitis, and perforation of a carcinoma, usually of the colon.
- The key signs of **extraperitoneal (retroperitoneal) air** are a streaky, linear appearance or a mottled, blotchy appearance outlining extraperitoneal structures and its relatively fixed position, moving little or at all with changes in patient positioning.
- Extraperitoneal air outlines extraperitoneal structures, such as the psoas muscles, kidneys, aorta, and inferior vena cava.
- Causes of extraperitoneal air include bowel perforation secondary to either inflammatory or ulcerative disease, blunt or penetrating trauma, iatrogenic manipulation, and foreign body ingestion.
- The key signs of **air in the bowel wall** include linear radiolucencies paralleling the contour of air in the adjacent bowel lumen, a mottled appearance

- that resembles air mixed with fecal material or, uncommonly, globular, cyst-like collections of air that parallel the contour of the bowel.
- Causes of air in the bowel wall (**pneumatosis intestinalis**) include a rare primary form called **pneumatosis cystoides intestinalis.** A more common secondary form includes diseases in which there is **necrosis of the bowel** wall, such as necrotizing enterocolitis in infants; ischemic bowel disease in adults; and obstructing lesions of the bowel that raise intraluminal pressure, such as Hirschsprung disease in children and obstructing carcinomas in adults.
- Pneumatosis intestinalis associated with diseases that produce necrosis of bowel is usually a **more ominous** prognostic sign than pneumatosis associated with obstructing lesions of the bowel or chronic obstructive pulmonary disease.
- Signs of **air in the biliary system** include tube-like, branching lucencies in the right upper quadrant overlying the liver that are central in location and few in number and gas in the lumen of the gallbladder.
- Causes of pneumobilia include incompetence of the sphincter of Oddi, prior sphincterotomy, prior surgery that resulted in the reimplantation of the common bile duct into another part of the bowel, and gallstone ileus.
- The triad of findings in **gallstone ileus** are air in the biliary system, small bowel obstruction, and visualization of the gallstone itself.

📶 More information on recognizing extraluminal air in the abdomen is available to registered users online.

17

Recognizing Abnormal Calcifications and Their Causes

- Soft-tissue calcifications lend themselves to a systematic approach that ties together a diverse group of diseases. Although this chapter focuses primarily on abdominal calcifications, the same principles and approach apply to dystrophic calcification found anywhere in the body.
- Most soft-tissue calcification occurs in tissue that is already abnormal. Such calcification is called ***dystrophic calcification.***
- The **nature of most calcifications can be determined by examining two of their characteristics:**
  - Their **pattern of calcification**
  - Their **anatomic location**
    - CT can easily identify the location of such calcifications.

PATTERNS OF CALCIFICATION

> ### ▶▶ IMPORTANT POINTS
>
> - Calcifications **tend to occur in one of four distinct patterns,** depending on the type of structure that has calcified.
> - The patterns are:
>   - **Rim-like**
>   - **Linear or track-like**
>   - **Lamellar (or laminar)**
>   - **Cloud-like, amorphous, or popcorn**

Rim-Like Calcification

- Rim-like calcification implies calcification that has occurred **in the wall of a hollow viscus.** A "hollow viscus" in this context means a structure containing fluid, fat, or air and is enclosed by an outer wall.
- Examples of structures that manifest rim-like calcifications include:
  - **Cysts:** calcification in any one of the following is relatively uncommon.
    - **Renal cysts**
    - **Splenic cysts**
    - And **extraabdominal sites,** such as:
      - Mediastinal cysts, such as pericardial and bronchial cysts (Fig. 17.1)
      - Popliteal cysts
  - **Aneurysms**
    - **Aortic aneurysms**
      - These can sometimes be recognized on radiographs of the lumbar spine, especially in the lateral projection.
      - The abdominal aorta should **normally** measure less than **3 cm in diameter**, a measurement that usually requires both opposing walls be visible (Fig. 17.2).

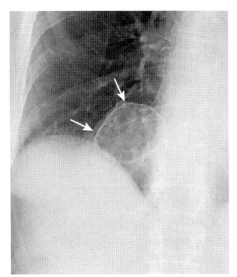

Fig. 17.1 Calcified Pericardial Cyst. A rim-like calcification (*white arrows*) identifies the structure containing the calcification as cystic or saccular. The calcification's location is ideal for a pericardial cyst. Pericardial cysts almost always occur on the right side and are usually asymptomatic, discovered when a chest radiograph is obtained for another reason.

Fig. 17.2 Calcified Aortic Aneurysm. Calcification in the wall of the abdominal aorta is a common finding in atherosclerosis, especially in those with diabetes mellitus. In this patient, the aorta demonstrates a rim-like calcification (*white arrows*). The opposite wall is also calcified, but overlaps the spine which is why aortic calcifications are usually easier to identify on lateral abdominal radiographs. When the diameter of the abdominal aorta exceeds its normal diameter by more than 50%, an aneurysm is present.

- **Splenic artery** or **renal artery** aneurysms
- And **extraabdominal sites** like:
  - Femoral artery aneurysms
  - Cerebral aneurysms
- **Saccular organs,** such as the gallbladder or urinary bladder
  - **Porcelain gallbladder**
    - This uncommon entity (named after the porcelain-like gross appearance of the gallbladder) that occurs with **chronic inflammation** and **stasis** of the gallbladder is associated with **gallstones** in over 90% of cases. It may possibly be associated with an increased incidence of carcinoma of the gallbladder (Fig. 17.3).
  - **Urinary bladder**
    - Calcification of the bladder wall is an uncommon occurrence in diseases such as **schistosomiasis, bladder cancer,** and **tuberculosis.**
- Table 17.1 highlights key facts about rim-like calcifications.

Linear or Track-Like Calcification

- Linear or track-like calcification implies **calcification that has occurred in the walls of tubular structures** (Fig. 17.4).
- Examples include calcifications in the walls of:
  - **Arteries**
    - **Common in atherosclerosis** and can be seen anywhere in the body
  - **Walls of veins do not calcify.**
    - In veins, **long, linear thrombi or small, focal thrombi** (the latter called *phleboliths*) may calcify (see Fig. 13.18).
  - **Tubular structures**
    - **Fallopian tubes and vas deferens**
      - Seen more often in diabetics (Fig. 17.5)

TABLE 17.1	Rim-Like Calcifications
Organ of Origin	**Remarks**
Renal cyst	Thick and irregular calcifications, although uncommon, may indicate the presence of renal cell carcinoma
Splenic cysts	May be a manifestation of hydatid cyst, old trauma, or prior infection
Aortic aneurysms	Occurs more often in diabetics with advanced atherosclerosis
Gallbladder	Associated with chronic stasis; called *porcelain gallbladder* for its gross appearance; possible slightly higher incidence of carcinoma of the gallbladder

Fig. 17.4 Calcified Arterial Wall. A linear or track-like calcification present in the thigh (*black arrows*) implies calcification that has occurred in the walls of tubular structures. In this location, this is calcification of the femoral artery. Such wall calcification occurs in arteries, not veins, and is usually secondary to atherosclerosis, frequently associated with diabetes, or in patients with chronic renal disease. This patient obviously suffered one of the complications of diabetes and has had an above-the-knee amputation (*white arrow*) of a previously gangrenous leg.

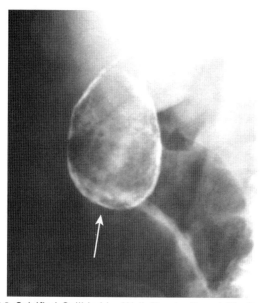

Fig. 17.3 Calcified Gallbladder Wall. The rim-like calcification (*white arrow*) identifies this as one that occurs in the wall of a cyst or saccular organ. The calcification is in the right upper quadrant, the location of the gallbladder. This is a ***porcelain gallbladder***, so-named because of its bluish color and brittle nature at the time of surgery.

Fig. 17.5 Calcification of the Vas Deferens. This male patient manifests two, track-like calcifications (*black arrows*) symmetrically located on each side of the urinary bladder that end in the urethra. The type of calcification identifies it as occurring in the wall of a tubular structure. The location identifies it as calcification in the walls of the vas deferens, which occurs more commonly and earlier in diabetics than as a natural, degenerative process.

- **Ureter**
  - Uncommon finding seen in schistosomiasis and even more rarely in tuberculosis (TB)
- Table 17.2 highlights key facts about linear or track-like calcifications.

Lamellar or Laminar Calcification

- Lamellar (or laminar) calcification implies calcification that **forms around a nidus inside a hollow lumen.** A "hollow lumen" refers to a structure such as the gallbladder or urinary bladder, which contains a fluid.

> ### ⟫ IMPORTANT POINTS
>
> - **Calcification in concentric layers** begins with a central nidus around which alternating layers of calcified and noncalcified material form because of the prolonged movement of the stone within the hollow viscus (Fig. 17.6).

- Lamellar or laminated calcifications are usually called **stones** or **calculi** (singular: calculus) and include:
  - **Renal calculi**

TABLE 17.2   Linear or Track-Like Calcifications

Organ of Origin	Remarks
Walls of smaller arteries	Mostly seen in atherosclerosis accelerated by diabetes and renal disease
Fallopian tubes or vas deferens	Usually accelerated by diabetes
Ureters	Uncommon occurrence described with schistosomiasis and, rarely, tuberculosis

- CT is the study of choice for the detection of renal and ureteral calculi.
- Conventional radiographs are only about 50% to 60% sensitive for displaying renal calculi despite the fact that about 90% of renal calculi contain calcium (Fig. 17.7).

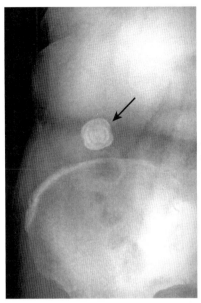

Fig. 17.6 Gallstone With Lamellated Calcification. A lamellated calcification is seen in the right upper quadrant (*black arrow*). The alternating bands of calcium and less-dense material identify it as a calculus that has formed in a viscus in this region. The anatomic location places it in the region of the gallbladder. Ultrasound is the most accurate imaging modality to detect gallstones.

Fig. 17.7 Renal Calculus: Conventional Radiograph and Axial CT Scan. (A) A calcification (*white arrow*) overlies the shadow of the left kidney (*black arrow*). Although it is too small for recognition of lamination, its location suggests a renal calculus. (B) In a different patient, an image from an unenhanced axial CT called a "stone search" reveals a large calcification in the proximal right ureter (*black arrow*) and several smaller calcifications in the left intrarenal collecting system (*white arrow*). Because of its greater sensitivity, a CT stone search done without intravenous contrast has mostly replaced conventional radiography for the identification of renal and ureteral calculi.

- **Gallstones**
  - **Ultrasound** is the study of choice for the detection of gallstones.
  - Only about 10% to 15% of gallstones contain enough calcification to be visible on conventional radiographs (Fig. 17.8).

- **Bladder stones**
  - Bladder stones usually develop secondary to **chronic bladder outlet obstruction**; they are very susceptible to developing lamination. (Fig. 17.9).
- Table 17.3 highlights key facts about laminated or lamellar calcifications.

Fig. 17.8 Gallstones: Conventional Radiographs and Axial CT Scan. (A) Multiple lamellar calcifications (*white circle*) have interlocking edges, suggesting that they all formed in a hollow viscus in proximity to each other. These are called ***faceted stones*** for their characteristic shapes. (B) In a different patient, a close-up view of an unenhanced axial CT scan of the right upper quadrant shows several gallstones (*white arrow*), two of which clearly have a central nidus surrounded by laminated, concentric rings of noncalcified and calcified material. The gallbladder (*black arrow*) contains bile fats and is less dense than the adjacent liver.

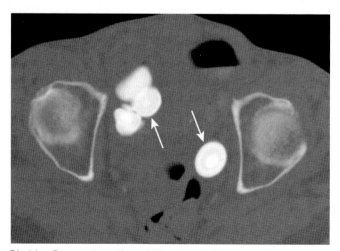

Fig. 17.9 Urinary Bladder Stones. Lamellar calcifications (*white arrows*) are seen on this axial CT scan through the level of the pelvis and windowed to show the laminations better. The laminations imply that these calcifications have formed inside of a hollow viscus. The anatomic location of these calculi places them in the urinary bladder.

TABLE 17.3 Laminar or Lamellated Calcifications

Organ of Origin	Remarks
Kidney	Most calcified renal stones are composed of calcium oxalate crystals; mostly form because of stasis, infection
Gallbladder	Most calcified gallstones are calcium bilirubinate; form because of chronic infection and stasis
Urinary bladder	Most bladder calculi contain urate crystals; form most often from outlet obstruction

Cloud-Like, Amorphous, or "Popcorn" Calcification

- Cloud-like, amorphous, or popcorn calcification is a calcification that has **formed inside of a solid organ or tumor** and examples include:

- **Body of the pancreas**
  - Pathognomonic for chronic pancreatitis (Fig. 17.10)
- **Leiomyomas of uterus**
  - Uterine fibroids or leiomyomas very commonly degenerate and calcify over time (Fig. 17.11).

Fig. 17.10 Chronic Calcific Pancreatitis: Conventional Radiograph and Axial CT Scan. (A) A close-up view of the upper abdomen on a conventional radiograph shows amorphous calcifications (*black arrows*) implying calcification in a solid organ or tumor. The anatomic distribution of the calcification corresponds to the location of the pancreas. (B) In another patient, a nonenhanced image of the upper abdomen shows calcifications distributed along the course of the body and tail of the pancreas (*white arrows*). There is oral contrast in the stomach (S). These calcifications are pathognomonic of chronic pancreatitis, an irreversible disease occurring mostly secondary to alcoholism that leads to atrophy of the gland and diabetes.

Fig. 17.11 Calcified Uterine Leiomyoma (Fibroid) on Conventional Radiograph and CT. (A) There is an amorphous or "popcorn" calcification (*white arrow*) in the pelvis of this 48-year-old female patient. The type of calcification suggests formation in a solid organ or tumor. This is the anatomic location and the classical appearance of calcified uterine leiomyomas (fibroids). (B) CT on another patient shows large uterine fibroids (*solid white arrows*), portions of which have necrosed (*solid black arrows*) and calcified (*dotted white arrow*). Ultrasound is the study of choice in diagnosing uterine fibroids.

! **DIAGNOSTIC PITFALLS**

- Sometimes a **solid tumor will outgrow its blood supply and the center of the tumor will undergo necrosis** leaving only a viable "outer shell." The subsequent calcification will be **more rim-like than amorphous.** Uterine fibroids are especially likely to have this appearance (Fig. 17.12).

- **Lymph nodes**
  - Can calcify anywhere in the body, mostly from prior granulomatous infection, such as old TB (**see Fig. 11.15A**).
- **Kidneys**
  - **Medullary nephrocalcinosis** is macroscopic calcification deposited in the pyramids of the renal medulla, usually secondary to a metabolic derangement such as hyperparathyroidism (Fig. 17.13)
  - **Mucin-producing adenocarcinomas** of the stomach, ovary, and colon may calcify in both their primary tumors and in metastatic deposits (Fig. 17.14).
  - And, outside of the abdomen, in structures like:
    - **Meningiomas** (see Fig. 27.29).
- Table 17.4 highlights key facts about amorphous, cloud-like, or popcorn calcifications.
- Table 17.5 summarizes the key findings of the four patterns of abnormal calcification.

▶▶ **IMPORTANT POINTS**

- **No matter what its cause, the presence of calcification implies a process that is subacute or chronic.**

Fig. 17.13 Medullary Nephrocalcinosis (Hypercalcemic Nephropathy). Cloud-like calcifications are seen bilaterally (*white arrows*), suggesting these calcifications have formed within a solid organ or tumor. The calcifications conform to the anatomic locations of the renal collecting systems. This is medullary nephrocalcinosis, a condition associated with hypercalcemia. This patient had primary hyperparathyroidism, the most common cause of nephrocalcinosis in adults.

Fig. 17.12 Calcified Rim in Uterine Leiomyoma. This is a rim-like calcification (*black arrows*) in the pelvis of a female patient so that it would be appropriate to consider that this calcification formed in the wall of a hollow viscus or saccular structure, such as a cyst. In fact, this is a characteristic pattern of calcification in the outer wall of a degenerated uterine leiomyoma (fibroid). It is a rim-like calcification, but the structure in which it originally formed was solid. Cystic lesions of the ovary might produce a similar appearance and ultrasound of the pelvis would be the study of choice to identify the organ of origin.

Fig. 17.14 Calcified Ovarian Metastases. An unenhanced axial CT scan of the upper abdomen shows multiple amorphous calcifications, some within the liver (*white arrows*) and others that stud the peritoneal surface of the abdomen (*black arrows*). This patient had a mucin-producing adenocarcinoma of the ovary that had metastasized to the peritoneum and liver. Mucin-producing tumors of the stomach and colon can also produce calcified metastases, but ovarian malignancy would be the most common to metastasize to the peritoneum. There is oral contrast in the stomach (S).

TABLE 17.4   Amorphous, Cloud-Like, or Popcorn Calcifications

Organ of Origin	Remarks
Pancreas	Chronic pancreatitis, frequently secondary to alcoholism
Uterine fibroids (leiomyomas)	Degenerating fibroids calcify
Mucin-producing tumors	Mucin-producing tumors of the ovary, stomach, or colon may calcify as can their metastases
Meningioma	Benign, extra-axial brain tumor of older individuals that calcifies about 20% of the time

TABLE 17.5   Identifying the Four Types of Abnormal Calcification

Type of Calcification	Implies	Examples
Rim-like	Formed in wall of hollow viscus	Cysts, aneurysms, gallbladder wall
Linear or track-like	Formed in walls of tubular structures	Ureters, arteries
Lamellar or laminar	Formed in stones	Renal, gallbladder, and bladder calculi
Amorphous, cloud-like, popcorn	Formed in a solid organ or tumor	Uterine fibroids; some mucin-producing tumors

LOCATION OF CALCIFICATION

- Identifying the **pattern** of calcification helps in identifying its **type.**
- Identifying the anatomic **location** of the calcification helps to identify its **organ or tissue of origin.**

TABLE 17.6   Location, Location, Location

Anatomic Quadrant in the Abdomen	Pattern of Calcification	Possible Organ of Origin	Cause
RUQ	Rim-like	Gallbladder wall	Chronic infection
	Track-like	Hepatic artery	Atherosclerosis
	Laminated	Gallbladder	Gallstones
	Amorphous	Head of pancreas	Chronic pancreatitis
LUQ	Rim-like	Splenic cyst	Amebic infection
	Track-like	Splenic artery	Atherosclerosis
	Laminated	Kidney	Renal stone
	Amorphous	Tail of pancreas	Chronic pancreatitis
RLQ	Rim-like	Iliac artery	Iliac artery aneurysm
	Track-like	Iliac artery	Atherosclerosis
	Laminated	Appendix	Appendicolith
	Amorphous	Uterus	Fibroids
LLQ	Rim-like	Iliac artery	Iliac artery aneurysm
	Track-like	Iliac artery	Atherosclerosis
	Laminated		
	Amorphous	Uterus or ovaries	Ovarian tumor

LLQ, Left lower quadrant; *LUQ,* left upper quadrant; *RLQ,* right lower quadrant; *RUQ,* right upper quadrant.

- Combining the **type** of calcification with its **anatomic location** should provide the key to the **cause** of most pathologic calcifications.
- Table 17.6 summarizes some of the possible locations of calcification in the abdomen.

🏠 TAKE HOME POINTS

- Soft-tissue calcifications can be characterized by the pattern of their calcification and their anatomic location.
- There are four distinct patterns: (1) rim-like, (2) linear or track-like, (3) lamellar (or laminar), and (4) cloud-like, amorphous, or popcorn.
- **Rim-like calcifications** imply calcification that has occurred in the wall of a hollow viscus (i.e., a saccular structure containing fluid).
- Examples of rim-like calcifications include the walls of cysts, aneurysms, or saccular organs, such as the gallbladder.
- **Linear or track-like calcifications** imply calcification that has occurred in the walls of tubular structures.
- Examples of track-like calcifications include the walls of arteries and tubular structures, such as the ureters, fallopian tubes, and vas deferens.
- **Lamellar (or laminar) calcifications** imply calcification that forms around a nidus inside a hollow (usually fluid-containing) lumen.
- Examples of lamellar calcifications include renal calculi, gallstones, and bladder stones.
- **Cloud-like, amorphous, or popcorn calcification** is calcification that has formed inside a solid organ or tumor.
- Examples of amorphous or popcorn calcifications include pancreatitis, leiomyomas of the uterus, old inflammatory disease in lymph nodes, and mucin-producing adenocarcinomas.
- Combining the type of calcification with its anatomic location should provide the key to the causes of most pathologic calcifications. CT scans will demonstrate the anatomic location easily.

 More information on recognizing abnormal calcifications and their causes is available to registered users online.

18

Recognizing Gastrointestinal, Hepatobiliary, and Urinary Tract Abnormalities

- In this chapter, you will learn how to recognize some of the most common abnormalities in the abdomen. We will also discuss selected hepatic abnormalities. Chapter 19, on ultrasound, describes some of the more common biliary and pelvic abnormalities.

BARIUM STUDIES OF THE GASTROINTESTINAL TRACT

- CT, ultrasound, and MRI have essentially replaced conventional radiography and, in many instances, barium studies for the evaluation of the gastrointestinal (GI) tract and the visceral abdominal organs.
- To review some of the terminology used for fluoroscopic studies of the GI tract, see the online glossary.

ESOPHAGUS

- Single and/or double-contrast examinations of the esophagus are performed with the patient drinking liquid barium, either by itself (**single contrast**) or accompanied by a gas-producing agent that provides the "air" in a **double-contrast examination.** Because both the single and double-contrast techniques have their own strengths, many esophagrams are routinely performed with **both** techniques, called a **biphasic examination.**
- **Video esophagography (video swallowing function)** is a study of the **swallowing mechanism,** usually performed with fluoroscopy and frequently captured dynamically either digitally, on videotape, or on film. This is the study of choice for diagnosing and documenting **aspiration,** in which ingested substances pass into the trachea below the level of the vocal cords (Fig. 18.1). (eVideo 18.1).
- **Fluoroscopic observation** of the esophagus can also **reveal abnormalities in esophageal motility.** For example, **tertiary waves** are a common but nonspecific abnormality of esophageal motility, representing disordered and nonpropulsive contractions of the esophagus. They can be observed fluoroscopically and captured on spot films (eVideo 18.2).

Esophageal Carcinoma

- Esophageal carcinoma continues to have a very **poor prognosis** as more than **50% of patients will have metastases on** initial presentation. The **lack of an esophageal serosa** and a **rich supply of lymphatics** aid in the extension and dissemination of esophageal carcinoma. Long-term alcohol and tobacco use are associated with a higher risk of esophageal carcinoma.
- Esophageal malignancies are either **squamous cell carcinomas** or **adenocarcinomas,** the latter of which is **increasing in prevalence. Adenocarcinomas** arise in esophageal epithelium that has undergone metaplasia from **squamous to columnar epithelium** (Barrett esophagus), a process in which **gastroesophageal reflux (GERD) plays a major role.**
- Barium esophagrams are **frequently the initial study** in patients with symptoms, such as dysphagia, which suggest this diagnosis.
- Esophageal carcinomas may **appear in one or more of several forms** (Fig. 18.2). Most often, they present as a mixture of several of these patterns.

Fig. 18.1 Aspiration. Barium, which was aspirated into the trachea at the start of an upper gastrointestinal series, outlines the bronchial tree in both lower lobes (*white arrows*). Barium is inert and did not cause any additional symptoms the patient was not already experiencing from aspirating his own secretions. It took some time, but almost all of this barium was reabsorbed with only a small amount remaining.

Fig. 18.2 Esophageal Carcinomas. Three different patients' barium esophagrams are shown with different appearances of esophageal carcinoma. (A) There is an **annular constricting** lesion of the mid-esophagus (*dotted black arrow*). The tumor encircles the normal lumen and almost completely obstructs it, in this case. (B) A **polypoid mass** arises from the right lateral wall of the esophagus and displaces the barium around it (*solid black arrow*). (C) This carcinoma appears more superficial, making the wall contour **irregular** and **rigid** (*dotted white arrow*). It contains a small **ulceration** (*solid white arrow*). Note that throughout this chapter, barium may be depicted as either white or black.

Hiatal Hernia and Gastroesophageal Reflux (GERD)

- Hiatal hernias are divided into the **sliding type** (almost all) in which the **esophagogastric junction lies above the diaphragm** or the **paraesophageal type (1%)** in which a **portion of the stomach herniates through the esophageal hiatus, but the esophagogastric junction remains below the diaphragm.** In general, hiatal hernia increases in incidence with age.
- **Most hiatal hernias are asymptomatic,** but there is an association between the presence of some hiatal hernias and clinically significant **gastroesophageal reflux.**
  - Gastroesophageal reflux also occurs in patients without any visible hiatal hernia, usually because of some dysfunction of the lower esophageal sphincter that normally acts to prevent gastric acid from repeatedly refluxing into the esophagus.

Fig. 18.3 Hiatal Hernia. The stomach (S) extends above the level of the diaphragm (*white line*) as a hiatal hernia (HH). Gastric folds are seen radiating from the stomach into the hernia. Notice that the esophagus does not narrow as it normally does when passing through the esophageal hiatus. A **Schatzki ring,** (*solid white arrow*) marks the position of the esophagogastric junction so that its appearance above the diaphragm automatically indicates the presence of a sliding hiatal hernia.

▶▶ IMPORTANT POINTS

- **The radiologic findings of hiatal hernia include:**
  - **A bulbous area** of the distal esophagus containing oral contrast at the level of the diaphragm with **failure of the esophagus to narrow** on multiple images **as it passes through the esophageal hiatus** of the diaphragm
  - **Extension of multiple gastric folds above the diaphragm**
  - Sometimes, visualization of a thin, circumferential filling defect in the distal esophagus called a **Schatzki Ring** (Fig. 18.3)

- **Gastroesophageal reflux may be evident during fluoroscopy** when barium is seen to move from the stomach retrograde into the esophagus, but reflux is intermittent so that it may not occur during the course of the examination. The absence of reflux during the study **does not exclude reflux** and demonstration of reflux **does not necessarily indicate the patient has the complications of GERD (i.e., esophagitis, stricture, and Barrett esophagus).**

STOMACH AND DUODENUM

- Today, the lumen of the stomach is most often studied by upper endoscopy and the wall thickness and structures outside of the stomach are studied by CT examination of the abdomen with oral contrast. Nevertheless, biphasic upper gastrointestinal (UGI) examinations, which include a study of the esophagus, stomach, and duodenum, remain a sensitive, cost-effective, readily available and noninvasive examination.

Gastric Ulcers

- In the United States, the incidence of **gastric ulcer disease has been declining.** In adults, infection with *Helicobacter pylori* accounts for almost three out of four cases of gastric ulcer disease. **Nonsteroidal anti-inflammatory agents** account for most of the rest.

> **IMPORTANT POINTS**
>
> - Most ulcers occur on the **lesser curvature** or **posterior wall** in the region of the **body or antrum.** About **95% of all gastric ulcers are benign.** The other **5% will represent ulcerations in gastric malignancies** (Fig. 18.4).

Gastric Carcinoma

- There has been a dramatic **decline in the incidence of gastric carcinoma in the United States.** The **mortality, however,** remains quite high as gastric carcinomas are frequently not diagnosed until after they have spread. Most gastric carcinomas (actually, they are adenocarcinomas) **occur in the distal third of the stomach** along the **lesser curvature.**

- Double-contrast UGI images and CT scans of the abdomen can demonstrate gastric carcinomas. CT is used for staging the extent of the tumor and degree of spread.
- Gastric carcinomas may be **polypoid, infiltrating** (i.e., **linitis plastica), or ulcerative,** in form (Fig. 18.5).
- Other mass lesions may resemble gastric carcinoma, including **leiomyomas,** a benign, wall lesion that characteristically ulcerates, and **lymphoma,** which may produce diffusely thickened folds or multiple masses in the stomach.

Duodenal Ulcers

> **IMPORTANT POINTS**
>
> - **Duodenal ulcers are two to three times more common than gastric ulcers.** Almost all duodenal ulcers occur in the **duodenal bulb,** the majority on the **anterior wall** of the bulb. They are **overwhelmingly caused by *H. pylori* infection (85% to 95%).**

- A double-contrast UGI series has a sensitivity that exceeds 90% in detecting duodenal ulcers (Fig. 18.6).
- **Complications** of duodenal ulcers, best demonstrated by CT, include **obstruction, perforation** (into the peritoneal cavity), **penetration** (e.g., into the pancreas), or **hemorrhage** (Fig. 18.7).

SMALL AND LARGE BOWEL

General Considerations

- Opacification and distension of the bowel lumen is necessary for proper evaluation of the bowel no matter what modality is used.

Fig. 18.4 Benign Lesser Curvature Gastric Ulcer. Note that the barium is depicted as black in these images. (A) Seen in profile is a large collection of barium that protrudes beyond the expected contour of the normal body of the stomach along the lesser curvature representing a gastric ulcer (*solid white arrow*). A mound of edematous tissue, called an **ulcer collar**, surrounds the ulcer (*dotted white arrow*). (B) Seen *en face*, are numerous gastric folds (*dashed white arrow*) that radiate to the ulcer margin as well as a central collection (*black arrow*) representing the ulcer itself. This was a benign gastric ulcer.

Fig. 18.5 Carcinomas of the Stomach. (A) A large, polypoid and ulcerating filling defect in the antrum of the stomach displaces the barium around it (*solid black arrows*). This was an adenocarcinoma of the stomach. (B) The entire body of the stomach displays a lack of distensibility, losing the motility that every portion of the GI tract normally demonstrates when filled with enough barium and/or air. Instead, the walls of the stomach are concave (*white arrows*) and **rigid**, a sign of malignancy. This is the typical appearance for **linitis plastica**, caused by an infiltrating adenocarcinoma of the stomach.

Fig. 18.6 Acute Duodenal Ulcer. Contained within the duodenal bulb on its anterior wall is a collection of barium (*black arrow*), shown to be **persistent** on a number of other images, surrounded by a **zone of edema** (*white arrow*) that displaces the barium from around the base of the ulcer. This collection is characteristic of an acute duodenal ulcer. When duodenal ulcers heal, they are likely to do so with scarring that deforms the normal triangular contour of the bulb.

Fig. 18.7 Perforated Duodenal Ulcer. Axial CT scan of the upper abdomen done with oral and intravenous contrast shows a tract of extraluminal oral contrast (*solid white arrow*) originating from the duodenum into the peritoneal cavity (*dotted white arrow*). The patient had a perforated duodenal ulcer repaired at surgery.

❗ DIAGNOSTIC PITFALLS

- **Collapsed or unopacified loops of bowel can introduce errors of diagnosis** related to an inability to **visualize** and **differentiate** real from artifactual findings or to accurately characterize the abnormality even if recognized. On CT scans of the abdomen and pelvis, unopacified loops of bowel may mimic masses or adenopathy and wall thickness is difficult to assess if the bowel is not distended.

- Therefore, **orally-administered contrast,** frequently given in doses divided over time to allow earlier contrast to reach the colon while later contrast opacifies the stomach, **is routinely utilized for most abdominal CT scans.** Exceptions might include those studies performed for **trauma,** the **stone search study,** and studies specifically directed toward evaluating vascular structures, such as the **aorta.** Oral contrast used for CT examinations is either a dilute solution containing barium or iodinated contrast.

> ## »» IMPORTANT POINTS
>
> - **Several important findings** are common to any part of the bowel and they are key to the diagnosis of bowel abnormalities by CT. All are demonstrated in Fig. 18.8. They include:
>   - **Thickening of the bowel wall** (Fig. 18.8A).
>   - **Submucosal edema or hemorrhage.** Submucosal infiltration produces varying degrees of **thumbprinting,** nodular indentations into the bowel lumen representing focal areas of submucosal infiltration by edema, hemorrhage, inflammatory cells, tumor (lymphoma), or amyloid (Fig. 18.8B).
>   - **Hazy or strand-like infiltration of the surrounding fat.** Extension of inflammatory reaction outside of the bowel into the adjacent fat is a sentinel finding that points to associated disease (Fig. 18.8C).
>   - **Extraluminal contrast or extraluminal air** indicates the presence of a bowel perforation (see Fig. 18.8C).

Small Bowel: Crohn Disease

- Crohn disease is a **chronic, relapsing granulomatous inflammation of the small bowel and colon** resulting in ulceration, obstruction, and fistula formation. Crohn disease **typically involves the ileum and right colon,** presents with **skip areas** (abnormal bowel interposed between normal bowel), is **prone** to fistula formation and has a **propensity for recurring** following surgical resection and reanastomosis in whatever loop of bowel becomes the new terminal ileum.

- Crohn disease may be imaged either with a barium **small bowel follow-through** (series) or **CT of the abdomen and pelvis.**

> ## »» IMPORTANT POINTS
>
> - Imaging findings in Crohn disease include:
>   - **Narrowing, irregularity, and ulceration of the terminal ileum,** frequently with proximal small bowel dilatation
>   - **Separation of the loops of bowel** due to fatty infiltration of the mesentery surrounding the ileum making the affected loop(s) stand apart from the surrounding loops of small bowel (called a **proud loop**)
>   - The **string-sign,** narrowing of the terminal ileum into a near slit-like opening by spasm and fibrosis
>   - **Fistulae,** especially between the ileum and colon but also to the skin, vagina, and urinary bladder (Fig. 18.9).

LARGE BOWEL

- The intraluminal surface of the colon is most often studied with optical colonoscopy or CT colonography, and/or double contrast barium enema examination. Structures outside of the colon are usually studied by CT examination of the abdomen and pelvis with oral or rectal contrast.

Diverticulosis

- **Colonic diverticula,** like most diverticula of the GI tract, represent herniation of the mucosa and submucosa through a defect in the muscular layer (**false diverticula**).

Fig. 18.8 Key Findings on CT of the GI Tract. These are findings applicable to any part of the bowel that are key to the diagnosis of bowel abnormalities on CT. (A) There is **thickening and enhancement** of the wall of the bowel (*white circle*). When distended, as these loops of large bowel are, the bowel wall is normally very thin, no greater than 3 mm. The small bowel **wall** is also usually **no thicker than 3 mm.** (B) **Submucosal infiltration** is producing irregularity of the wall (*white arrow*). In this case of ischemic colitis, it most likely represents edema with some hemorrhage. (C) There is **infiltration of the surrounding fat** (*dotted white arrow*), a sentinel finding that usually heralds adjacent inflammation. There is also **extraluminal air** (*white circle*), a sign of bowel perforation.

Fig. 18.9 Crohn Disease. (A) The terminal ileum (*black arrow*) is markedly narrowed **(string sign)** and stands apart from other loops of small bowel **(proud loop).** (B) A close-up image of the right lower quadrant from a small bowel follow-through study in another patient shows multiple streaks of barium (*solid white arrows*) representing multiple enteric fistulae connecting two adjacent abnormal loops of small bowel (*dotted white arrows*). Fistula formation is a common complication of this disease.

Fig. 18.10 Diverticulosis. (A) In this CT scan of the pelvis, diverticula contain air and appear as small, usually round outpouchings, especially in the region of the sigmoid colon (*white oval*). (B) Numerous diverticula are seen in the sigmoid colon of this air-contrast barium enema examination. Some diverticula are filled with barium (*solid black arrow*), whereas others contain air outlined with barium (*dotted white arrow*). Where an air-containing diverticulum is seen *en face*, it produces a circular density (*solid white arrow*) that can mimic the appearance of a polyp.

> ## ⟩⟩ IMPORTANT POINTS
>
> - They occur more frequently with increasing age and may be caused, at least in part, by an increase in intraluminal pressure and weakening of the colonic wall. They are **usually multiple (diverticulosis)**, are almost always **asymptomatic** (≈90% of the time), but **can become inflamed** or **bleed. Diverticulosis is the most common cause of massive lower GI bleeding.** When they bleed, the **right-sided** diverticula seem to bleed more than those on the left.

- They occur most often in the sigmoid colon and are readily **identified on either barium enema or CT examination as small spikes or smoothly contoured pouches attached to the colon containing either air and/or contrast** (Fig. 18.10).

Diverticulitis

- Diverticula can become **inflamed** and **perforate (diverticulitis)**, most often secondary to mechanical irritation and/or obstruction. **CT is the modality of choice** for the **diagnosis**

of diverticulitis because the pericolonic soft tissues can be visualized with CT, which is impossible with either a barium enema or optical endoscopy.

IMPORTANT POINTS

- CT findings of diverticulitis start with the **presence of diverticula** and include:
  - **Thickening** of the adjacent colonic wall (> 4 mm)
  - **Pericolonic inflammation**: hazy areas of increased attenuation and/or streaky and disorganized linear and amorphous densities in the pericolonic fat
  - **Abscess formation**: multiple small bubbles of air or pockets of fluid contained within a pericolonic soft-tissue, mass-like density
  - **Perforation of the colon**: extraluminal air or contrast, either around the site of the perforation or, less likely, free in the peritoneal cavity (Fig. 18.11)

Colonic Polyps

- The **incidence of polyps increases with age** and the **incidence of malignancy increases with the size** of the polyp. Patients with **polyposis syndromes**, in which multiple adenomatous polyps are present, have a much higher risk of developing a colonic malignancy.

IMPORTANT POINTS

- Most colonic polyps are **hyperplastic polyps** that have **no malignant potential. Adenomatous polyps** carry a **low potential** for malignancy that **increases with the size of the polyp** so that those greater than **1.5 cm in size** have about a **10% chance of being malignant.** Therefore, the early detection and removal of adenomatous polyps will decrease the chances of malignant transformation.

- Colonic polyps can be visualized using barium enema examination, CT colonography, or optical colonoscopy.
- **CT colonography** is a technique made possible by newer, faster CT and MRI scanners and complex computer algorithms that allow for the three-dimensional reconstruction of the appearance of the inside of the bowel lumen, including time-of-flight (motion) displays without the use of an endoscope. CT colonography also allows for visualization of the other abdominal structures outside of the colon (Fig. 18.12A); (eVideo 18.3).
- Polyps may be **sessile** (attach directly to the wall) or **pedunculated** (attach to the wall by a stalk) (Fig. 18.12B).
- Occasionally, a polyp may serve as a **lead point** for an **intussusception,** in which the polyp drags and prolapses one part of the bowel into the lumen of the bowel immediately ahead of it. The bowel proximal to the intussusception is usually obstructed and therefore dilated. Intussusception may produce a characteristic **coiled-spring** appearance on imaging studies (Fig. 18.13).

Colonic Carcinoma

IMPORTANT POINTS

- Colon cancer is the **most common cancer of the GI tract**. Most occur in the **rectosigmoid** region and take years to develop. **Risk factors** include adenomatous polyps, ulcerative colitis, Crohn disease, polyposis syndromes, a family history of colonic polyps or colon cancer, and prior pelvic irradiation.

- The **imaging findings** of carcinoma of the colon include:
  - The presence of a **persistent, large polypoid filling defect**
  - **Annular constriction** of the colonic lumen producing an *apple-core* lesion (Fig. 18.14).

Fig. 18.11 Diverticulitis: CT. (A) **Infiltration** of the pericolonic fat is demonstrated by a hazy increase in attenuation (*white arrow*) of the normal fat. Focal infiltration of fat is a common characteristic of inflammatory disease. (B) There is a large **abscess cavity** (A) in the left lower quadrant in this close-up of a CT scan of the lower abdomen. There are adjacent small bubbles of **extraluminal gas** and infiltration of the normal fat (*dotted white arrow*). These findings are secondary to a confined perforation with abscess formation from diverticulitis.

Fig. 18.12 Colonic Polyps. (A) **CT colonography** uses CT scanning of the abdomen to allow for the 3D reconstruction of the appearance of the **inside** of the bowel lumen without the use of an endoscope. A polyp in the descending colon (*black arrow*) is seen as a distinct mass, whereas the normal haustral folds (*white arrows*) are ridge-like structures present throughout the large bowel. (B) Example of an **air-contrast barium enema** on another patient with a filling-defect in the sigmoid colon outlined by barium (*dotted white arrow*). In this patient, the polyp is attached to the wall of the colon by a **stalk** (*solid white arrow*). Polyps on a stalk are called **pedunculated polyps**.

Fig. 18.13 Intussusception, Barium Enema and CT Scan. (A) When one loop of bowel prolapses inside the loop immediately distal to it, the resultant obstruction produces a **coiled-spring** appearance on barium enema examination as two loops of bowel are superimposed on one another (*white arrow*). (B) CT on another patient with an intussusception shows a loop of large bowel (*white arrow*) prolapsing into the loop distal to it (*black arrow*) producing a filling defect and obstructing the lumen.

Fig. 18.14 Annular Constricting Carcinoma of the Rectum. There is a characteristic **apple-core** lesion of the rectum caused by circumferential growth of a colonic carcinoma. The margins of the lesion (*black arrows*) demonstrate what is called an **overhanging edge** where tumor tissue projects into and overhangs the normal lumen, typical of this type of lesion. The "core" of the "apple" (*white arrow*) is composed of tumor tissue; all of the normal colonic mucosa has been replaced. Identification of such a lesion is pathognomonic for carcinoma.

- **Frank perforation or microperforation** manifest by infiltration of the pericolonic fat with streaky or hazy densities of increased attenuation with or without the presence of extraluminal air.
- **Other findings** of carcinoma of the colon can include **large bowel obstruction (see Fig. 15.15)** and **metastases**, especially to the liver and the lungs.

Colitis

- Colitis is **inflammation of the large bowel.** There are **numerous causes** of colitis, including infectious, ulcerative and granulomatous, ischemic, and radiation-induced and antibiotic-associated etiologies. Because many forms of colitis appear similar radiologically, **clinical history is of paramount importance.**

> ### ▶▶ IMPORTANT POINTS
>
> - **CT findings of colitis** include:
>   - Segmental **thickening of the bowel wall**
>   - Irregular **narrowing of the bowel lumen** due to edema (*i.e., thumbprinting* [Fig. 18.15])
>   - **Infiltration** of the surrounding fat

Appendicitis

- Pathophysiologically, the development of appendicitis is invariably preceded by **obstruction** of the **appendiceal lumen.** CT or ultrasound is now the modalities of choice in diagnosing appendicitis. Appendicitis may also be visualized with MRI.

Fig. 18.15 Colitis. The colon demonstrates **thumbprinting,** nodular indentations on the lumen (*white arrows*), and an overall pattern that is called the **accordion sign**. This patient had *Clostridium difficile* colitis, formerly called pseudomembranous colitis, and now known to be caused almost exclusively by toxins produced by *C. difficile*. It frequently follows antibiotic therapy. The diagnosis is usually made clinically by visualization of the pseudomembrane on endoscopy. The accordion sign represents contrast that is trapped between enlarged folds and indicates the presence of marked edema or inflammation, but it is not specific for *C. difficile* colitis.

- An **appendicolith is a calcified concretion found in the appendix** of about 15% of all people. It will be visible, especially on CT, as a calcification in the appendiceal lumen. The combination of **abdominal pain** and the **presence of an appendicolith** is associated with **appendicitis about 90% of the time** and indicates a higher probability for **perforation.**

> ### ▶▶ IMPORTANT POINTS
>
> - **The key CT findings of acute appendicitis** are:
>   - Identification of a **dilated appendix** (>6 mm) that does **not fill** with oral contrast
>   - **Periappendiceal inflammation,** which is evidenced by streaky, disorganized, linear high-attenuation densities in the surrounding fat (Fig. 18.16A)
>   - **Increased contrast enhancement of the wall of the appendix** due to inflammation
>   - **Perforation** occurs in up to 30% of cases and is **recognized by small quantities of periappendiceal, extraluminal air or a periappendiceal abscess.** Because obstruction of the appendiceal lumen is a prerequisite for appendicitis, the presence of a **large amount** of free intraperitoneal air should point to **another diagnosis** (Fig. 18.16B).

> ### ✳ IMAGE-GUIDED INTERVENTION
>
>
>
> This is a 34-year-old female with severe right lower quadrant pain determined to be perforated appendicitis with abscess formation *(arrow)*. How might an image-guided procedure benefit in this case? See the answer in Chapter 29.

- The use of ultrasound in appendicitis will be discussed in Chapter 19.
- The **appendix** of this book (not to be surgically removed) lists the **studies of first choice** for many **different clinical scenarios** relating to **abdominal pain.**

Lower Gastrointestinal Bleeding

- **Diverticulosis** is one of the main causes of lower gastrointestinal bleeding (LGIB). LGIB is defined as bleeding that originates from the ileocecal valve to the rectum. Other causes of LGIB include angiodysplasias, inflammatory bowel disease, and neoplasms.

Fig. 18.16 Appendicitis: CT. (A) There is infiltration of the periappendiceal fat in the right lower quadrant manifest by the increased attenuation in the mesenteric fat (*white arrow*). Focal infiltration of fat is a common characteristic of inflammatory diseases and helps in their localization. (B) Contained within the lumen of the appendix is a small calcification (*black arrow*) or **appendicolith,** in another patient. There is inflammatory infiltration of the surrounding fat producing high attenuation (*solid white arrow*). A very small amount of air is present outside of the appendiceal lumen from a confined perforation (*dotted white arrow*).

Fig. 18.17 CT Angiogram (CTA) of Lower GI Bleed. Active GI bleeding is diagnosed by demonstrating extravasation of intravenously injected contrast into the bowel lumen. (A) Axial image of the pelvis after intravenous, but no oral, contrast shows an amorphous collection of contrast **in the lumen** of the cecum (*white circle*), representing extravasated blood. (B) Coronal reconstruction on the same patient demonstrates several collections of intraluminal contrast in the cecum (*white circle*). The *white arrows* on both images identify opacified iliac arteries. The patient was bleeding from a vascular malformation of the cecum. *AC,* Ascending colon.

- In acute (overt) lower GI bleeding, there are several diagnostic approaches. **Colonoscopy, catheter angiography, and CT angiogram (CTA)** are the diagnostic studies most often employed for evaluation of acute LGIB. Radionuclide bleeding scans may also be used.
- Both **colonoscopy** and **catheter angiography** have the added benefit of allowing **treatment** of the cause of bleeding as well as identification of its site. Colonoscopy is frequently utilized as the initial modality in **hemodynamically stable** patients (with adequate bowel preparation). Angiography is especially helpful in those who are **hemodynamically unstable** and have massive lower GI bleeding.
- **CT angiography** requires a certain rate of active arterial bleeding (at least 0.5 mL/min) to effectively show **extravasation of contrast into the bowel lumen** to identify a bleeding site. It is less invasive than colonoscopy or catheter angiography; it is **readily available** and may demonstrate lesions in the **small bowel,** which colonoscopy cannot (Fig. 18.17).

✳ IMAGE-GUIDED INTERVENTION

A 36-year-old male presented to the emergency department with bright red blood per rectum. CT angiography of the abdomen and pelvis demonstrates focal, active extravasation of contrast in the terminal ileum *(white circle)*. How might an image-guided procedure benefit in this case? See the answer in Chapter 29.

Fig. 18.18 Acute Pancreatitis. The pancreas is markedly enlarged and irregular in appearance (*black arrow*). There is extensive infiltration of the peripancreatic fat (*white arrows*). Severe abdominal pain, often radiating to the back, is an almost universal symptom of acute pancreatitis. This patient had a markedly elevated amylase and lipase. *GB*, Gallbladder.

- **Nuclear scintigraphy bleeding scans** are a sensitive diagnostic tool for GI hemorrhage but suffer from a relatively low specificity because of its limited resolution compared with endoscopy or angiography.

PANCREAS

Pancreatitis

- The two **most common causes of pancreatitis** are **alcoholism** and **gallstones.** Inflammation of pancreatic tissue leading to disruption of the ducts and spillage of pancreatic juices occurs readily, in part because of the lack of a capsule surrounding the pancreas.

▶ IMPORTANT POINTS

- Pancreatitis is a **clinical diagnosis** with CT serving to document either a **cause** (e.g., gallstones) or a **complication** (e.g., pseudocyst formation).

- **Recognizing acute pancreatitis on CT:**
  - **Enlargement** of all or part of the pancreas (normal measurements for the pancreas are **3 cm for the head, 2.5 cm for the body,** and **2 cm for the tail**).
  - **Peripancreatic stranding** or **fluid collections** (Fig. 18.18).
  - **Low-attenuation** lesions in the pancreas from **necrosis** may represent areas of nonviable pancreas and have a poorer prognostic significance. They usually develop **early** in the course of the disease and require intravenous contrast administration for visualization.
  - **Pseudocyst formation.** Fibrous tissue can encapsulate a walled-off collection of pancreatic juices released from the

Fig. 18.19 Pancreatic Pseudocyst. A pseudocyst (P) of the pancreas is a collection of fluid, usually high in pancreatic enzymes, outside of the pancreas and enclosed by a wall of fibrous and granulation tissue. The wall may contrast-enhance (*white arrows*). The cyst is indenting a loop of adjacent bowel, in this case the posterior wall of the stomach (S). The type of indentation on a loop of bowel by an extrinsic mass, whatever its origin, is called a **pad sign** (*black arrow*).

inflamed pancreas. The **wall of a pseudocyst is usually visible by CT** and **may contrast-enhance** (Fig. 18.19).

Chronic Pancreatitis

- Chronic pancreatitis is a continuous and irreversible disease of the pancreas, most often secondary to **alcohol abuse,** leading to **fibrosis, atrophy of the gland, ductal dilatation,** and, frequently, **diabetes.**

>> IMPORTANT POINTS

- The **hallmarks** of the disease are **multiple, amorphous calcifications** that form within the **dilated ducts** of the **atrophied gland** (see Fig. 17.10).

Pancreatic Adenocarcinoma

- Risk factors for pancreatic adenocarcinoma include **alcoholism, cigarette smoking, chronic pancreatitis,** and **diabetes.** Pancreatic adenocarcinoma has an **exceedingly poor prognosis:** most tumors are unresectable and incurable at the time of diagnosis. **Most of the time** (75%), the tumor is located in the **head** of the pancreas; about 10% occur in the body and 5% in the tail. About half of the patients present with **jaundice** and, most of the time, **there is associated pain.**
  - **Ultrasound is the study of choice in the initial work-up of the jaundiced patient** (see Chapter 19).

>> IMPORTANT POINTS

- **Recognizing pancreatic adenocarcinoma on CT:**
  - **Focal pancreatic mass,** usually **hypodense** to the remainder the gland (Fig. 18.20).
  - **Ductal dilatation,** usually involving **both** the **pancreatic and biliary ducts.** The normal **pancreatic duct** measures **less than 4 mm** in the head and tapers to the tail; the **common duct** should be **less than 7 mm** in diameter.
  - Other findings of pancreatic carcinoma include spread to contiguous organs, enlarged lymph nodes, and/or ascites.

HEPATOBILIARY ABNORMALITIES

Liver: General Considerations

- CT evaluation of **liver masses** is usually done with a **sequence** of scans obtained **before** and then **twice after intravenous contrast** injection, which is called a **triple-phase scan.** The combination of images helps to best define and characterize liver masses (Fig. 18.21).
- **MRI** is increasingly utilized as the modality of choice in the evaluation of both focal and diffuse liver disease. MRI can

often definitively characterize hepatic lesions described as indeterminate on CT, such as cysts, benign hepatic neoplasms such as hemangioma and focal nodular hyperplasia, hepatocellular carcinoma, and metastatic disease. It is **particularly useful in the evaluation of small (≤10 mm) lesions** compared with CT.

- For routine MRI imaging of the liver, an intravenous contrast agent called **gadolinium** is typically administered, and multiple postgadolinium-enhanced images are obtained. Gadolinium will be discussed in Chapter 21.

Fatty Infiltration

- The term **nonalcoholic fatty liver disease** refers to a spectrum of diseases of the liver ranging from **hepatic steatosis** (fatty infiltration of the liver) to **nonalcoholic steatohepatitis (NASH)** to **cirrhosis.**

Fig. 18.20 Pancreatic Adenocarcinoma. The head of the pancreas is enlarged by a mass (*white arrow*). Normally, the head of the pancreas should roughly be the same size as the width of the lumbar vertebral body nearest to it. The symptoms of pancreatic adenocarcinomas are frequently vague, laboratory findings are nonspecific, and pancreatic adenocarcinomas are difficult to image, especially in patients with concomitant changes of chronic pancreatitis.

Fig. 18.21 Triple-Phase CT Scan of the Liver: Hepatocellular Carcinoma. Evaluation of liver masses is usually done with a combination of scans, including an **unenhanced** scan (A) and then two postcontrast scans: one obtained quickly (B), called the **hepatic-arterial phase,** and a second about a minute later (C), called the **portal-venous phase.** This case shows the typical findings of a focal hepatocellular carcinoma. Most are low density (hypodense) or the same density as normal liver (isodense) **without contrast** (*white arrow* in A), **enhance** on the arterial phase with intravenous contrast (hyperdense) (*dotted arrow* in B) and then return to **hypodense or isodense** on the venous phase (*dashed arrow* in C).

- **Fatty infiltration of the liver** (hepatic steatosis) is a **very common** abnormality in which there is fat accumulation in the hepatocytes in such diseases as obesity, diabetes, hepatitis, or cirrhosis. Most patients with a fatty liver are **asymptomatic**. The **fatty infiltration** may be **diffuse** or **focal**, and focal lesions may be **solitary** or **multiple**.

- Normally on noncontrast CT scans, the liver is always denser than or equal to the density of the spleen. With **fatty infiltration of the liver, the spleen is denser than the liver without intravenous contrast** (Fig. 18.22).
- When diffuse, the **liver is usually slightly enlarged.** The **blood vessels stand out prominently,** but are usually **neither obstructed nor displaced.**

⚠ **DIAGNOSTIC PITFALLS**

- **Focal** fatty infiltration can produce an appearance that **mimics tumor.** Fatty infiltration usually produces **no mass effect** and has the ability to **appear and disappear** in a matter of weeks, quite unlike tumor masses.

- **MRI is the most accurate modality in the evaluation of a fatty liver,** using a phenomenon called *chemical shift imaging* to detect the presence of microscopic, intracellular lipid present in such a liver. Chemical shift relates to the way that lipid and water protons behave in the magnetic field (Fig. 18.23).

Cirrhosis

- Cirrhosis is a chronic, irreversible disease of the liver that features destruction of normal liver cells and diffuse fibrosis that appears to be the final common pathway of many abnormalities, including **hepatitis B** and **C, alcoholism, nonalcoholic fatty infiltration of the liver,** and miscellaneous diseases such as **hemochromatosis** and **Wilson disease.** Complications of cirrhosis include **portal hypertension, ascites, renal dysfunction, hepatocellular carcinoma, hepatic failure,** and **death.**

Fig. 18.22 Diffuse Fatty Liver: Unenhanced CT. In this patient with diffuse fatty infiltration of an enlarged liver (L), the spleen (S) is denser than the liver, the reverse of normal on an unenhanced scan. In this case, the degree of fatty infiltration is such that the vessels stand out in the fatty liver (*solid white arrows*). K, Kidneys.

- **Recognizing cirrhosis of the liver on CT:**
  - **Early** in the disease, the liver may demonstrate **diffuse fatty infiltration.** As the disease progresses, the liver **contour becomes lobulated.** The **liver shrinks in volume** with the **right lobe** characteristically becoming **smaller** whereas the **caudate lobe and left lobe become disproportionately larger,** especially in alcoholic cirrhosis (Fig. 18.24A).
  - There is a **mottled, inhomogeneous** appearance to the liver parenchyma following intravenous contrast enhancement due to a mixture of regenerating nodules, focal fatty infiltration, and fibrosis.
  - **Portal hypertension** may develop, which can lead to **dilated vessels** around the stomach, splenic hilum, and esophagus, representing **varices.**
  - **Splenomegaly** may result (Fig. 18.24).
  - **Ascites** may be present. Sometimes it can be difficult to differentiate between ascites and pleural effusion on CT examinations (Box 18.1).

✳ **IMAGE-GUIDED INTERVENTION**

A 48-year-old female presented with cirrhosis, refractory ascites, and a history of variceal bleeding. Sequelae of portal hypertension are present and demonstrated by large-volume ascites (A), liver that is nodular and heterogeneous in attenuation (L), and the presence of gastric varices (circle). How might an image-guided procedure benefit in this case? See the answer in Chapter 29.

BOX 18.1   Differentiating Ascites From Pleural Effusion

- Patients may have a combination of ascites and pleural effusion for a number of reasons, including cirrhosis, ovarian tumors, metastatic disease, hypoproteinemia, and congestive heart failure.
- Differentiation between ascitic fluid and pleural fluid at the lung base on axial CT examinations may be difficult because **both may appear posterior to the liver.**
- **Ascitic fluid** will appear **anterior to the hemidiaphragm** in the axial plane. **Pleural effusion** will be located **posterior to the hemidiaphragm** (Fig. 18.25A).
- Ascitic fluid **will not spread to the "bare" area of the liver posteriorly** where there is no peritoneal lining (see Fig. 14.2).
- Therefore, **fluid that appears posterior to the bare area of the liver is pleural in location** (Fig. 18.25B).

Fig. 18.23 Fatty Liver: MRI. Using a phenomenon called **chemical shift imaging** to detect the presence of intracellular lipid present in a fatty liver, MRI provides the most accurate identification of a fatty liver. (A) The liver (*white arrow*) appears normal, brighter than the spleen (S). (B) This is called an **opposed-phase image** and it demonstrates marked signal loss (signal dropout) throughout the liver (*dotted white arrow*) indicating a fatty liver. Most of the liver is now darker than the spleen (S), except for the caudate lobe (C), which is normal.

Fig. 18.24 Cirrhosis, Portal Hypertension, and Varices: CT. (A) The spleen (S) is enlarged from portal hypertension secondary to cirrhosis. There is characteristic enlargement of the caudate lobe (C) relative to the right lobe of the liver (*black arrow*). Several contrast-enhanced dilated veins (varices) are seen around the stomach and splenic hilum (*white arrows*). (B) Another patient shows the typical nodular and shrunken appearance of the cirrhotic liver (*white arrows*) along with numerous contrast-enhanced, periesophageal varices (*white circle*). *Ao,* Descending aorta.

Fig. 18.25 Differentiating Pleural Effusion from Ascites. (A) Patients may have a combination of ascites and pleural effusions for a number of reasons, cirrhosis being one of them. Ascitic fluid **(As)** will appear anterior to the hemidiaphragm (*white arrow*) in the axial plane. Pleural effusion **(P)** will be located posterior to the hemidiaphragm. (B) Ascites will never completely encircle the dome of the liver because of the **"bare area"** (*black arrow*), not covered by peritoneum (see Fig. 14.2). Fluid posterior to the bare area must be in the pleural space **(P)**.

Space-Occupying Lesions of the Liver

- One of the primary aims of imaging studies, no matter the body part, is to accurately differentiate between benign and malignant processes with techniques that do not place patients in danger or subject them to unnecessary pain. This is the central goal in evaluating liver masses as well.
- CT studies are best at demonstrating liver masses when performed **both with and without contrast** as either study alone may fail to reveal an **isodense** mass (i.e., one that appears identical in attenuation to the surrounding normal tissue), therefore hiding its presence.
- **MRI is useful in characterizing liver masses,** particularly small lesions 10 mm or less.

Metastases

> ### IMPORTANT POINTS
>
> - Metastases are the **most common malignant hepatic masses.** Although **most are multiple**, metastases also represent the **most common cause** of a **solitary** malignant mass in the liver.

- **Most liver metastases originate in the GI tract,** in particular the **colon,** and almost all reach the liver via the bloodstream. Other primary sites of metastatic spread to the liver include the stomach, pancreas, esophagus, lung, breast, and malignant melanoma.
- **Recognizing liver metastases on CT and MRI:**
  - Metastases are usually **multiple, low attenuation masses** (Fig. 18.26). **Larger metastases** may demonstrate areas of necrosis that can be recognized as mottled areas of low attenuation within the mass. **Mucin-producing carcinomas,** such as might originate in the stomach, colon, or ovary, can **calcify** in both the primary tumor and the metastases (see Fig. 17.14).

Fig. 18.26 Metastases to the Liver and Spleen. Multiple, low-attenuation masses fill the liver (*solid black arrows*) on this contrast-enhanced CT scan. There are also low-attenuation metastatic lesions in the spleen (*dotted black arrows*). The patient had a primary adenocarcinoma of the colon.

- **MRI is as sensitive** as CT in detecting liver metastases, but it is usually used in a **problem-solving role.** In general, MRI is more expensive than CT scanning and may suffer from more motion artifact than CT.

Hepatocellular Carcinoma (Hepatoma)

- Hepatocellular carcinoma is the **most common primary malignancy** of the liver. Virtually all arise in livers with pre-existing abnormalities such as **cirrhosis** and/or **hepatitis. Most are solitary,** but up to one out of five can be multiple, mimicking metastases. **Vascular invasion is common,** particularly of the portal system.

> ### IMPORTANT POINTS
>
> - **Recognizing hepatocellular carcinoma on CT and MRI:**
>   - Hepatocellular carcinomas (HCC) can be **solitary** (see Fig. 18.21), **multiple masses**, or **diffusely infiltrating.**
>   - On CT, most HCCs are **low density (hypodense)** or the same density as normal liver **(isodense) without contrast**, **enhance** on the **arterial phase** with intravenous contrast **(hyperdense)** and then return to **hypodense** or **isodense** on the **venous phase** (Fig. 18.27).
>   - Low attenuation areas from **necrosis** are common. **Calcification** occurs relatively frequently.
>   - **MRI** can demonstrate certain features that are fairly specific for **hepatocellular carcinoma,** as well as detect intrahepatic metastases and venous invasion. Unlike benign lesions, such as hemangiomas of the liver which tend to retain intravenously administered gadolinium contrast, hepatocellular carcinomas **show washout** of the contrast material.

> ### ✳ IMAGE-GUIDED INTERVENTION
>
>
>
> This image is from an MRI on a 62-year-male with a mass in the liver *(white circle)*. The mass was biopsied and returned as hepatocellular carcinoma. How might an image-guided procedure benefit in this case? See the answer in Chapter 29.

Cavernous Hemangiomas

- Cavernous hemangiomas are the **most common primary liver tumor** and **second in frequency to metastases for localized liver masses.** More common in **women,** they are usually

solitary and are almost always **asymptomatic.** They are complex structures composed of multiple, large vascular channels lined by a single layer of endothelial cells.

IMPORTANT POINTS

- **Recognizing cavernous hemangiomas of the liver on CT and MRI:**
  - **Cavernous hemangiomas** have a characteristic appearance on triple-phase, unenhanced and enhanced CT scans of the liver (Fig. 18.28).

- **MRI is frequently the preferred modality** in the evaluation of hemangiomas; it is **more sensitive** than nuclear medicine tagged red blood cell scans and more specific than a multiphase CT scan.
- Similar to CT, **hemangiomas on MRI** usually have a characteristic nodular **enhancement from the periphery inward** following injection of intravenous contrast. Contrast tends to be retained within the numerous vascular spaces of hemangiomas so that they typically appear brighter than the rest of the liver on delayed (10 minute) scans (Fig. 18.29); (eVideo 18.4).

Fig. 18.27 Diffuse Hepatocellular Carcinoma of the Liver: CT. The three major patterns of appearance for hepatocellular carcinoma are **solitary mass** (see Fig. 18.21), **multiple nodules,** and **diffuse infiltration** throughout a segment or lobe (as in this case) or the entire liver. (A) A typical low-attenuation lesion is seen in the right lobe of the liver on the unenhanced scan (*white arrow*). (B) The arterial phase demonstrates patchy enhancement (*black arrow*) indicating the probability of tumor necrosis in the low-attenuation areas. Ascites is present **(As).** The overall volume of the liver is decreased and the contour is lobulated from underlying cirrhosis.

Fig. 18.28 Cavernous Hemangioma of the Liver: Triple-Phase CT Study. (A) Cavernous hemangiomas (*white arrows* on all images) are usually **hypodense** lesions on unenhanced scans. (B) They characteristically **enhance from the periphery** inward following injection of intravenous contrast during the **arterial phase** and eventually become isodense. (C) Contrast then tends to be retained within the numerous vascular spaces of the lesion so that they characteristically appear **denser** than the rest of the liver on **delayed scans**.

Fig. 18.29 Cavernous Hemangioma of the Liver: MRI. (A) This image (an axial T1-weighted image) demonstrates a well-circumscribed, slightly lobular dark mass in the right hepatic lobe (*white arrow* in all images). (B) Subsequent images following the administration of intravenous contrast (gadolinium), show peripheral-to-central enhancement, until the entire mass homogeneously enhances on a delayed 10 minute image (C). The combination of this enhancement pattern and the signal characteristics of the lesion allows an unequivocal diagnosis of hemangioma.

Fig. 18.30 Hepatic Cysts: CT. Believed to be **congenital** in origin, hepatic cysts are easily identified as **sharply marginated** lesions of **low attenuation (fluid density)** compared with the remainder of the liver, on both unenhanced and enhanced CT scans. MRI is much better than CT at characterizing cysts. They are usually **solitary** and are **homogeneous** in density (*black arrows*).

Hepatic Cysts

- See Fig. 18.30.

BILIARY SYSTEM

Magnetic Resonance Cholangiopancreatography

- Magnetic resonance cholangiopancreatography (MRCP) is a **noninvasive** way to image the biliary tree **without requiring injection of contrast material.** MRCP uses MRI imaging sequences that make fluid-filled structures such as the bile ducts, pancreatic ducts, and gallbladder extremely bright, and everything else dark. Patients are imaged during a single-breath hold (Fig. 18.31).
- MRCP is excellent at depicting **biliary or ductal strictures, ductal dilatation, stones in the bile ducts (choledocholithiasis), gallstones, adenomyomatosis of the gallbladder, choledochal cysts, and pancreas divisum.**
- If there is a concern for malignancy (e.g., pancreatic adenocarcinoma or cholangiocarcinoma) as the cause of pancreaticobiliary ductal dilatation, then additional pulse sequences following the administration of gadolinium contrast can be

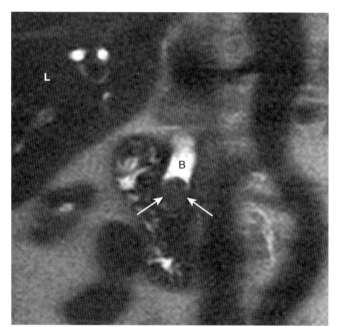

Fig. 18.31. Choledocholithiasis and Biliary Ductal Dilatation on Magnetic Resonance Cholangiopancreatography (MRCP). This is a coronal close-up of the right upper quadrant with MR imaging. There is a large obstructing gallstone (*white arrows*) in the distal common bile duct (B), the latter of which is dilated to 13 mm. Because of the signal characteristics of bile, an MRCP can be done **without** the need for the injection of contrast. *L,* Liver.

obtained. Contrast administration allows better detection of malignancy.

URINARY TRACT

Kidneys: General Considerations

- The kidneys are retroperitoneal organs, encircled by varying amounts of fat and enclosed within a fibrous capsule. So long as they are functioning properly, the **kidneys are the route through which intravenously injected, iodinated contrast (and gadolinium-based MRI contrast) agents are excreted from the body.** Following injection of iodinated contrast agents, the kidneys will therefore **enhance.**

Space-Occupying Lesions
Renal Cysts

- Simple renal cysts are a **very common** finding on CT and ultrasound (US) scans of the abdomen; they occur in more than half of the population over 55 years of age.

>> **IMPORTANT POINTS**

- Simple cysts are **benign, fluid-filled** structures that are frequently **multiple** and **bilateral**. On CT scans, they tend to have a **sharp margin** where they meet the normal renal parenchyma. They have density measurements (Hounsfield numbers) of **water density** (−10 to +20). They **do not contrast-enhance** (Fig. 18.32A).

Fig. 18.32 Renal Cysts: CT Urogram and US. (A) This coronal image from a CT urogram demonstrates a low attenuation mass (*white arrow*) in the upper pole of the right kidney, which is homogeneous in density and sharply marginated from the rest of the kidney. These findings are characteristic of a simple cyst. (B) A sagittal ultrasound of the kidney (*dotted white arrows*) in another patient demonstrates an anechoic mass (C) with strong through transmission (*solid white arrow*), features consistent with a simple cyst of the lower pole.

Fig. 18.33 Renal Cell Carcinomas: CT and US. (A) There is a low-density mass involving the anterior portion of the left kidney (*white arrow*). The tumor extends directly into the left renal vein (*black arrow*), a feature of renal cell carcinomas. (B) Sagittal ultrasound on another patient with renal cell carcinoma shows an echogenic mass (M) occupying the midportion of the kidney (*dotted white arrows*). Contrast the absence of internal echoes for the renal cyst (see Fig. 18.32B) and the echo-density of this renal cell carcinoma.

- On **ultrasound examinations,** simple cysts are **echo-free** (anechoic) masses with **strong through transmission** of the ultrasound signal; they have **sharp borders** where they meet the renal parenchyma and **round or oval shapes.** Thickening of the wall or dense internal echoes raise suspicion for a malignant lesion (Fig. 18.32B).

Renal Cell Carcinoma (Hypernephroma)

- Renal cell carcinoma is the **most common primary renal malignancy** in **adults.** Solid masses in the kidneys of adults are usually renal cell carcinomas. They have a propensity for

extending into the renal veins, into the **inferior vena cava** and metastasizing via the bloodstream to produce **nodules in the lung.** When they metastasize to bone, they are **purely lytic** and **often expansile.**

- Ultrasound is used in the characterization of renal masses, particularly in assessing their cystic or solid nature and involvement of the collecting system or surrounding vessels.

- On **ultrasound,** smaller renal cell carcinomas are **usually hyperechoic;** as the lesion increases in size and undergoes necrosis it may be hypoechoic. Its wall, however, should be thicker and more irregular than a simple cyst (Fig. 18.33B).

>> **IMPORTANT POINTS**

- **Recognizing renal cell carcinoma on CT:**
  - A dedicated CT scan for renal cell carcinoma usually consists of images obtained before and after intravenous contrast administration.
  - Ranging from **completely solid** to **completely cystic**, renal cell carcinomas are **usually solid lesions that may contain low-attenuation areas of necrosis.** Even though renal cell carcinomas **enhance with intravenous contrast,** they still tend to remain **lower in density than the surrounding normal kidney.**
  - **Renal vein invasion** occurs in up to one in three cases and may produce filling defects in the lumen of the renal veins (see Fig. 18.33A).

Fig. 18.34 Transitional Cell Carcinoma of the Bladder: CT Urogram. There is a filling defect in the left lateral wall of the contrast-filled bladder (*solid white arrow*) representing a bladder tumor. The defect at the base of the bladder (*black arrow*) is caused by the prostate gland. The calyceal collecting systems (*dotted white arrows*) are normal.

- The primary role of **MRI of the kidneys** is in the evaluation of **small masses** less than 1.5 cm or in any renal mass characterized as **indeterminate** for malignancy by either CT or US.

PELVIS

General Considerations
- **Ultrasound is the study of first choice in evaluation of suspected abnormalities of the female pelvis** (see Chapter 19).
- **MRI** has assumed an increasingly important role in defining the anatomy of the uterus and ovaries and in clarifying questions in patients in whom US findings are confusing. MRI is also used in staging and surgical planning.
- MRI can be particularly useful in evaluating ovarian dermoid cysts, endometriosis, hydrosalpinges (fluid-filled fallopian tubes), and in determining whether an ovarian cystic lesion is simple (benign) or contains a solid component (often malignant) (see Fig. 21.5).

URINARY BLADDER

Bladder Tumors
- Most malignant bladder tumors are **transitional cell tumors.** Transitional cell tumors may occur simultaneously from uroepithelium anywhere from the bladder to the ureter to the kidney. The **primary tumor** appears as **focal thickening of the bladder wall** and/or produces a **filling defect in the contrast-filled bladder** (Fig. 18.34).

ADENOPATHY

Lymphoma
- Lymphoma can involve any part of the GI or genitourinary tract. Thoracic lymphoma is almost always caused by Hodgkin disease, whereas **the stomach is the most common extranodal site of gastrointestinal non-Hodgkin lymphoma.**

- **Extranodal involvement** and **noncontiguous spread** to other organs or nodes are features of non-Hodgkin lymphoma.

>> **IMPORTANT POINTS**

- **Recognizing the CT findings of abdominal lymphoma:**
  - **Multiple enlarged lymph nodes.** Pelvic lymph nodes are considered pathologically enlarged if they exceed 1 cm in their shortest dimension.
  - **Conglomerate masses of coalesced nodes.** Bulky tumor masses that can encase and obstruct vessels.
  - Lymphadenopathy will classically **displace the aorta and/or vena cava anteriorly** (Fig. 18.35).

- Other malignancies can produce abdominal and/or pelvic adenopathy besides lymphoma and even benign disease like sarcoid can produce abdominal adenopathy.

Fig. 18.35 Massive Lymphadenopathy: Lymphoma. Massive abdominal lymphadenopathy occupies most of the abdomen (*white arrows*) and displaces the kidneys (K) laterally and the aorta (A) anteriorly (*black arrow*) far from its normal location next to the spine. The patient had non-Hodgkin lymphoma.

🏠 TAKE HOME POINTS

- CT, US, and MRI have essentially replaced conventional radiography and, in many instances, barium studies for the evaluation of the GI tract.
- **Esophageal carcinoma** has a poor prognosis, with an increasing incidence of adenocarcinomas forming in Barrett esophagus, a condition in which gastroesophageal reflux plays a major role in stimulating metaplasia of the squamous to columnar epithelium.
- Esophageal carcinomas appear in one or more of several forms, including an annular-constricting lesion, a polypoid mass, and a superficial, infiltrating type lesion.
- **Hiatal hernias** are a common abnormality that may be associated with GERD, although GERD can occur even in the absence of a demonstrable hernia; they are usually of the **sliding** variety in which the esophagogastric junction lies above the diaphragm.
- The radiologic findings of **gastric ulcer** include a persistent collection of barium that extends outward from the lumen beyond the normal contours of the stomach, usually along the lesser curvature or posterior wall in the region of the body or antrum; the ulcer may have radiating folds that extend to the ulcer margin and a surrounding margin of edema.
- The key finding in **gastric carcinoma** is a mass that protrudes into the lumen and produces a filling defect, displacing barium; gastric carcinomas may be associated with rigidity of the wall and nondistensibility of the lumen as well as irregular ulceration or thickening of the gastric folds (>1 cm), especially localized to one area of the stomach.
- The radiologic findings of **duodenal ulcers** include a persistent collection of contrast, more often seen *en face* with surrounding spasm and edema. Healing of duodenal ulcers produces scarring and deformity of the duodenal bulb.
- Any imaging evaluation of the bowel should ideally be carried out with the bowel distended with air or contrast because collapsed and unopacified loops of bowel can introduce artifactual errors of diagnosis.

- Key abnormal findings of bowel disease on CT are **thickening** of the bowel wall, **submucosal edema or hemorrhage**, **hazy infiltration** of fat, and **extraluminal air** or contrast.
- **Crohn disease** is a chronic, relapsing, granulomatous inflammation of the small bowel and colon, usually involving the terminal ileum, resulting in ulceration, obstruction, and fistula formation; it may have skip areas and has a propensity for recurring following surgical removal of an involved segment.
- Colonic **diverticulosis** increases in incidence with increasing age; it most often involves the sigmoid colon and is almost always asymptomatic, although it can lead to diverticulitis or massive GI bleeding, especially from right-sided diverticula.
- CT is the study of choice for imaging **diverticulitis** and the findings include pericolonic inflammation, thickening of the adjacent colonic wall (>4 mm), abscess formation, and/or confined perforation of the colon.
- Most **colonic polyps** are hyperplastic and have no malignant potential; adenomatous polyps carry a malignant potential that is related, in part, to their size. Colonic polyps can be visualized with barium enema examination, CT colonography, or optical colonoscopy.
- Imaging signs of colonic polyps include a persistent filling defect in the colon, with or without a stalk.
- The imaging findings of **colonic carcinoma** are a persistent, polypoid, or annular constricting filling defect of the colon that may have frank or microperforation or large bowel obstruction and metastases, especially to the liver and the lungs.
- **Colitis** of any etiology can cause thickening of the bowel wall, narrowing of the lumen, and infiltration of the surrounding fat.
- CT or ultrasound are the studies of choice in diagnosing **appendicitis.** Findings include a dilated appendix (>6 mm) that does not fill with oral contrast, periappendiceal inflammation, increased enhancement of the wall of the appendix with intravenous contrast, and sometimes identification of an appendicolith (fecalith).

Continued

TAKE HOME POINTS—cont'd

- **Lower gastrointestinal bleeding** is frequently caused by diverticulosis. CT angiography, tagged-red blood cell bleeding scans, catheter angiography, and colonoscopy can be used to visualize the site of bleeding with the latter two also capable of treating the cause.

- The two most common causes of **pancreatitis** are gallstones and alcoholism; pancreatitis is a clinical diagnosis with CT serving to document a cause or a complication of the disease; CT findings include enlargement of the pancreas, peripancreatic stranding, pancreatic necrosis, and pseudocyst formation.

- **Pancreatic adenocarcinoma** has a very unfavorable prognosis; it occurs most often in the pancreatic head and usually manifests as a focal hypodense mass that may be associated with dilatation of the pancreatic and/or biliary ducts.

- **Fatty infiltration** of the liver is very common and can produce focal or diffuse areas of decreased attenuation that characteristically do not displace or obstruct the hepatic vessels; the liver appears less dense than the spleen on unenhanced CT scans.

- In its later stages, **cirrhosis** produces a small liver (especially the right lobe) with a lobulated contour, inhomogeneous appearance of the parenchyma, prominent left and caudate lobes, splenomegaly, varices, and ascites.

- Evaluation of liver masses is frequently done with a **triple-phase CT scan** that includes a precontrast scan and two postcontrast scans, one in the hepatic-arterial phase and then another in the portal-venous phase.

- **Metastases** are the most common malignant hepatic masses and they mostly originate in the GI tract; they appear as multiple, low density masses that may necrose as they become larger.

- **Hepatocellular carcinoma** is the most common primary hepatic malignancy; these lesions are usually solitary and typically enhance with intravenous contrast on CT.

- **Cavernous hemangiomas** are usually solitary, more common in females, and typically produce no symptoms; they have a characteristic "outside-in" pattern of enhancement and frequently retain contrast longer than the remainder of the liver.

- **MRCP** is a noninvasive way to image the biliary tree without requiring injection of contrast material; it can be used to demonstrate biliary strictures, gallstones, and congenital anomalies.

- **Renal cysts** are a very common finding; they are frequently multiple and bilateral, do not enhance, and typically have sharp margins where they meet the normal renal parenchyma. On US, simple cysts are well-defined anechoic masses.

- **Renal cell carcinoma**, the most common primary renal malignancy, shows a propensity for extension into the renal vein and for metastasizing to lung and bone; on CT, it is usually a solid mass that enhances with intravenous contrast, but remains less dense than the normal kidney. On US, they are frequently echogenic masses.

- **Ultrasound** is the imaging study of first choice in evaluating the **female pelvis.**

- **Abdominal and/or pelvic adenopathy** may be caused by lymphoma, other malignancies, or benign diseases such as sarcoid; multiple enlarged nodes or conglomerate masses of nodes may be seen on CT.

 More information on recognizing gastrointestinal, hepatobiliary and urinary tract abnormalities is available to registered users online.

Ultrasonography: Understanding the Principles and Its Uses in Abdominal and Pelvic Imaging

Peter Wang, MD

- **Ultrasound (US)** is a diagnostic imaging tool that makes use of **probes (transducers)** that can produce an acoustical frequency that is hundreds of times greater than humans can hear and which uses that acoustical energy to localize and characterize human tissues.

HOW IT WORKS

- Ultrasonography is performed by placing the transducer on a body surface and sweeping back and forth while real-time images are displayed on a monitor. Adequate contact between the transducer and the body surface is essential to obtain a good sonographic image. Therefore, a **coupling gel** is applied to produce the best contact between the transducer and the body surface by eliminating air gaps.
- The body surface that is scanned may be **external, such** as in **transabdominal** sonography, **or internal,** such as in **transvaginal, transrectal, transesophageal,** and **endovascular** sonography.

> ## ⟫ IMPORTANT POINTS
>
> - The creation of a sonographic image *(sonogram)* depends on three major components: the production of **high-frequency sound waves**, the reception of a **reflected wave** or **echo,** and the conversion of that echo into the actual **image.**

- The sound wave is produced by the **probe** or **transducer,** which sends out extremely short bursts of acoustical energy at a given frequency.
- As with all sound waves, the pulses produced by the transducer travel at different speeds depending on the **density** of the medium through which they are traveling.
- Where the wave strikes an **interface** between tissues of **differing densities,** some of the sound wave will be **transmitted forward** while some will be **reflected back** to the transducer (Fig. 19.1).
- How much sound is transmitted versus how much is reflected depends on the property of the tissues that make up the interface and is called *acoustical impedance.* **Small differences** in acoustical impedance will result in **greater sound transmission; large differences** in acoustical impedance will result in **greater sound reflection.**

- For example, if the pulse encounters a gallstone, the acoustical impedance is **high** and most of the acoustical energy is **reflected** back. If the tissue that is encountered is extremely dense, such as bone, so much of the energy is reflected that there are not enough transmitted sound waves to define tissues deeper to the bone (see Fig. 19.1A).
- If a pulse traveling through soft tissue encounters fluid, the acoustical impedance (difference in densities) is relatively **low** and most of the acoustical energy is **transmitted** (see Fig. 19.1C).
- As the sound waves pass through tissue, their intensity decreases as they are absorbed by the tissue and converted into heat energy.

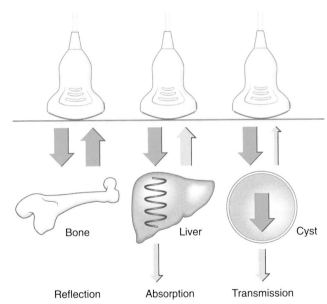

Fig. 19.1 Diagram of Three "Probes" on "Skin Surface." The amount of sound that is transmitted or reflected depends on the acoustic impedance of the tissues. (A) Large differences in acoustic impedance are encountered with bone and result in predominant **reflection** of the sound with little or no transmission. (B) As the sound passes through tissues, such as the liver, its intensity decreases as some of it is **absorbed** and transformed to heat while some may be transmitted. (C) Small differences in acoustic impedance such as encountered in a fluid-filled cyst result in predominant **transmission** of the sound.

Bone / Liver / Cyst labels and Reflection / Absorption / Transmission in figure.

19

- When the reflected echo arrives back at the transducer (a matter of microseconds), it is converted from **sound** into **electrical pulses** that are then sent to the scanner itself.
- Using an on-board computer, the scanner determines the **length of time** it took for the echo to be received, the **frequency** of the reflected echo, and the **magnitude (amplitude)** of the signal.
- With this information, a sonographic image of the scanned body part can be generated by the computer and displayed on the screen. The images may then be captured as **single, static images** or recorded as a **cine loop**, which is composed of a set of images that can be played as a video. Both this chapter and the next incorporate numerous cine loops of US studies that can be viewed online by registered users of this text.

Echogenicity

- The **echogenicity (brightness or darkness)** of a tissue on US is determined by the amount of sound waves the tissue transmits or reflects.

▶▶ IMPORTANT POINTS

- A tissue that **reflects more** echoes is depicted **brighter or whiter** on the sonogram; it is called **echogenic (hyperechoic)**.
- A tissue that **transmits more** echoes (resulting in less echoes reflected back to the transducer) is depicted **darker** on the image; it is called **sonolucent (hypoechoic)**.
- A tissue that essentially transmits **all** the echoes is depicted as **black** on the sonogram; it is called **anechoic**.
- When a very dense structure, such as a gallstone or bone, reflects so many echoes that virtually no sound waves are transmitted, the tissue deeper to this structure is displayed as hypoechoic and this phenomenon is called **posterior acoustic shadowing**.
- When a structure transmits more echoes than the surrounding tissues, such as a cyst in the liver might, the sound waves deeper to this structure (compared with surrounding structures) are depicted as hyperechoic and this phenomenon is called **posterior acoustic enhancement**.

- The typical appearances of different types of commonly encountered tissues and structures are described in Table 19.1.

Imaging Planes

- Images can be produced in any plane of the body by adjusting the direction of the probe. By convention, two common imaging planes are used.
  - The **sagittal or longitudinal plane** is obtained along the **long axis** of the body or body part being scanned and is **viewed** with the **patient's head toward the left** and **feet toward the right**. The **upper part** of the image is more **superficial or closer to the transducer** and the **lower part** of the image is **deeper and farther from the probe** (Fig. 19.2A).
  - The **transverse plane** is obtained **perpendicular to the long axis** of the body or body part being scanned and is conventionally viewed with the patient's right on your left side and the patient's left on your right side (Fig. 19.2B).

TABLE 19.1	Appearance of Commonly Encountered Tissues on Ultrasound	
Tissue	**Appearance**	**Examples**
Fluid	Hypoechoic or anechoic, depending whether the fluid is **simple** or **complex** (containing debris, pus, or blood); may have **posterior acoustic enhancement**	Cysts, abscesses, gallbladder, urinary bladder, spinal fluid, blood in vessels
Calcium	Hyperechoic; may have **posterior acoustic shadowing**	Gallstones, renal stones, bones, calcifications in soft tissue
Air	Hyperechoic foci; may cause **posterior acoustic shadowing**	Gas-forming infections (abscesses, Fournier's gangrene, endometritis), intraperitoneal air, necrotizing enterocolitis, portal venous gas, pneumobilia

Fig. 19.2 Sagittal and Transverse US Images of the Right Kidney. (A) The sagittal plane is along the long-axis of the body or long-axis of the body part being scanned and is viewed with the patient's head toward the left and feet toward the right. (B) The transverse plane is perpendicular to the sagittal plane and is typically viewed with the patient's right side on the left of the image and the patient's left side on the right of the image, just as most radiologic images are. In both planes, the **upper** part of the image is more **superficial** and closer to the transducer probe and the **lower** part of the image is **deeper** and farther from the probe. Throughout the next two chapters, many figures will have one or more of the following abbreviations to help your orientation: Ant, anterior; F, foot of the patient; H, head of the patient; L, left; Post, posterior; R, right.

Frequency and Resolution

- The **frequency of the soundwaves** used in any given US study plays an integral role in the **resolution** of the US images.
  - **Higher frequencies** result in **higher resolution** images and **more detail.** However, the higher the frequency, the shorter the penetration distance. Therefore, although higher frequencies will provide more detail, they cannot display deeper tissues because of their shorter penetration.
- US transducers are designed to produce inherently different frequencies of sound waves, usually labeled on the probe. Choosing the proper transducer for the type of study is important in order to provide as much **detail** as possible while providing enough **penetration** to reach the desired tissue.
- In general, higher frequency transducers are appropriate for superficial structures or those that require fine detail and lower frequency transducers are appropriate for deep structures.
- Several types of US are used in medical imaging. They are described in Table 19.2.

TYPES OF ULTRASOUND

TABLE 19.2	Types of Ultrasound
A-Mode	Simplest; spikes along a line represent the signal amplitude at a certain depth; used mainly in ophthalmology.
B-Mode	Mode most often used in diagnostic imaging; each echo is depicted as a dot and the **sonogram** is made up of thousands of these dots; can depict real-time motion.
M-Mode	Used to show moving structures, such as blood flow or motion of the heart valves
Doppler	Uses the Doppler effect to assess blood flow; used for vascular US. **Pulsed Doppler** devices emit short bursts of energy that allow for an accurate localization of the echo source.
Duplex ultrasonography	Used in vascular studies; refers to the simultaneous use of both gray-scale (or color Doppler) to visualize the structure of, and flow within, a vessel and spectral (waveform) Doppler to quantitate flow (eVideo 19.1).

Doppler Ultrasonography

- You are probably familiar with the common examples of the **Doppler effect** illustrated by a passing train whistle or police siren. The effect generally states that sound **changes in frequency** as the object producing the sound **approaches** or **recedes** from your ear (eAudio 19.2).
- Sonography makes use of the Doppler effect to determine if an object, usually blood, is **moving toward** or **away** from the transducer and at what velocity it is moving. Here is how it works:
  - The transducer sends out a signal of **known frequency;** the frequency of the echo returned is **compared** with the frequency of the original signal.

TABLE 19.3	Advantages and Disadvantages of Ultrasonography	
Advantages	**Disadvantages**
No ionizing radiation	Difficulty penetrating through bone
No known long-term side effects	Gas-filled structures reduce its utility
"Real-time" images	Obese patients may be difficult to penetrate
Produces little or no patient discomfort	Dependent on the skills of the operator scanning
Small, portable, inexpensive, ubiquitous	

- If the returning echo has a **lower frequency** than the original, then the object is **moving away** from the transducer. If the returning echo has a **higher frequency** than the original, then the object is **moving toward** the transducer.

> ## IMPORTANT POINTS
>
> - The **direction of flow** is represented by the colors red and blue. By convention, **red indicates flow toward** and **blue indicates flow away** from the transducer.

ADVERSE EFFECTS OR SAFETY ISSUES

- US procedures are **well-tolerated.** Scans can be obtained relatively quickly, done at the bedside if necessary and, for the most part, require no patient preparation other than abstinence from food before abdominal studies.
- US has the short-term potential of causing **minor elevation of heat** in the area being scanned, although not at levels used in diagnostic imaging.
- **No known long-term side effects** have been scientifically demonstrated from the use of medical US in humans. Nevertheless, like all medical procedures, it should be used only when medically necessary. The United States Food and Drug Administration warns against the use of US during pregnancy to produce "keepsake photos or videos."
- The **advantages of US** over CT and conventional angiography include the **lack of ionizing radiation, lack of intravenous iodinated contrast, and portability** (Table 19.3).

MEDICAL USES OF ULTRASONOGRAPHY

- We will look at several common abnormalities in which US plays a primary imaging role.

Biliary System

- US is the **study of first choice** for abnormalities of the biliary system. Patients who present with the relatively common complaint of right upper quadrant abdominal pain usually undergo an US examination as their first imaging study. CT may be helpful in cases with difficult or unusual anatomy, for detecting masses, or in determining the extent of disease already diagnosed, but **CT is less sensitive than US in detecting gallstones.**

Fig. 19.3 Normal Gallbladder, Sagittal View. The gallbladder (GB) is normally filled with bile and is sonolucent. The wall of the gallbladder is >3 mm in size and slightly echogenic (*white arrow*). *Ant,* Anterior; *F,* foot; *H,* head; *Post,* posterior.

Fig. 19.4 Gallstones and Posterior Acoustical Shadowing. Multiple echogenic stones (*dotted arrows*) are seen in the gallbladder (GB). The gallstones reflect most of the sound waves back toward the transducer. The paucity of sound waves that penetrate the stones results in **posterior acoustic shadowing** (*solid white arrow*), which is helpful in the diagnosis of gallstones.

Normal Gallbladder Anatomy: Ultrasound

- The **gallbladder** is an elliptical sac that lies between the right and left lobes of the liver in the interlobar fissure. Although different layers of its wall have different echogenic properties, the gallbladder overall consists of a **fluid-filled sonolucent lumen** surrounded by an **echogenic wall**. In the fasting patient, the gallbladder is about **4 × 10 cm in size** and the **wall** is normally **no thicker than 3 mm** (Fig. 19.3).

Gallstones and Acute Cholecystitis

- **Cholelithiasis** is estimated to affect more than 20 million people in the United States. In almost all cases, acute cholecystitis starts with a **gallstone impacted in the neck of the gallbladder or cystic duct.** The presence of gallstones does not, by itself, mean that the source of a patient's pain is the gallbladder because asymptomatic gallstones are common. Cholecystitis can also occur, although less commonly, in the absence of stones (**acalculous cholecystitis**).
- Because of the force of gravity, **gallstones usually fall to the most dependent part of the gallbladder,** which will be influenced by the patient's position at the time of the scan. This helps to differentiate gallstones from polyps or tumors that may be attached to a nondependent surface. Gallstones are characteristically **echogenic** and produce **posterior acoustical shadowing** (Fig. 19.4).
- **Biliary sludge** can be found in the lumen of the gallbladder and is an aggregation that may contain cholesterol crystals, bilirubin, and glycoproteins. It is often associated with biliary stasis. Although it may be echogenic, **sludge does not produce acoustical shadowing** as gallstones do (Fig. 19.5). Sludge layers along the dependent gallbladder wall or may appear as a rounded, mobile "mass," which is called *tumefactive sludge.*

Fig. 19.5 Sludge in the Gallbladder. Sludge (*white arrow*) in the gallbladder (GB) is associated with biliary stasis. Although it may be echogenic, sludge **does not** produce acoustical shadowing as do gallstones (the **absence** of shadowing is shown by black arrow).

> ## IMPORTANT POINTS

- **Recognizing acute cholecystitis on US:**
  - **Thickening of the gallbladder wall** (>3 mm) (Fig. 19.6A)
  - **Pericholecystic fluid** (fluid around the gallbladder) (Fig. 19.6B)
  - A **positive sonographic Murphy sign** (i.e., pain that is elicited by the compression of the gallbladder with the US probe).

Fig. 19.6 Acute Cholecystitis, Sagittal Views, Two Patients. (A) There is thickening of gallbladder (GB) wall (*white arrows*). The wall is normally 3 mm or less. This wall is markedly thickened at 6 mm. (B) An echo-free crescent (dotted white arrow) surrounds a thickened gallbladder (GB) wall representing pericholecystic fluid. The patient had a **positive sonographic Murphy's sign.**

- If gallstones are present (see Fig. 19.4) in addition to these features, the diagnosis of **acute calculous cholecystitis** can be made. In the presence of gallstones and gallbladder wall thickening, US has a positive predictive value for acute cholecystitis as high as 94%.
- If these features exist in the absence of gallstones, the patient may have **acalculous cholecystitis**, which typically tends to occur in critically ill patients.
- Radionuclide scans (**hepatoiminodiacetic acid [HIDA] scans**) are also used in the diagnosis of acute cholecystitis.
  - Hepatoiminodiacetic acid, which is physiologically absorbed by the liver and excreted into the biliary system, is tagged with a radioactive tracer (**technetium-99m**) and injected intravenously. The tagged HIDA can then be imaged with a special camera to demonstrate its normal physiologic uptake by the liver and subsequent excretion into the bile ducts, gallbladder, and small intestine.
  - In patients with **obstruction of the cystic duct,** the tracer will **not appear** in the **gallbladder;** in patients with **obstruction of the common bile duct,** the tracer will **not appear** in the **small intestine.** Either finding is typically caused by an obstructing stone (Fig. 19.7).

Normal Bile Duct Anatomy: Ultrasound

- **US plays a key role in the evaluation of the intrahepatic and extrahepatic bile ducts and the pancreatic duct.** The intrahepatic biliary radicals drain into the left and right hepatic ducts, which join to form the common hepatic duct (CHD). The common bile duct (CBD) begins where the cystic duct from the gallbladder joins with the CHD. It drains into the

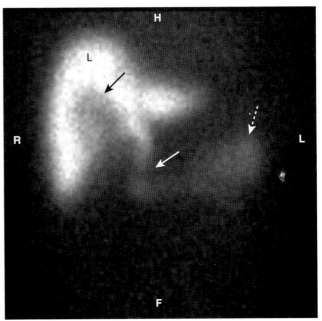

Fig. 19.7 HIDA Scan in Cystic Duct Obstruction. HIDA, a radioactive labeled isotope, concentrates in the liver (L) and is then excreted into the biliary ducts. On this delayed image, the common bile duct (solid white arrow) and small bowel (*dotted white arrow*) fill normally because the common bile duct is patent. The cystic duct and gallbladder do not fill, however, because the cystic duct is obstructed, by a stone in this case. There is a tracer-free (photopenic) area in the gallbladder fossa because the nuclide cannot fill the gallbladder lumen, as it normally would with a patent cystic duct (*solid black arrow*). *HIDA,* Hepatoiminodiacetic acid.

second portion of the duodenum, either within or adjacent to the head of the pancreas, via the ampulla of Vater.

- **The CBD lies anterior to the portal vein and lateral to the hepatic artery in the porta hepatis** (Fig. 19.8A).
- The CHD and proximal CBD can be visualized on virtually all US studies of the right upper quadrant. The **CHD** measures **no more than 4 mm** (inner wall to inner wall) in diameter, and the **CBD** measures **no more than 6 mm** in diameter (Fig. 19.8B). The **pancreatic duct** measures **less than 2 mm.**
- Normally, the **intrahepatic bile ducts** are **not visible** on US. However, they may become dilated over time when there is prolonged CBD obstruction. Dilated intrahepatic ducts appear as additional, tubular sonolucent structures adjacent

to the portal veins that results in a **"tram-track"** appearance (Fig. 19.9).
- **Causes of bile duct obstruction** include gallstones, pancreatic carcinoma, strictures, sclerosing cholangitis, cholangiocarcinoma, and metastatic disease.

Urinary Tract
Normal Renal Anatomy: Ultrasound
- The kidneys normally measure **9 to 12 cm in length, 4 to 5 cm in width, and 3 to 4 cm in thickness.** The **renal sinus** is home to the renal pelvis and the major branches of the renal artery and vein. Because the renal sinus contains fat, it normally appears **brightly echogenic.** The **calyces** are

Fig. 19.8 Normal Common Bile Duct, Portal Vein, and Hepatic Artery: Illustration and Sagittal view. (A) The illustration demonstrates the normal relationships of some of the structures in the porta hepatis. (B) A sagittal view of the right upper quadrant shows the **common bile duct (CBD),** which measures 3 mm (normal <6 mm). The white arrow points to the **hepatic artery (HA),** seen on end. The **portal vein (PV)** is posterior to the common duct and the **inferior vena cava (IVC)** is seen posterior to the portal vein. The pancreas (P) is anterior to the CBD. *CD,* Common duct; *CHD,* common hepatic duct.

Fig. 19.9 Dilated Intrahepatic and Extrahepatic Ducts in Two different Patients: Sagittal Images. (A) The intrahepatic biliary ducts are normally not visible by US. In this case, they are dilated (*white arrow*) from obstruction by a pancreatic carcinoma (not shown). (B) The CBD is dilated at 15 mm (*dotted white arrows*), and the gallbladder (GB) is distended from an obstructing stone (not shown). *CBD,* Common bile duct; *L,* liver.

Fig. 19.10 Normal Right Kidney: Longitudinal. The renal sinus (S) is home to the renal pelvis and the major branches of the renal artery and vein. Because the renal sinus contains fat, it normally appears brightly echogenic. The normal renal pelvis is not visible in the renal sinus. The renal parenchyma (*white arrow*) has uniformly low echogenicity and is usually **less echogenic than the adjacent liver (L) or spleen**.

Fig. 19.11 Hydronephrosis: Sagittal View, Right Kidney. The renal sinus contains a markedly dilated, fluid-filled and anechoic renal pelvis (P) in this patient with hydronephrosis. The renal parenchyma remains normal in size and echogenicity (*dotted white arrows*). The patient had an obstructing stone at the ureteropelvic junction.

normally not visible. The **pyramids** are **hypoechoic.** The **renal parenchyma** has **uniformly low echogenicity,** which is usually **less** than that of the **adjacent liver and spleen** (Fig. 19.10).

- Renal masses are discussed in **Chapter 18.**

Hydronephrosis

- **Hydronephrosis** is defined as **dilatation of the renal pelvis and calyces.** Renal pelvis dilatation by itself is called **pelviectasis** and calyceal dilatation alone is called **caliectasis.**

✳ IMAGE-GUIDED INTERVENTION

This is a 75-year-old female with flank pain and hematuria with obstructive hydronephrosis (*solid arrow*) whose noncontrast CT also shows renal calculi (*dotted arrows*). How might an image-guided procedure benefit in this case? See the answer in Chapter 29.

- In patients experiencing **renal colic,** US is used primarily to evaluate for the **presence of hydronephrosis.** Because the ureters may be difficult to visualize on US, "stone searches" are usually carried out by CT scanning (see Fig. 17.07).
- However, in the hands of an experienced sonographer, even stones in the ureter can often be found, eliminating the additional expense and radiation associated with a CT scan.

▷▷ IMPORTANT POINTS

- The typical appearance of obstructive uropathy is a **dilated calyceal system.** The echogenic renal sinus contains a **dilated, fluid-filled, and therefore anechoic renal pelvis.**
- The **ureter** may be **dilated** to the level of the obstructing stone.
- Severe hydronephrosis may distort the appearance of the kidney (Fig. 19.11).

Medical Renal Disease

- **Medical renal disease** refers to a host of diseases that primarily affect the **renal parenchyma.** They include such diseases as glomerulonephritis, diseases that cause the nephrotic syndrome, and renal involvement in collagen vascular diseases.
- In the early stages of medical renal disease, the kidneys may appear normal on US. As the disease advances, the **renal parenchyma becomes more echogenic (brighter) than the liver and spleen,** the reverse of the normal echo pattern. However, these changes usually cannot differentiate between the numerous causes of medical renal disease. A biopsy with

US guidance may be performed to determine the etiology of the disease (Fig. 19.12).

- **Renal size** may be a helpful indicator of disease chronicity; when associated with abnormal renal parenchymal echotexture, **renal sizes smaller than normal indicate more chronic disease.**

Urinary Bladder

- As a fluid-filled structure, the urinary bladder lends itself well to US evaluation. US of a fluid-distended bladder can be used to assess bladder wall thickness and the presence of bladder **tumors, stones, and diverticula.** The **post void residual bladder volume** can also be estimated, which is helpful in the assessment of **urinary incontinence, bladder outlet obstruction, and in patients with a neurogenic bladder** (Fig. 19.13).

- A full, fluid-filled bladder is also used as an **acoustic window** to avoid image-degrading, air-filled bowel to assess the prostate in men and pelvic structures in women.

Scrotal Ultrasound

- Differential diagnosis of **acute scrotal pain** includes epididymitis, orchitis, testicular torsion, testicular trauma, and herniation of abdominal contents into the scrotum. Prompt intervention is required in cases of testicular torsion and trauma to salvage the affected testis.

- **Testicular torsion**, which usually occurs in adolescents, is an especially important diagnosis because **timely detorsion is curative**, whereas a missed torsion can result in loss of the testicle. **Color Doppler US** (which can reveal scrotal blood flow) is used in the assessment of suspected torsion; there is usually **no flow in the torsed testis** (Fig. 19.14). Adjacent to

Fig. 19.12 Chronic Medical Renal Disease: Sagittal View. The right kidney (K) is small, measuring 6× 3 cm (cursor marks). The renal parenchyma (*black arrow*) is more echogenic (brighter) than the adjacent liver (L), the reverse of the normal echo pattern. This patient had chronic glomerulonephritis from long-standing diabetes.

Fig. 19.13 Bladder Tumor. This is a sagittal US image of the urinary bladder (B) that demonstrates a large, polypoid mass arising from the anterior bladder wall (*white arrows*). A bladder stone would unlikely come to rest on the nondependent surface of the bladder. On biopsy, this was a transitional cell carcinoma, which comprise 90% of bladder tumors.

Fig. 19.14 Scrotal US: Torsion of the Left Testicle. Color Doppler images of both testicles were obtained. (A) The right testicle (*black arrow*) demonstrates normal blood flow (*white arrows*). (B) The torsed left testicle is enlarged and demonstrates no blood flow because of the vessels leading into the testicle are occluded by the torsion (*dotted arrow*).

Fig. 19.15 Abdominal Aortic Aneurysm: Sagittal View. This fusiform dilatation of the abdominal aorta (Ao) measures 4.9 cm between marks (*dotted white arrows*). There is hypoechoic thrombus in the aneurysm (*solid black and white arrows*). For aneurysms 4 to 5 cm in diameter, the risk of rupture increases to almost 25%.

✳ IMAGE-GUIDED INTERVENTION

The image is from a contrast-enhanced, sagittal CT angiogram of the abdomen and pelvis in an 80-year-old male with a pulsatile abdominal mass (*dotted arrow*) that measures 6 cm. How might an image-guided procedure benefit in this case? See the answer in Chapter 29.

the testicle, identification of a twisted vascular pedicle (which has a swirling appearance) *(whirlpool sign)* confirms the diagnosis (eVideo 19.3).

Abdominal Aortic Aneurysms

- An **aneurysm** is defined as a localized dilation of an artery by **50% or more above its normal size.** Most aortic aneurysms occur in the abdominal aorta **inferior to the origin of the renal arteries and frequently extend into one or both common iliac arteries.**
- Most aortic aneurysms are either **fusiform** in shape or produce uniform dilatation of the entire vessel.

> ### ▶▶ IMPORTANT POINTS
>
> - The **abdominal aorta normally measures no more than 3 cm in diameter** (outer wall to outer wall).

- The **size** of an aneurysm is directly related to its **risk of rupture.** For aneurysms **less than 4 cm** in diameter, there is a **less than 10% chance** of rupture; aneurysms **4 to 5 cm** in diameter have almost a **25% risk of rupture.**
- **Recognizing an abdominal aortic aneurysm:**
  - US is the **screening study of choice** when there is an asymptomatic, **pulsatile abdominal mass.**
  - **Moving blood** within the lumen of the aorta will appear **anechoic; thrombus** in the wall of the aneurysm will appear **echogenic** (Fig. 19.15).

- Unenhanced CT has the advantage of depicting the absolute size of the aneurysm, but to define the extent of mural thrombus and the presence of dissection, intravenous contrast must be used.

FEMALE PELVIC ORGANS

- **US is the imaging study of choice in evaluating a pelvic mass or pelvic pain in the female patient. Leiomyomas** confined to the myometrium are the most common tumors of the uterus. **Endometrial carcinomas** are usually confined to the uterus at the time of discovery. The most common mass in the ovary is a **functional cyst.** In general, **uterine masses** are **solid** and **ovarian masses** are **cystic.**

Normal Uterine Anatomy: Ultrasound

- The uterus is made up of a thick muscular layer (**myometrium**) and a mucous surface (**endometrium**). It is divided into a **body** (with **cornu** to receive the **fallopian tubes**) and the **cervix.** Anterior to the uterus is the peritoneal space called the **anterior cul-de-sac.** The **posterior cul-de-sac** is also called the **rectouterine recess.**
- The position of the uterus in the body is described by its *version* (i.e., the angle of the cervix relative to the vagina) and *flexion* (i.e., the angle of the uterine body relative to

the cervix). These relationships are shown in Fig. 19.16. **Usually, the uterus is anteverted and anteflexed**

- In the adult, the uterus has a **pear-shape** with maximum dimensions of approximately **8 cm in length, 5 cm in width, and 4 cm in the anteroposterior dimension.** The size of the normal uterus increases with multiparity; with aging, the uterus decreases in size (Fig. 19.17).
- The **normal endometrial cavity** is in a collapsed state, forming a **thin, echogenic stripe or line** between the apposing surfaces of the endometrium. By convention, the endometrial thickness is measured by including both walls on a sagittal view of the mid-uterus. The appearance of both the endometrium and the ovaries varies, depending on the phase of the menstrual cycle.
- Normal **fallopian tubes** are collapsed and not usually visualized on US.

- The standard **transabdominal (through the abdominal wall)** study of the uterus is done with a **full urinary bladder.** The full bladder provides an **acoustical window** to the uterus by pushing bowel loops upward out of the pelvis and it helps to delineate the bladder itself.
- **Transvaginal** studies are done with higher frequency probes and thus provide better resolution images. They are done with the **bladder empty.** Transabdominal and transvaginal studies are considered complementary techniques.
- **Sonohysterography** is a procedure in which saline is instilled in the endometrial cavity while transvaginal US images are obtained. The saline distends the normally collapsed endometrial cavity and separates the endometrial walls to allow the delineation of **endometrial polyps, submucosal myomas, and adhesions** (eVideo 19.4).

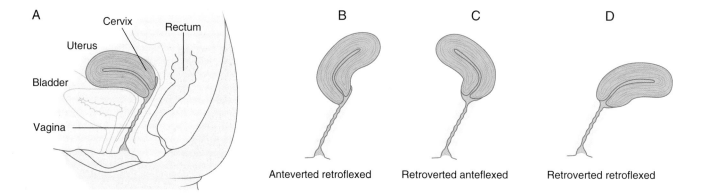

Anteverted retroflexed   Retroverted anteflexed   Retroverted retroflexed

Anteverted anteflexed

Fig. 19.16 Normal Variations in Uterine Position. The position of the uterus in the body is described by its **version** (i.e., the angle of the cervix relative to the **vagina**) and **flexion** (i.e., the angle of the **uterine body** relative to the **cervix**). Anteversion (A and B) occurs when the cervix is angled anteriorly relative to the vagina. Anteflexion (A and C) occurs when the uterine body is angled anteriorly relative to the cervix. In retroversion (C and D) and retroflexion (B and D), the cervix and body are angled posteriorly relative to the vagina and cervix, respectively. **Usually, the uterus is anteverted and anteflexed** as in (A).

Fig. 19.17 Normal Uterus: Longitudinal (A) and Transverse (B). (A) The uterus is shown in the longitudinal plane (*solid white arrows*). The endometrium lines the uterine cavity and would be measured in a longitudinal view, such as this (*black arrows*). (B) In the transverse plane, the uterus has a rounded appearance (*solid white arrows*). The collapsed uterine cavity is within the center and is visualized as a thin, echogenic line (*dotted white arrow*).

Uterine Leiomyomas (Fibroids)

- **Leiomyomas** are **benign smooth muscle tumors** of the uterus that occur in up to 50% of women over the age of 30. Most women with fibroids are asymptomatic. When symptoms occur, it is usually because of the size of the fibroid and can include pain, infertility, menorrhagia, and urinary and bowel symptoms.
- **Pelvic US is the imaging study of choice in evaluating uterine fibroids.** Magnetic resonance imaging (MRI) may be used to evaluate complicated cases or in surgical planning.
- **Recognizing uterine leiomyomas on US:**

⟫ IMPORTANT POINTS

- They are **heterogeneously hypoechoic, solid masses,** meaning they may display areas of varying echogenicity (brightness or darkness) (Fig. 19.18).
- Fibroids may undergo **degeneration** and **calcify.** These calcifications may reflect enough sound to produce **acoustical shadowing.** Fibroid degeneration may also manifest as cystic or fatty components.

- **Recognizing uterine leiomyomas on CT scans:**
  - Fibroids typically appear as **rounded, lobulated soft-tissue uterine masses.** They may contain **amorphous or popcorn calcifications,** indicating degeneration, or they may undergo central necrosis, which manifests as low-attenuation areas (see Fig. 17.11).
  - Although fibroids are frequently visualized on CT scans, their extent may be more difficult to assess on CT than on US or MRI because they have a similar density to normal uterine myometrium and endometrium.
- The **location** of fibroids is important to aid in treatment planning (either surgical or interventional). Fibroids can be characterized as **submucosal** (which has implications for

bleeding and infertility), **myometrial** (most common), or **subserosal.** When subserosal fibroids are attached to the uterus by a stalk of tissue, they are characterized as **pedunculated.**

Adenomyosis

- **Adenomyosis** refers to **ectopic endometrial tissue within the myometrium.** It usually occurs in women 35 to 50 years of age and may be the cause of **dysmenorrhea** and **menorrhagia.** It can be associated with ectopic endometrial tissue **outside** of the uterus (i.e., **endometriosis**). Symptoms will usually abate after menopause.
- The findings of adenomyosis are shown in Fig. 19.19.

✳ IMAGE-GUIDED INTERVENTION

The image is from a postcontrast MRI of the pelvis in a 44-year-old female with pain and menorrhagia. The arrows point to large uterine fibroids. How might an image-guided procedure benefit in this case? See the answer in Chapter 29.

Fig. 19.18 Leiomyoma of the Uterus: Sagittal View. A heterogeneously hypoechoic mass (*solid white arrows*) is seen in the uterus (U). Uterine leiomyomas may display some areas that contain many echoes and others that demonstrate few echoes. They frequently absorb enough sound to produce acoustical shadowing (*dotted white arrow*).

Fig. 19.19 Adenomyosis of the Uterus. This sagittal, transvaginal image of the uterus demonstrates some sonographic findings of adenomyosis, including a markedly thickened myometrium (*double white arrows*) and a myometrial cyst (*dotted white arrow*). Other findings of adenomyosis include a globular uterine shape, a heterogenous myometrial echotexture, and asymmetric uterine wall thickening (more often posterior wall). *A,* Anterior; *P,* posterior.

Normal Ovarian Anatomy/Physiology: Ultrasound

- US is the **imaging study of choice** for evaluating the **ovaries.**
- In **premenopausal women,** the ovaries are approximately **2 × 3 × 4 cm in size** (≈ 5 to 15 mL in volume), frequently containing **cystic follicles.** The ovaries atrophy after menopause (Fig. 19.20).
- The normal ovary changes in appearance not only with age, but also with the phases of each menstrual cycle. Under normal hormonal stimulation, one, egg-containing **follicle** becomes **dominant** and attains a size of about 2.5 cm at the time of ovulation (Fig. 19.21).

Ovarian Cysts

- The **majority** of ovarian cysts in **premenopausal women** are **functional cysts,** which include **follicular cysts** and **corpus luteal cysts.** These cysts occur as a result of the hormonal stimuli associated with ovulation and usually involute within one or two menstrual cycles.
- A **follicular cyst** forms when a nondominant follicle fills with fluid and does not rupture.
- A **corpus luteum** forms after an egg is expunged from a dominant ovarian follicle. If the corpus luteum fills with fluid, it then becomes a **corpus luteal cyst.**

▶ IMPORTANT POINTS

- **Functional cysts** are characteristically **well-defined, thin-walled, anechoic** structures with **homogenous internal fluid echogenicity** (Fig. 19.22). These cysts are **physiologic** and **do not require follow-up** or other imaging in the asymptomatic patient. Occasionally, a functional cyst may contain blood, which will appear as lacy reticular echoes (Fig. 19.23).

Fig. 19.22 Simple Ovarian Cyst: Sagittal View. Contained within the left ovary (*white arrows*) is a well-defined, thin-walled, anechoic structure representing a simple ovarian cyst (C). Ovarian cysts may contain echogenic material if hemorrhage occurs into the cyst.

Fig. 19.20 Normal Right Ovary, Sagittal View. In premenopausal women, the ovary is approximately 2 × 3 × 4 cm in size (*white arrows*), usually containing small cystic follicles (C) as shown here.

Fig. 19.21 Dominant Follicle Ruptures During Scan. Under normal hormonal stimulation, one egg-containing follicle becomes dominant and attains a size of about 2.5 cm at the time of ovulation. (A) The dominant follicle is 3.3 × 2.8 cm at the start of the study (*white arrow*). (B) A few minutes later, **during the study**, the follicle ruptures (ovulation occurs) and the follicle shrinks dramatically in size (*solid white arrow*). A small, physiologic amount of free fluid appears in the peritoneal cavity (*dashed white arrow*).

Fig. 19.23 Hemorrhagic Ovarian Cyst. Sagittal US image of the left ovary (Ov) demonstrates a cystic mass containing lacy reticular echoes (*white arrow*) consistent with a hemorrhagic cyst.

Fig. 19.25 Ovarian Dermoid Cyst. A large, solid echogenic mass (*solid white arrows*) is seen in the right ovary (O) with acoustical shadowing (*dotted white arrow*). Dermoid cysts, also called teratomas, are almost always benign.

Fig. 19.24 Polycystic Ovarian Disease. Polycystic Ovarian Disease is an endocrine abnormality that allows for numerous ovarian follicles to develop in various stages of hormonal growth and atresia. This ovary is enlarged (*white arrows*) and contains multiple peripheral cysts, some of which are labeled (C). When associated with oligomenorrhea, hirsutism, and obesity, polycystic ovarian disease is called the **Stein-Leventhal syndrome**.

Fig. 19.26 Endometrioma. Transverse US image of the right ovary demonstrates a cystic mass containing diffuse, low-level echoes creating a **"snow-storm"** appearance that is typical of an endometrioma (*white arrow*).

- **Polycystic ovarian disease** is an endocrine abnormality that allows for numerous ovarian follicles (>25/ovary) to develop in various stages of hormonal growth and atresia. When associated with **oligomenorrhea, hirsutism, and obesity,** the constellation is called the **Stein-Leventhal syndrome** (Fig. 19.24).
- **Nonfunctional cystic lesions** of the ovary include **dermoid cysts** and **endometriomas.** A specific diagnosis can usually be made with US.
  - **Dermoid cysts** are **mature teratomas** composed of cells from all three germ layers that can produce hair, bone, teeth, and fat in the cyst. They are most commonly found in **women of reproductive age,** are **bilateral** in up to 25% of cases, and may serve as a lead point for **ovarian torsion** (Fig. 19.25).
- **Endometriomas,** part of the disease **endometriosis,** are cystic ovarian lesions, sometimes called **"chocolate cysts"** because they are filled with brownish-red blood. They are frequently bilateral. Endometriomas can become large and multilocular (Fig. 19.26).

Fig. 19.27 Ovarian Tumor: US and CT. (A) A transverse scan through the right adnexa demonstrates a large, solid ovarian mass (*solid white arrows*). (B) CT of the same patient shows this large, heterogeneous mass arising from the right adnexa (*solid black arrow*). A small amount of ascites is seen (*dotted white arrow*). This patient had a fibroma of the ovary, a tumor sometimes associated with ascites and pleural effusion (**Meig syndrome**).

Ovarian Tumors

- **Most ovarian tumors are cystic;** they arise from the **surface epithelium** that covers the ovary and include **serous or mucinous tumors.** The **majority** of serous tumors (**serous cystadenomas**) and the overwhelming number of mucinous tumors (**mucinous cystadenomas**) are **benign.** Malignant tumors are designated **serous or mucinous adenocarcinomas. Staging** of ovarian cancer is best done with **CT or MRI.**

> ## ⟫ IMPORTANT POINTS
>
> - In contrast to benign ovarian cysts, features of **malignant ovarian cysts** include **thick and irregular walls, thick and irregular septations, internal vascular flow,** and **solid papillary projections in the tumors** (Fig. 19.27).

Ovarian Torsion

- Like testicular torsion, **ovarian torsion is a surgical emergency** and its timely diagnosis and treatment is essential to prevent loss of the ovary. The typical presentation is the **acute onset of excruciating adnexal pain.**
- Unlike testicular torsion, the **diagnosis of ovarian torsion** largely depends on the **morphologic appearance of the ovary.** The torsed ovary will appear **asymmetrically enlarged** and may have **increased stromal echogenicity** (Fig. 19.28).

Pelvic Inflammatory Disease

- Pelvic inflammatory disease (PID) is a term used to describe a group of **infections affecting the uterus, fallopian tubes, and ovaries.** Most cases of PID **begin** as a **transient endometritis** and **ascend** to infection of the tubes and ovaries. Patients can have **pain, vaginal discharge, adnexal tenderness, fever,** and **elevated white blood cell counts.** Complications include infertility, chronic pain, or ectopic pregnancy.

Fig. 19.28 Ovarian Torsion. Sagittal US image of a markedly enlarged right ovary which contains several cysts (*white arrows*) and has an echogenic central stroma (*asterisk*). In the setting of severe right pelvic pain, these findings are diagnostic of ovarian torsion, even if color and spectral Doppler flow can still be demonstrated in the ovary.

> ## ⟫ IMPORTANT POINTS
>
> - **Recognizing PID on US:**
>   - The **ovaries are enlarged** with **multiple cysts** and periovarian inflammation.
>   - The fallopian tubes may be **fluid-filled** and **dilated (pyosalpinx)** (Fig. 19.29A).
>   - There may be **fusion of the dilated fallopian tube and ovary (tubo-ovarian complex)** (Fig. 19.29B).
>   - A **multiloculated mass** with septations (**tubo-ovarian abscess**) may be present.
> - CT can be used for cases of complicated PID or for patients whose history may not suggest the diagnosis.

Fig. 19.29 Pelvic Inflammatory Disease, Longitudinal and Transverse Views: US. (A) There is a fluid-filled and dilated fallopian tube (FT) containing pus and debris (*solid black arrow*) representing a pyosalpinx. (B) Because of progressive inflammation, there is fusion of a dilated and tortuous fallopian tube (*solid black arrow*) and the adjacent ovary (*solid white arrow*) producing a **tubo-ovarian complex**.

BOX 19.1 **Uses of Ultrasound During Pregnancy**

- Fetal presence and gestational age
- Fetal abnormalities and viability
- The presence of multiple pregnancies
- Placental localization
- Amniotic fluid volume
- Intrauterine growth retardation
- Helping guide invasive studies, such as amniocentesis, chorionic villus sampling and intrauterine transfusions

---

PREGNANCY

- US has provided a **safe and reliable** means of visualizing the fetus in utero and the ability to do so repeatedly during the course of a pregnancy, if necessary. The overwhelming majority of pregnant women in North America and Western Europe undergo at least one US evaluation sometime during pregnancy.
- Even before pregnancy, US can be used to determine ovulation time to aid in the process of successful fertilization.
- The uses of US during pregnancy are outlined in Box 19.1.
- The goals of sonography during pregnancy may differ, depending on the timing of the scan.
  - During the **first trimester**, goals are to exclude an ectopic pregnancy, estimate the age of the pregnancy, to determine viability and the number of embryos.
  - During the **second and third trimesters**, goals may include estimates of amniotic fluid volume, detection of fetal anomalies, determination of placental and fetal positioning, or guidance for invasive studies to determine the likelihood of fetal viability in the event of a premature birth (eVideo 19.5).
- We will look at three important uses of US during pregnancy.

Ectopic Pregnancy

- Most ectopic pregnancies are **tubal in location** and occur near the **fimbriated (ovarian) end**. The classical clinical findings of **pain, abnormal vaginal bleeding, and a palpable adnexal mass** occur in only about half of cases. The incidence

Fig. 19.30 Early Intrauterine Pregnancy. A single, live intrauterine pregnancy (*white arrows*) is contained within the gestational sac (*solid black arrow*) inside the uterus (U). With a measurement called the crown-rump length (between the white arrows), the embryo was estimated at 9 weeks of age. Sonographic gestational age begins on the **first day** of the **last normal menstrual cycle** because, for most individuals, that is a more certain date than the date of ovulation.

of ectopic pregnancies is increasing, most likely because of increasing risk factors, but the mortality rate has declined, in part because of early diagnosis by US.
- Using transvaginal scanning, **US is best at identifying the presence** of an **intrauterine pregnancy** and is less effective at visualizing the actual ectopic pregnancy itself.

▶▶ **IMPORTANT POINTS**

- If a **gestational sac** (the earliest sonographic findings in pregnancy, appearing at about 4 to 5 weeks gestational age), or a **yolk sac** (the first structure to be seen normally in the gestational sac) or **embryo** is identified **in the uterine cavity**, an ectopic pregnancy is effectively **excluded**. Endovaginal examinations are usually performed to find the gestational sac (Fig. 19.30).
- Simultaneous intrauterine and extrauterine pregnancies, also called **heterotopic pregnancies**, are **extremely rare** except in those undergoing fertility treatment. Therefore, **identification of an intrauterine pregnancy effectively excludes an ectopic pregnancy.**

Fig. 19.31 Ectopic Pregnancy. (A) A normal endometrial stripe (*solid black arrow*) is seen with no evidence of a pregnancy in the uterus (U). (B) In the same patient, there is an adnexal mass (*solid white arrow*) containing an embryo (E). There is fluid in the cul-de-sac (C). The demonstration of an embryo outside of the uterus is diagnostic of an ectopic pregnancy.

- Conversely, the demonstration of a **live embryo outside of the uterus is diagnostic of an ectopic pregnancy.** However, this is not a common occurrence with most ectopic pregnancies (Fig. 19.31).

IMPORTANT POINTS

- Most often, the ectopic location is diagnosed by a combination of findings that includes **absence of an identifiable intrauterine pregnancy**, often with an **extrauterine, extraovarian solid or cystic mass.**

- **Serum human chorionic gonadotropin hormone (β-HCG)** is produced by placental tissue shortly after the implantation of a fertilized ovum in the uterus. Combined with US, the β-HCG level may be helpful in distinguishing between intrauterine pregnancy, ectopic pregnancy, and early abortion (Fig. 19.32).
- An ectopic pregnancy is presumed present when there are **large amounts of free fluid (blood) inside the abdominal cavity.** **Small amounts** of free fluid can occur from other causes, such as spontaneous abortion, ruptured ovarian cysts, and normal ovulation.
- Ectopic pregnancies are **managed** either **surgically** (usually laparoscopic surgery) or **medically** with an abortifacient, such as methotrexate. Some spontaneously resolve.

Fetal Abnormalities

- US is used extensively to monitor normal **fetal growth** and **development.**
- US can recognize certain fetal anomalies in utero that are known to be universally fatal after birth, such as **anencephaly** (Fig. 19.33) or complete **ectopia cordis.** The accurate

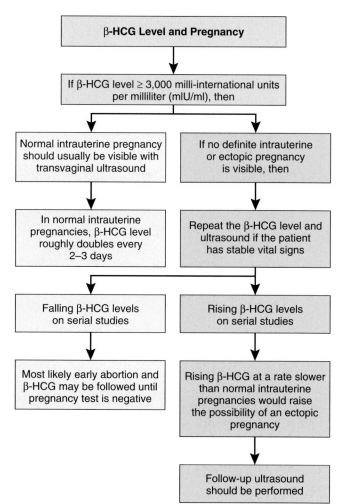

Fig. 19.32 Serum Human Chorionic Gonadotropin Hormone (β-HCG) and Pregnancy.

Fig. 19.33 Anencephaly: Sagittal View. There is a single, live intrauterine pregnancy. The body (B) and face (F) are present, but the cranium and all of the cerebrum and cerebellum are absent (*white arrow*). Anencephaly involves a failure of closure of the neural tube during the third to fourth weeks of development. It virtually always leads to fetal demise, stillbirth, or neonatal death.

TABLE 19.4	**In Utero Abnormalities Diagnosable by Ultrasound**
Organ System	**Abnormalities**
Central nervous system	Hydrocephalus, abnormalities of the prosencephalon, agenesis of the corpus callosum, intrauterine infections, cysts, meningomyelocele, anencephaly (see Fig. 19.32)
Skeletal anomalies	Dwarfism, skeletal dysplasias, achondroplasia, osteogenesis imperfecta, asphyxiating thoracic dysplasia, limb anomalies
Gastrointestinal abnormalities	Esophageal atresia and tracheoesophageal fistula, duodenal atresia, small and large bowel obstruction, abdominal wall defects, congenital diaphragmatic hernias, choledochal cyst
Genitourinary tract abnormalities	Renal agenesis, congenital ureteropelvic junction and ureterovesical junction obstruction, bladder outlet obstruction, multicystic dysplastic kidney, polycystic kidney disease
Cardiac anomalies	Hypoplastic left heart syndrome, tricuspid atresia, endocardial cushion defects, Ebstein's anomaly, tetralogy of Fallot, transposition of the great vessels, coarctation of the aorta, cardiac arrhythmias

interpretation of sonograms by someone trained and experienced in obstetric US is important in detecting such anomalies.

- Some of the many fetal anomalies that can be diagnosed by US in utero are shown in Table 19.4.
- In detecting fetal anomalies, US has played a major role in obstetric management of pregnancy. As more reliable markers for chromosome abnormalities that can be quickly assessed without prolonged waiting periods become available, its role may increase.

Molar Pregnancy

- **Molar pregnancy** is the most common of a group of disorders of the **placenta** that also includes **invasive mole** and **choriocarcinoma.** Pathologically, molar pregnancies feature **cystic (grape-like or hydatidiform) degeneration of chorionic villi** and proliferation of the placental trophoblast.

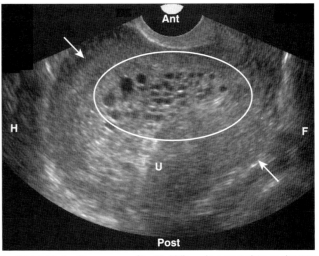

Fig. 19.34 Molar Pregnancy: Sagittal View. In a complete molar pregnancy, as in this patient, there is no fetus. Typical US findings of a molar pregnancy include innumerable, uniform-sized cystic spaces that represent hydropic villi (*white oval*) and an enlarged uterus (U) filled with echogenic tissue that thickens the endometrium (*white arrows*). The ovaries may also be enlarged and cyst-filled (not shown).

> ### IMPORTANT POINTS
>
> - A molar pregnancy is suggested by uterine size that is **disproportionately large** for the gestational age, β-HCG levels in **excess of 100,000 mIU/mL** (normal pregnancies are less than 60,000 mIU/mL), **vomiting, vaginal bleeding,** and **toxemia.**

- The sonographic findings of molar pregnancy are shown in Fig. 19.34.
- Treatment is **uterine evacuation.** About 20% of those with complete molar pregnancies may harbor persistent trophoblastic tissue, so follow-up is carried out with serial HCG determinations.

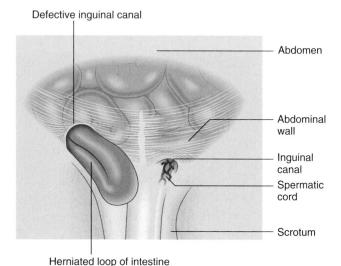

Defective inguinal canal

Abdomen

Abdominal wall

Inguinal canal

Spermatic cord

Scrotum

Herniated loop of intestine

Fig. 19.35 Graphic Representation of a Right Inguinal Hernia. The most common location of an abdominal wall hernia is in the inguinal region. The herniated tissue may contain a combination of fat, bowel (as shown here), and/or visceral organs. The defect in the abdominal wall may pinch the herniated bowel, causing bowel obstruction or compress blood vessels supplying the bowel causing bowel ischemia (strangulation).

ABDOMINAL HERNIAS

- An abdominal hernia is a protuberance of tissue, usually bowel, through a defect or hole in the abdominal wall (Fig. 19.35).
- US evaluation for inguinal hernias is initially performed with the patient supine. Under real-time US, the patient performs the **Valsalva maneuver,** which increases the intraabdominal pressure and may elicit a hernia that is not normally present at rest (eVideo 19.6).
  - If a hernia is not detected in the supine position, having the patient **stand** while performing the Valsalva maneuver further increases the intraabdominal pressure and improves elicitation of a hernia. The ability of US to evaluate the inguinal region under real-time imaging either in the supine or standing position affords it an advantage over other imaging modalities.

APPENDICITIS

- The appendix is a blind-ending tube that arises from the cecum. The **normal diameter** of the appendix is **less than 6 mm.** When visible, the normal appendix **will compress** when pressure is applied with the transducer.
- The **pathophysiology** of acute appendicitis begins with obstruction of the appendiceal lumen, followed by progressive distension of the obstructed appendix until perforation occurs and a periappendiceal abscess forms.

> ### ▶▶ IMPORTANT POINTS
>
> - In **acute appendicitis,** the abnormal appendix may be recognized on US as a blind-ending, aperistaltic tube with a diameter of **6 mm or more.** The inflamed appendix is **noncompressible** (using a technique called **graded compression**). It may also be tender when palpated with the probe. In about one-third of appendicitis cases, a **fecalith** will be present (Fig. 19.36).

Fig. 19.36 Acute Appendicitis: Longitudinal View. There is a blind-ending (*solid black arrow*) tubular structure (*solid white arrows*) with a thick wall and a distended lumen representing an inflamed and distended appendix. Two echogenic structures with posterior acoustic shadowing are contained within the appendix, consistent with **appendicoliths** (*dotted white arrows*).

- The CT findings of appendicitis are discussed in **Chapter 18.**
- In addition to appendicitis and abdominal wall hernias, US can be used for other gastrointestinal abnormalities, such as bowel wall thickening, masses and intussusception.
- Endoscopic US allows for further characterization of the bowel wall and helps in guidance for biopsies.

ASCITES

- Normally, the peritoneal cavity contains only a few milliliters of fluid. Excessive accumulation of fluid in the cavity is called **ascites.** When a large amount of ascites is present, it is easily identified in all four quadrants of the abdomen on US.
- However, smaller amounts may only be detectable where such fluid typically accumulates. The **right upper quadrant** between the liver and diaphragm is one of the first locations that ascites collects, because the fluid flows up the right paracolic gutter to the right subphrenic space in the recumbent position.
- Other common locations for the detection of ascitic fluid are the **pouch of Douglas** in women and **rectovesical pouch** in men, which are the most dependent locations of the peritoneal cavity.
  - Ascitic fluid that is a **transudate** is primarily **sonolucent or anechoic.** Fluid collections that are **exudates** or contain hemorrhage or pus **may contain echoes** (Fig. 19.37).
- US is frequently used to identify the largest pocket of fluid that, in turn, provides image guidance for the safe removal of the fluid via **paracentesis.**

MUSCULOSKELETAL SYSTEM

- Although the musculoskeletal system is typically assessed with MRI, US is increasingly used to evaluate musculoskeletal structures.
- US has the advantages of **real-time imaging, lower cost,** and **lack of contraindications** associated with the strong magnetic field used in MRI.

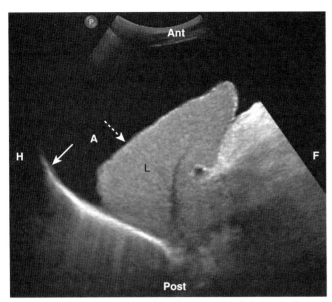

Fig. 19.37 Ascites: US. Ascitic fluid flows up the right paracolic gutter to the right subphrenic space so ascites (A) is generally easier to detect by US in the right upper quadrant between the liver (L) and the diaphragm (*solid white arrow*). The liver is contracted and has a nodular margin (*dotted white arrow*), both features of cirrhosis. If the fluid is a transudate, as in this case of ascites caused by cirrhosis, the fluid will be anechoic. Exudates will produce internal echoes.

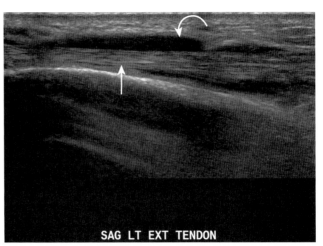

Fig. 19.38 Extensor Pollicis Longus Tendon: Sagittal US. The normal tendon appears as a band of echogenic striations (*straight arrow*). There is anechoic fluid (*curved arrow*) surrounding this tendon which is consistent with tenosynovitis.

- **Real-time US imaging** allows a structure to be evaluated in **different positions,** including the position that elicits the patient's pain. For example, tendon subluxation may only occur in certain positions and subtle tendon or ligament tears may only be seen when they are stretched in certain positions.

> ## » IMPORTANT POINTS
>
> - **Tendinopathy** can be diagnosed by US when the tendon appears thickened or when there is fluid around the tendon (Fig. 19.38). A **tendon tear** appears as **fluid** in the tendon or **discontinuity** of the tendon fibers.

- US is also useful at the **point of care** to identify **foreign bodies** in the superficial soft tissues. Wood splinters, which may not be visible on conventional radiographs, can be **echogenic** on US and readily visible. Other materials, such as metal, glass, and plastic, can also appear as echogenic structures and may be visible on US (Fig. 19.39).
- Musculoskeletal US can also be used to evaluate joint effusions, superficial ligaments, musculature, and small joints in the hands and feet. It can also be used to guide therapeutic and diagnostic injections.

CONTRAST-ENHANCED ULTRASOUND

- Contrast-enhanced US is increasingly used in the United States to aid in the diagnosis of a wide variety of pathologies. It involves the use of a **microbubble contrast agent** with

Fig. 19.39 Foreign Body in the Ear Lobe. The patient complained of swelling and redness in the left earlobe. An US image of the earlobe demonstrates a linear echogenic structure (*white arrow*) corresponding to the plastic backing of an earring accidentally pulled into the earring tract of the earlobe. (Courtesy Ryan K. Cunningham, MD.)

specialized US imaging software to demonstrate **vascular flow and soft-tissue perfusion.**

- The enhancement pattern of masses in abdominal organs such as the liver and kidneys can be assessed on contrast-enhanced US (eVideo 19.7). The presence or lack of enhancement as well as the enhancement pattern itself aids in the diagnosis, especially of soft tissue tumors.
- The microbubble contrast agent is safe with no nephrotoxicity or risk of nephrogenic systemic fibrosis as might accompany the contrast agents used for CT and MRI, respectively.

Fig. 19.40 Contrast-Enhanced US. (A in color and B in grayscale) This enhancing mass in the kidney is consistent with renal cell carcinoma. The mass (*solid arrows*) is predominantly hypoechoic but demonstrates enhancement depicted as the brighter echoes (*dotted arrows*). The enhancement is more prominent when visualized in real-time (eVideo 9.7). (Courtesy Shuchi K. Rodgers, MD.)

TAKE HOME POINTS

- Creation of a sonographic image **(sonogram)** depends on three major components: the production of a high-frequency sound wave, the reception of a reflected wave or echo, and the conversion of that echo into an image.
- **Echogenic (hyperechoic)** is a sonographic term used to describe tissue that reflects many echoes and appears bright or white on the sonogram. **Hypoechoic or anechoic** are sonographic terms used to describe tissue that reflects few or no echoes and appears dark or black on the sonogram.
- The **Doppler effect** is used in US to determine and display the direction and velocity of a moving object, usually blood.
- No known long-term side effects have been scientifically demonstrated to be caused by the medical use of US in humans.
- **Gallstones** are characteristically echogenic and produce an **acoustical shadow** because they reflect most of the sound waves.
- **Biliary sludge** can also be seen in the gallbladder. Although sludge may also appear echogenic, it does not produce acoustic shadowing as gallstones do.
- **Obstructive uropathy** typically appears as a dilated calyceal system and is depicted as a fluid-filled, dilated, hypoechoic collecting system on US.
- In **medical renal disease,** the renal parenchyma becomes more echogenic than the liver and spleen, which is the reverse of the normal echo pattern.
- **Scrotal torsion** is a medical emergency and appears as an absence of blood flow on color Doppler imaging in the torsed testicle.
- US is the study of choice to screen for **abdominal aortic aneurysms** when an asymptomatic, pulsatile abdominal mass is palpated.
- **Leiomyomas (fibroids),** the most common tumor of the uterus, appear as heterogeneously hypoechoic, solid masses. **Adenomyosis** refers to ectopic endometrial tissue in the myometrium and presents as small, cystic spaces in the myometrium of an enlarged, globular uterus.
- The most common ovarian mass is a **functional cyst,** which appears as a thin-walled anechoic structure on US. The cyst may be echogenic if it contains hemorrhage.

- **Nonfunctional ovarian cysts** include dermoid cysts and endometriomas.
- **Ovarian tumors** most often arise from the surface epithelium and are either serous or mucinous.
- **Pelvic inflammatory disease (PID)** is a term used to describe a group of infectious diseases affecting the uterus, fallopian tubes, and ovaries, with most beginning as transient endometritis.
- US is a safe and reliable means of visualizing the fetus in utero and provides the ability to do so repeatedly during the source of a pregnancy, if necessary.
- Most **ectopic pregnancies** are tubal in location and can be effectively excluded if an intrauterine pregnancy is present and included if the extrauterine pregnancy is demonstrated.
- A **molar pregnancy** is suggested by uterine size that is disproportionately large for the dates of gestation and markedly elevated β-HCG levels of greater than 100,000 mIU/mL.
- An **abdominal hernia** is a protuberance of tissue through a defect in the abdominal wall. It can be diagnosed on US by visualizing the intraabdominal contents (usually fat and/or bowel) herniated through abdominal wall, with detection improved if intraabdominal pressure is increased by having the patient stand and perform the Valsalva maneuver.
- The appendix is a blind-ending, aperistaltic tube that can become inflamed in **acute appendicitis.** On US, the appendix appears thickened (diameter >6 mm) and noncompressible in acute appendicitis. The patient's right lower quadrant may be tender when palpated with the US probe.
- US may be used to evaluate superficial tendons, ligaments, and musculature and for the presence of joint effusions. Superficial foreign bodies may also be detected by US as echogenic structures, even when they cannot be visualized on radiographs.
- **Contrast-enhanced US** is increasingly used in the United States and involves the injection of a microbubble contrast agent to determine vascular flow and tissue perfusion.

More information on ultrasonography and understanding the principles and its uses in abdominal and pelvic imaging is available to registered users online.

20

Vascular, Pediatric, and Point-of-Care Ultrasound

Peter Wang, MD

In this chapter, we will discuss some additional applications of ultrasound, including vascular ultrasound, pediatric applications of ultrasound, and point-of-care ultrasound.

VASCULAR ULTRASOUND

- **Vascular ultrasound** uses both **B-mode (gray-scale) ultrasound** and **Doppler ultrasonography**—a combination called **duplex sonography**—to display the morphologic appearance of vessels while recording the **flow direction** and **velocity of moving blood** in those vessels.
- Duplex sonography ensures that the direction and flow measurements are made in the exact anatomic location of interest (eVideo 20.1).
- The two most common types of Doppler ultrasound are **color Doppler** and **spectral Doppler.**
  - Color flow imaging can provide specific, but limited information over a relatively large region, whereas spectral Doppler provides more precise information about a smaller region. The two modes are complementary.

> **▶▶ IMPORTANT POINTS**
>
> - **Color Doppler ultrasound superimposes** color on the gray-scale image to indicate the presence and direction of moving blood. By convention, **red** indicates **movement toward the transducer** and **blue** indicates **movement away from transducer** (Fig. 20.1).

- **Spectral Doppler ultrasound** is displayed as a **waveform,** which is a graphic representation of the **velocity of flow** measured **over time** within a **focused area.** It is depicted along an **X** (**time**) and **Y** (**velocity**) axis. By convention, **flow toward** the transducer is displayed **above the baseline** and **flow away** is **below the baseline** (Fig. 20.2).

Fig. 20.1 Color Doppler Image. By convention, color Doppler depicts flow toward the transducer as red and flow away from the transducer as blue. This is an image of the **splenic vein** (*straight arrow*) posterior to the pancreas (P). The normal flow direction in the splenic vein is shown (*curved arrow*). When imaged anteriorly at the midline, the splenic vein has blood flowing anteriorly toward the transducer on the left (your right) and posteriorly away from the transducer on the right (your left). Therefore, color Doppler depicts flow both as red (toward the transducer) and blue (away from the transducer) in same vessel. Throughout this chapter, many figures will have one or more of the following abbreviations to help your orientation: *Ant,* anterior; *F,* foot of the patient; *H,* head of the patient; *L,* left; *Post,* posterior.

Fig. 20.2 Normal Color and Spectral Doppler Images. (A) This image is of the portal vein. Flow toward the transducer in the portal vein is depicted as red. (B) This is the common femoral vein. Flow away from the transducer in the common femoral vein is blue. The spectral Doppler waveforms are located below the color portions of the ultrasound images and are drawn on a time-velocity scale with the x-axis depicting time and the y-axis depicting velocities. The portal vein waveform in (A) is **above** the baseline (the baseline is the *thin, horizontal white line*) indicating blood flow **toward** the transducer. The waveform in the common femoral vein in (B) is **below** the baseline, indicating blood flow **away** from the transducer.

Fig. 20.3 Normal Color and Spectral Doppler Images of the Hepatic Artery. End organs, such as the liver, require **continuous** blood flow and therefore have a vascular bed with **low resistance** to the flowing blood from its supplying artery. Hence, flow in the hepatic artery is normally **always toward** the liver (in this case red and above the base-line) during both systole (*curved arrow*) and diastole (*straight arrow*).

Fig. 20.4 Normal Color and Spectral Doppler Images of Popliteal Artery. An extremity at rest usually does not require continuous blood flow and has a vascular bed with **high resistance** to flow from its sup-plying peripheral artery. Hence, flow in the popliteal artery (which supplies the calf and foot) typically has interrupted flow. The flow is **toward** the foot (above the baseline) during the **high pressures of systole** (*curved arrow*) and may **stop or reverse** (below the baseline) during the **low pressures of diastole** (*straight arrow*).

- There are distinctive arterial spectral Doppler waveforms, depending on the **resistance** to blood flow in the vascular bed that the artery supplies (Figs. 20.3 and 20.4) Venous waveforms can also vary depending on their proximity to the heart, the cardiac function, and phase of respiration (see Fig. 20.2).
- If an ultrasound signal is reflected from a **stationary object**, the returning signal should theoretically retain the **same frequency** with which it was transmitted. But based on the principles of Doppler ultrasound, the frequency of a signal reflected from **moving objects**, such as blood cells, will **change** in proportion to the **velocity** of the target.
- With this information, we can **interrogate vessels** to determine if they are **narrowed** or **occluded** because an **arterial stenosis** leads to an **increase in blood velocity** through the area of narrowing. If we gradually advance the Doppler probe along the path of a blood vessel, we can identify a stenotic lesion and its location.
- This is analogous to the velocity of water flowing through the open end of a garden hose. When the opening of the garden hose is narrowed, the velocity of the flowing water must increase for the same volume of water to flow through the smaller lumen (Fig. 20.5).

- Because of changes in blood flow, abnormalities in the spectral waveforms can also suggest narrowing or occlusion that occurs in a part of the vessel that is more **proximal** or **distal** to the area being studied.

ARTERIAL STENOSIS

Carotid Arteries

- **Carotid ultrasonography** has become the study of choice for the non-invasive assessment of **extracranial atherosclerotic disease.** Carotid ultrasound is also used to evaluate bruits, as preoperative screening prior to other major vascular surgery, and to assess the patency of the vessel after endarterectomy.
- When there is **greater than 50% stenosis** of the carotid artery lumen, the **velocity** of flow becomes **elevated.** Significant stenosis alters the Doppler waveform at points **proximal, at,** and **distal** to the stenosis.
- Ultrasound is also used to assess the **thickness of the vessel wall** (it gets thicker with atherosclerosis) and the **presence and nature of plaque.**

Fig. 20.5 Color and Spectral Doppler Image of a Narrowed Superficial Femoral Artery. (A) Significant narrowing of the superficial femoral artery (*arrow*) results in markedly elevated velocities (depicted on the y-axis) on spectral Doppler imaging, much like water flows faster when the opening of a garden hose is narrowed (B) because the same volume of water must travel through a smaller opening. In addition, the arterial waveform at a stenosis may change to **monophasic,** which are waveforms that remain on one side of the spectral Doppler baseline and have a similar appearance to the waveforms in arteries feeding end-organs (see Fig. 20.3).

Peripheral Arteries

- Peripheral artery disease occurs when **atherosclerotic plaques** are deposited in the arteries feeding the extremities. Significant narrowing or occlusion of the peripheral arteries usually occurs in the **lower extremities** and can result in **claudication** (i.e., leg pain during exertion) or pain at rest.
  - **Risk factors** include smoking, diabetes, hypertension, hyperlipidemia, male gender, and black ethnicity.
- The peripheral arteries in the extremities normally have what is called a **high-resistance waveform** because **at rest,** the vascular bed in the muscles they supply are constricted (see Fig. 20.4).
- **Significant narrowing of a peripheral artery** will cause an **elevation in the velocities** of the flowing blood.

> ## ⟫ IMPORTANT POINTS
>
> - **Screening** for peripheral arterial disease typically involves obtaining the **ankle-brachial index (ABI)**, which is the **ratio** of the systolic blood pressure in the **ankle** divided by the systolic blood pressure in the **arm** (brachial artery).
>
> $$ABI = \frac{\text{Systolic blood pressure in ankle}}{\text{Systolic blood pressure in arm}}$$

- Blood pressures are measured by **detecting arterial flow** with a **Doppler probe** on the artery instead of with a stethoscope. Pressures are usually taken in **both arms**, and the posterior tibial and dorsalis pedis arteries on **each leg** by inflating blood pressure cuffs past the point where flow and Doppler sounds **cease,** then slowly deflating the cuffs until flow and Doppler sounds **return.**
- **Normally, the systolic blood pressures in the ankle should be equal to that in the arm** resulting in an ABI of 1. As the blood pressure in the ankle falls due to peripheral vascular disease in the legs and because ankle pressures are the numerator for the ABI, there will be a **decrease** in the value of the ABI and an **ABI of 0.5 or less** usually indicates **severe arterial disease.**

PSEUDOANEURYSM

- One of the complications following an invasive vascular procedure, such as cardiac catheterization, is the development of a *pseudoaneurysm,* most often at the **catheter entrance site,** which is usually in the **groin** at the common femoral artery or in the **arm** at the brachial artery.
- A **pseudoaneurysm** forms when there is a **rupture or injury to the arterial wall**, but the blood leaking through the defect

remains confined either by an intact, thin outer layer of the arterial wall itself or by the surrounding perivascular tissues. Because the wall or perivascular tissue containing the pseudoaneurysm is thin, it is at **high risk for additional rupture and extravasation.** A **true aneurysm's** arterial walls are intact, in contradistinction, but the caliber of the artery is abnormally dilated.

> #### ▶▶ IMPORTANT POINTS
>
> - On ultrasound, a pseudoaneurysm appears as a **hypoechoic outpouching** arising from an artery (eVideo 20.2). Occasionally, the pseudoaneurysm may be connected to the artery by a thin neck or stalk. **Blood flowing into and out of a pseudoaneurysm** results in a **distinctive appearance** on color and spectral Doppler images (Fig. 20.6).

- Ultrasound is also used for the **treatment of pseudoaneurysms** by applying direct **compression with the ultrasound probe** to occlude the aneurysm sac, especially if the sac is small. Ultrasound can also be used to guide thrombin injection resulting in thrombosis or occlusion of the pseudoaneurysm.

DEEP VEIN THROMBOSIS (DVT)

- Ultrasound is the **study of choice** when **deep vein thrombosis** is suspected in the upper or lower extremities. **Local symptoms** can include pain, tenderness, and warmth in the affected area, although most patients with DVT are asymptomatic. The most serious complication of DVT is **pulmonary embolism.**

- The highest-yield sonographic examination for DVT in the leg occurs in the **symptomatic patient** who manifests local symptoms **above the knee.** Ultrasound has a much lower sensitivity in asymptomatic patients.
- Sonographic evaluation for deep venous thrombosis of the legs and arms involves the use of the transducer to systematically **compress** the deep veins while scanning the leg along **certain anatomic landmarks, including** the common femoral vein, proximal deep femoral vein, greater saphenous vein, femoral vein, popliteal vein, and the posterior tibial and peroneal veins.

> #### ▶▶ IMPORTANT POINTS
>
> - **Normal** venous structures have **elastic walls** and will **easily compress** and **completely collapse** when pressure is applied by the transducer. Veins containing **thrombus will not completely collapse.** The echogenic thrombus itself may be visualized on gray-scale imaging. Duplex sonography can be used to determine the presence or absence of flow in the vein (Fig. 20.7).

PEDIATRICS

- Ultrasound's **lack of ionizing radiation** is especially important in pediatric patients because younger and developing patients are more susceptible to the effects of radiation and have a relatively longer lifespan to develop potential complications. In addition, the smaller body habitus of a child allows better

Fig. 20.6 Color and Spectral Doppler Images of a Pseudoaneurysm. (A) This color Doppler image demonstrates a pseudoaneurysm (*curved arrow*) arising from the common femoral artery (*straight arrow*) via a thin neck. Due to flow into and out of the pseudoaneurysm, a typical pattern of red and blue color Doppler flow similar to a **yin-yang** symbol is displayed. (B) Spectral Doppler interrogation of the pseudoaneurysm neck (*solid arrow*) demonstrates flow into and out of the pseudoaneurysm as flow above (*dotted white arrows*) and below the baseline. The pseudoaneurysm developed from the common femoral artery after cardiac catheterization.

Fig. 20.7 Normal and Thrombosed Femoral Veins. (A) When compression is applied by the ultrasound transducer, the normal femoral vein (V) because of its elastic walls, demonstrates collapsibility from its precompression (*solid arrow*) to its postcompression (*dotted arrow*) state. The adjacent femoral artery (A) does not collapse with pressure because its walls are more rigid. (B) In another patient, thrombus in the femoral vein (V) prevents its normal collapse between the precompression (*solid arrow*) and postcompression (*dotted arrow*) states. (C) Color Doppler imaging of the thrombosed femoral vein demonstrates hypoechoic thrombus (T) and lack of color flow in the vein. The adjacent artery (A) is patent and filled with color Doppler flow.

penetration of the ultrasound signal and the use of higher frequency transducers to provide higher resolution images.
- Many uses of ultrasound are specific to the pediatric age group, several of which are discussed below.

Germinal Matrix Hemorrhage

- A **sonographic window** describes a pathway for the ultrasound signal to travel that is relatively free of bone or gas, both of which would degrade the US image. The intracranial contents of the neonate are particularly accessible by US because of the sonographic windows provided by the **open fontanelles.**
- Many of the structures in the supratentorial and infratentorial spaces, including the brain parenchyma and extraaxial spaces, can be evaluated. In the neonate, one such use is for the evaluation of intracranial hemorrhage.
- **Neonatal intracranial hemorrhage** can cause significant morbidity and mortality, particularly in **premature infants.** These **hemorrhages most commonly occur in the germinal matrix** that is only transiently present before 34 weeks of gestation. It occurs in the vessel-rich **caudothalamic groove,** which is in the subependymal region between the caudate nucleus and thalamus (Fig. 20.8A).
- Germinal matrix hemorrhages are divided into four grades, usually by US imaging, with increasing predicted mortality

> **IMPORTANT POINTS**
>
> - The hemorrhage appears as an area of **echogenic material** in the caudothalamic groove that can expand into the ventricle and brain parenchyma (Fig. 20.8B).

as the grade increases. Injury to the germinal matrix has substantial mortality and morbidity consequences.

Developmental Dysplasia of the Hip (DDH)

- Developmental dysplasia of the hip is a common disorder of newborns that can result in **dislocation or subluxation of the hip.** It is more common in females, first-born children, breech presentation, and children whose parents had DDH. The left hip is also more commonly affected.
- Physical examination findings that suggest DDH include positive **Ortolani and Barlow tests.**
  - In the **Ortolani test,** the hip is **externally rotated** and **abducted.** A positive test occurs when a "click" or "clunk" is felt or heard during this test owing to **reduction** of the dislocated or subluxed hip.
  - In the **Barlow test,** the hip is **flexed, internally rotated, and adducted** with posterior pressure on the femoral head. A positive test occurs when a "click" or "clunk" is felt from the **hip dislocating.**
- In infants with a high risk of DDH or abnormal physical examination findings, the morphology of the acetabulum may

Fig. 20.8 Germinal Matrix Hemorrhage. Sagittal, ultrasound images of the brain demonstrate both the right and left caudothalamic grooves. (A) The normal right caudothalamic groove is depicted as a thin, echogenic line straight (*arrow*) between the thalamus (T) and caudate (C). (B) On the other side of the brain, globular, echogenic material (*curved arrow*) located in the caudothalamic groove represents a germinal matrix hemorrhage.

be assessed by ultrasound at 4 to 6 weeks of age while the femoral head epiphysis is still cartilaginous. An **abnormal morphology of the acetabulum** or **frank dislocation** of the femoral head indicates DDH (Fig. 20.9). The Barlow maneuver can also be performed under real-time ultrasound to depict any subluxation or dislocation of the hip.

- **Once the epiphysis ossifies**, which occurs at approximately 3 to 4 months of age, **radiographs are needed** for assessment because ultrasound cannot penetrate the ossified bone to evaluate the acetabulum.

Necrotizing Enterocolitis (NEC)

- **Necrotizing enterocolitis** most commonly affects **premature infants** within the first weeks of life. It can be a life-threatening gastrointestinal condition in neonates. The pathophysiology has been postulated to involve the breakdown of the intestinal mucosa, translocation of intestinal bacteria, and an inflammatory response that can lead to **dissection of gas into the bowel wall** and **portal venous system.** Severe cases of NEC may result in bowel perforation and free intraperitoneal air (**see Chapter 28: Necrotizing Enterocolitis**).
- Although **conventional abdominal radiographs** are the **study of choice** for the diagnosis of NEC, ultrasound may be complementary.

⟫ **IMPORTANT POINTS**

- Ultrasound can depict **air dissecting into the bowel wall** (intramural gas or pneumatosis intestinalis) (Fig. 20.10), free **intraperitoneal gas, bowel wall thickening,** and **portal venous gas** (Fig. 20.11). Small amounts of gas difficult to detect on radiographs may be readily seen on ultrasound.

Fig. 20.9 Developmental Dysplasia of the Hip. Coronal ultrasound image of the right hip in a newborn with breech presentation. The femoral head (FH) normally sits in the acetabulum. Abnormal morphology of the acetabulum can be depicted by the **alpha angle,** which is formed by the cortex of the ilium (*dashed line pointed to by straight arrow*) and the acetabular roof (*solid line pointed to by curved arrow*). The alpha angle is normally greater than 60 degrees at 4 to 6 weeks of age and greater than 55 degrees in a newborn. This angle measured less. Alpha angles that are **less** indicate a **shallow shape of the acetabulum** that is consistent with developmental hip dysplasia and a higher risk of femoral head subluxation or dislocation.

Intussusception

- Intussusception occurs when a segment of bowel **telescopes forward** into the lumen of an adjacent bowel loop, causing

bowel obstruction (Fig. 20.12). In children, intussusception typically occurs between **6 months and 2 years** of age, is most frequently **ileocolic** (i.e., the ileum telescopes into the colon), and most often **idiopathic** in origin.

⟫ IMPORTANT POINTS

- On a transverse ultrasound image, intussusception may display a **target or donut** appearance as a result of the multiple alternating hypoechoic and hyperechoic layers of the bowel walls imaged tightly adjacent to each other. In the longitudinal plane, the intussusception might have a **bowel-within-bowel appearance** and may sometimes display the **pseudokidney** sign (Fig. 20.13).

A

Fig. 20.12 Intussusception. (A) Intussusception occurs when a loop of bowel telescopes into an adjacent bowel loop. The bowel loop that telescopes is called the ***intussusceptum*** (*straight blue arrow*). The bowel loop that receives the telescoping segment is called the ***intussuscipiens*** (*curved* blue *arrow*). B. Ultrasound image of the left abdomen demonstrating an intussusception of the small bowel, including the intussusceptum (*straight* white *arrow*) and intussuscipiens (*curved white arrow*). The intussusception occurred in the direction of the dotted white arrow.

Fig. 20.10 Pneumatosis Intestinalis. Ultrasound image of the left upper quadrant in a neonate demonstrates multiple, nondependent echogenic foci (*arrows*) in the bowel wall consistent with pneumatosis intestinalis. The echogenic foci represent gas.

Fig. 20.11 Portal Venous Gas. (A) Transverse ultrasound of the liver demonstrates multiple linear and branching echogenic foci (*straight arrow*) that extend to the periphery of the liver, which is consistent with portal venous gas. (B) Spectral Doppler interrogation of the main portal vein in the same patient demonstrates characteristic small spikes (*curved arrow*) along the spectral waveform from small air bubbles passing intermittently in the blood flowing through the portal vein.

Fig. 20.13 Intussusception, Transverse, and Sagittal Images. (A) On the transverse image, the intussusception has a **target** or **donut** appearance (*solid white arrows*) with the echogenic, mesenteric fat (F) of the intussusceptum in the center surrounded by the hypoechoic, bowel wall (W) of the intussuscipiens. (B) On the sagittal image, the ring of hypoechoic, bowel wall (W) is seen partially encasing the hyperechoic, mesenteric fat (F), creating what is called the **pseudokidney sign** (*solid white arrows*) because of its similarity with the sagittal image a normal kidney (see Fig. 19.10).

- Clinically, it is characterized by vomiting, intermittent and colicky abdominal pain, and passage of blood per rectum, although this classical triad occurs in only about a third of patients

Hypertrophic Pyloric Stenosis (HPS)

- Hypertrophic pyloric stenosis occurs when there is hypertrophy (thickening) of the gastric pyloric musculature that results in **gastric outlet obstruction.** It typically presents at **4 to 6 weeks of age** with **nonbilious vomiting** that becomes more **frequent** and **projectile** over time. The enlarged pylorus, called an *olive,* may be palpable in the right upper quadrant or epigastrium in about 60% to 80% of infants.

 IMPORTANT POINTS

- Ultrasound is the imaging study of choice. On US, **pyloric musculature that is thickened to more than 3 mm** or a **pyloric channel longer than 15 mm** is considered abnormal and indicative of hypertrophic pyloric stenosis (Fig. 20.14).

POINT-OF-CARE ULTRASOUND

- Ultrasound is increasingly being used at the **point-of-care** or **bedside** to help facilitate diagnoses and **direct management and therapy.** Point-of-care ultrasound (sometimes abbreviated POCUS) is a highly focused interrogation that quickly determines the presence or absence of a specific pathologic condition. Although extremely useful, **it does not replace detailed, routine sonographic evaluation.** Incidental findings that may be detected during point-of-care ultrasound often require follow-up detailed sonography to determine their etiology.

Focused Assessment With Sonography In Trauma (FAST)

- The **FAST examination** is part of the Advanced Trauma Life Support protocol and is performed simultaneously with other resuscitative measures in the trauma patient.

- The primary goal of the FAST examination is to identify **intraperitoneal bleeding** because the presence of **hemoperitoneum** in a hemodynamically **unstable patient** will generally lead to **emergent laparotomy.**
- The FAST examination has largely replaced the previously used diagnostic peritoneal lavage, but CT still remains much more sensitive for detecting abdominal and thoracic injuries.

 IMPORTANT POINTS

- A typical FAST examination involves the **search for blood or fluid in the pericardium and peritoneum.** The peritoneal search focuses on the area between the liver and right kidney and posterior pelvis (between the rectum and bladder in men and between the rectum and uterus in women) as they are the **most dependent portions of the abdominopelvic cavity** when the patient is supine (Fig. 20.15).

Pleural Effusion

- A pleural effusion is fluid that **accumulates between the visceral and parietal pleura (see Chapter 8).** Although radiographs and CTs are generally used to evaluate the presence of pleural effusions, US can detect **small amounts of pleural fluid** and is increasingly used at the point-of-care.
- Ultrasound can also help to determine if a radiographic opacity is due to **pleural fluid** and/or **parenchymal lung disease.** In addition, US may be used for **image-guided thoracentesis,** especially if the amount of fluid is small or the fluid is loculated.

IMPORTANT POINTS

- A simple effusion will be **anechoic** on ultrasound and is depicted as a fluid collection above the diaphragm. The diaphragm appears as a highly echogenic, curvilinear structure that abuts the liver (Fig. 20.16). The presence of **echoes within an effusion** suggests an **exudative effusion,** which may contain pus or blood.

Fig. 20.14 Hypertrophic Pyloric Stenosis. Sagittal ultrasound of the pylorus (P) in a 2-month-old baby with projectile vomiting. The stomach (ST) and gallbladder (GB) are also included in the image. The pylorus has a thickened wall (*double white arrow*) and elongated channel (*dashed white arrow*) consistent with hypertrophic pyloric stenosis.

Fig. 20.15 Ascites. Sagittal image of the right upper quadrant including the liver (L) and right kidney (K). There is anechoic fluid (*asterisk*) between the liver and kidney (Morrison's pouch) representing ascites.

Fig. 20.16 Pleural Effusion. This is a sagittal, gray-scale ultrasound image of the right upper quadrant, including the liver (L). The highly echogenic curvilinear structure abutting the liver is the diaphragm (*curved white arrow*). The pleural fluid is depicted as the anechoic fluid above the diaphragm (*asterisk*).

Fig. 20.17 Pneumothorax. This is a sagittal, gray-scale ultrasound image of the chest. The pleura is depicted as a highly echogenic line (*white arrow*) between the ribs (R) and lung (L). **eVideo 20.3** displays the **normal, sliding motion** of the pleural line during respiration. **eVideo 20.4** demonstrates the **absence** of the sliding motion of the pleural line when a pneumothorax is present.

Pneumothorax

- Ultrasound has become a useful and reliable modality in the diagnosis of pneumothorax. In the trauma patient, US has been shown to be **more sensitive than radiographs** for the diagnosis of **small pneumothoraces.** In the critical care patient, ultrasound is especially helpful because small pneumothoraces may be difficult or impossible to visualize radiographically in the supine patient (**see Chapter 25**).
- In a **supine patient,** air in a pneumothorax will **rise to the most superior** part of the chest that is located **anteriorly** between the **second and fourth intercostal spaces** near the **midclavicular line.**
- Normally the **pleura appears as an echogenic line** deep to and between the ribs (Fig. 20.17). During real-time ultrasound, the parietal and visceral pleurae can normally be seen **sliding** across each other as the patient breathes (eVideo 20.3).

> ≫ **IMPORTANT POINTS**
>
> - When a patient has a **pneumothorax**, air in the pleural cavity separates the parietal and visceral pleurae, which **prevents the sliding motion** and results in a **stationary echogenic pleural line** on ultrasound (eVideos 20.4 and 20.5).

Pericardial Effusion

- Ultrasound is a useful tool for the bedside diagnosis of pericardial effusions and cardiac tamponade.

> ≫ **IMPORTANT POINTS**
>
> - **Pericardial effusions** will appear as **anechoic fluid** collections surrounding the heart (Fig. 20.18; eVideo 20.6). Echoes within the fluid would suggest a **hemopericardium.**

Fig. 20.18 Pericardial Effusion. Gray-scale, ultrasound image demonstrates hypoechoic fluid (*inside the curved arrows*) around the heart from a pericardial effusion. If a diagnosis of cardiac tamponade is made, emergency drainage of the pericardial fluid by either pericardiocentesis or surgery is the usual course of treatment.

- **Cardiac tamponade** occurs when a pericardial effusion prevents blood from filling the **right atrium** and **right ventricle** during **diastole**. It can be caused by as little as 50 mL of fluid. Real-time sonography is useful in detecting tamponade by demonstrating complete **collapse of the right atrium or ventricle** or a **flattening or concavity of the right atrial or ventricular wall** during diastole.

Cardiac Function

- Cardiac function can be quickly assessed at the point-of-care and may be valuable in trauma and critical care patients.
- Bedside ultrasound can identify patients with poor cardiac output by allowing estimation of the **left ventricular ejection fraction,** which is the percentage of blood pumped out of the left ventricle during systole. Normally, the **ejection fraction is above 50%.**
- The ejection fraction may be estimated subjectively by **visual evaluation** during real-time ultrasound based on a **change in the size** of the left ventricle between end-diastole and end-systole. Severely decreased left ventricular function is present when there is **less than 30% difference** between the size of the left ventricle during end-diastole and end-systole.
  - Other methods of determining ejection fraction involve the use of additional software packages on the ultrasound machine that can calculate the left ventricular size during end-diastole and end-systole.
- **Right heart (right ventricular) strain** can also be assessed at the point-of-care. It refers to the presence of right ventricular dysfunction **without** an underlying cardiomyopathy as its cause. It might occur with pulmonary embolism, pulmonary hypertension, or chronic obstructive pulmonary disease.
  - Normally the **right ventricle** is **smaller** than the **left ventricle.** Enlargement of the right ventricle to the **same size or larger** than the left ventricle is **abnormal** and indicates right heart strain.

Central Venous Pressure

- Central venous pressure refers to the **blood pressure in the intrathoracic vena cava** and may be assessed via bedside ultrasound.
- Multiple etiologies can cause **elevated central venous pressure,** including heart failure, hypervolemia, massive pulmonary embolism, cardiac tamponade, tension pneumothorax, large pleural effusions, and mechanical ventilation itself. **Decreased central venous pressure** can occur with hypovolemia and shock.
- Because the vena cava is a thin-walled vessel, it normally **expands and contracts with respiration.**
  - During **inspiration,** the vena cava **decreases** in size because the **negative intrathoracic pressure** allows more blood to drain from the vena cava into the right atrium. Conversely, the vena cava **increases** in size during **expiration** as the blood flow out of the vena cava decreases with the **positive intrathoracic pressure.**

Fig. 20.19 Central Venous Pressure Elevation. This is a sagittal, gray-scale ultrasound image of the inferior vena cava (*straight white arrow*), heart, and hepatic veins (*curved white arrow*) obtained at end-inspiration in a patient with congestive heart failure. The inferior vena cava measured 2.5 cm at end-inspiration in this patient, which is consistent with an elevated central venous pressure.

- The inferior vena cava (IVC) typically averages about 2 cm in diameter during the respiratory cycle (in a nonventilated patient). An IVC diameter that is greater than 2 cm throughout the respiratory cycle and collapses less than 50% at end-inspiration suggests **elevated** central venous pressure (Fig. 20.19; eVideo 20.7). An IVC diameter that is less than 2 cm throughout the respiratory cycle and which collapses more than 50% at end-expiration suggests **decreased** central venous pressure.

Ocular Ultrasound

- Ophthalmologic emergencies account for approximately 3% of visits to the emergency department. Because the eye is a superficial, fluid-filled structure, ultrasound can be used to assess the internal structures of the eye at the point-of-care, especially if the **eyelid is swollen shut,** preventing direct visualization with an ophthalmoscope.
- Common indications for the performance of ocular US include **eye trauma, sudden decrease or loss of vision, ocular pain,** and **suspected foreign body.**
- The closed eye can be scanned gently with a high-frequency, linear transducer providing high-resolution sonographic images.
- Normal structures that can be visualized during ocular US include the **cornea, anterior chamber, iris and ciliary body, lens, vitreous chamber, retina,** and **optic nerve** (Fig. 20.20).
- Pathologic conditions in the orbit that can be diagnosed with point-of-care ocular US include globe perforation, retinal detachment, lens dislocation, vitreous hemorrhage, intraocular foreign body, and retrobulbar hematoma.

Fig. 20.20 Ultrasound of the Normal Eye. The **cornea** (*white arrow*) is depicted as a thin echogenic line just beneath the eyelid. The **anterior chamber** (*asterisk*) is an anechoic, fluid-filled space posterior to the cornea. The **lens** (*star*) is an ovoid, anechoic structure between the echogenic iris and ciliary body (*dashed white arrows*). The **vitreous chamber** is the large fluid-filled anechoic space posterior to the lens. The **retina** (*curved dashed line*) is located along the periphery of the vitreous chamber and cannot be differentiated from the choroidal layers on ultrasound. The **optic nerve** (*striped white arrow*) is located posterior to the globe.

🏠 TAKE HOME POINTS

- **Vascular ultrasound** uses gray-scale and Doppler ultrasonography to display the morphologic appearance of vessels and the direction and velocity of blood flow simultaneously.
- Significant **arterial narrowing** typically causes an elevation in blood flow velocities. Ultrasound is used to evaluate for carotid artery stenosis and for peripheral vascular disease, especially in the lower extremities.
- A **pseudoaneurysm** is formed when there is a rupture or injury to the arterial wall, but the blood leaking through the rupture is confined by an intact, thin outer layer of the arterial wall or the surrounding perivascular tissues. Pseudoaneurysms are at high risk of further rupture and bleeding.
- Sonographic evaluation of **deep venous thrombosis** is based on the principle that veins have thin, elastic walls that are easily compressible by the US probe. Thrombus in a vein will prevent it from being easily compressed. The echogenic thrombus itself may also be seen on gray-scale US imaging.
- Several uses of ultrasound that are specific to the pediatric patient are highlighted, including germinal matrix hemorrhage, developmental dysplasia of the hip, necrotizing enterocolitis, hypertrophic pyloric stenosis, and intussusception.
- The **germinal matrix** has a rich network of microscopic vessels that are at risk of bleeding in the premature infant. Germinal matrix hemorrhages appear as echogenic material in the caudothalamic groove and can extend into the ventricle and brain parenchyma with increasing morbidity and mortality.
- **Developmental dysplasia of the hip** can be evaluated on ultrasound at 4 to 6 weeks of age during which time the femoral head epiphysis is cartilaginous. Once the epiphysis ossifies, radiographs are needed to assess the acetabular morphology and femoral head location.
- **Necrotizing enterocolitis** is a life-threatening gastrointestinal condition in neonates that can result in bowel perforation. Ultrasound may be complementary to radiographs in the diagnosis of necrotizing enterocolitis and has the ability to visualize pneumatosis intestinalis, free intraperitoneal air, portal venous gas, and bowel wall thickening.
- **Intussusception** typically occurs between 6 months and 2 years of age and is most frequently ileocolic and idiopathic. Ultrasound may demonstrate a

bowel-within-bowel (pseudokidney) appearance or a target or donut appearance.
- **Hypertrophic pyloric stenosis** results in gastric outlet obstruction, leading to nonbilious projectile vomiting. The abnormally thickened pyloric musculature and elongated pyloric channel may be depicted on ultrasound.
- **Point-of-care ultrasound** is a highly focused interrogation that can quickly determine the presence or absence of a specific pathologic condition, facilitating treatment or often suggesting further, more extensive studies for evaluation.
- The **focused assessment with sonography in trauma (FAST) examination** is used in the trauma patient to detect intraperitoneal bleeding, especially in those hemodynamically unstable and unable to undergo more sensitive CT or US imaging.
- Ultrasound can detect a small amount of **pleural fluid** and can be used to guide thoracentesis.
- In the supine patient, **pneumothoraces** rise to the most superior part of the chest. Normally, the parietal and visceral pleurae can be seen sliding across each other on real-time US, but a pneumothorax prevents that sliding motion from occurring.
- **Pericardial effusions** are readily visible on US as hypoechoic or anechoic fluid around the heart. **Cardiac tamponade** occurs when the pericardial fluid prevents adequate filling of the right atrium and right ventricle.
- Cardiac function, including an estimate of the **left ventricular ejection fraction,** can be assessed at the bedside on US. Normally, the ejection fraction is above 50%.
- An elevated or decreased **central venous pressure** is depicted on US by the caliber of the inferior vena cava during inspiration and expiration. The normal inferior vena cava is usually around 2 cm throughout the respiratory cycle.
- As a superficial fluid-filled structure, the **eye** is readily assessed by ultrasound, especially if the eyelid is swollen closed preventing direct visualization. Point-of-care ocular US can be used to diagnose globe perforation, retinal detachment, lens dislocation, vitreous hemorrhage, foreign bodies, and retrobulbar hematoma.

📶 More information on ultrasonography: vascular, pediatric, and point-of-care ultrasound is available to registered users online.

21

Magnetic Resonance Imaging: Understanding the Principles and Recognizing the Basics

Daniel J. Kowal, MD

HOW MRI WORKS

- Because magnetic resonance imaging (MRI) uses the **molecular composition** of tissues, especially water, it is particularly sensitive to detecting **soft-tissue abnormalities** in much higher detail than CT scans, although the two imaging modalities are complementary. MRI produces no ionizing radiation, which is an advantage compared with CT, but MRI examinations take longer to acquire and are more expensive than CT scans.
- MRI uses a **very strong magnetic field** to manipulate the electromagnetic activity of atomic nuclei in a way that releases energy in the form of **radiofrequency signals,** which are recorded by the scanner's receiving coils and then computer-processed to form an image.
  - **Clinical MRI scanners** utilize the properties **of hydrogen nuclei** (which contain one proton) because of their abundance in the human body.
- Each proton has a **positive electrical charge** and because protons also have a **spin**, this charge is **constantly moving.** Remember that a **moving electrical charge** is also an **electrical current** and because an electrical current induces a **magnetic field,** each proton has its own small magnetic field (called a *magnetic moment*).
- When a patient enters an MRI scanner, the mini-magnet protons all align with the more powerful external magnetic field of the MRI magnet. Most of these protons will point **parallel to the field** and others point **antiparallel** to the field, but they will all align with the external magnetic field of the MRI.

- Protons do not like to be couch potatoes, so they **precess** (i.e., wobble like a spinning top) along the magnetic field lines of the MRI (Fig. 21.1).
- We will return to our little wobbling protons in a (magnetic) moment.

HARDWARE THAT MAKES UP AN MRI SCANNER

Main Magnet

- The main magnet in an MR scanner is usually a *superconducting magnet.*
- Superconducting magnets contain a conducting coil that is cooled down to **superconducting temperatures** (4° K or −269° Celsius) in order to carry the current. At temperatures that low (close to absolute zero), **resistance to the flow of electricity in the conductor practically disappears.**

> ### ▶▶ IMPORTANT POINTS
>
> - Therefore, an electric current sent once through this ultra-cold conducting material will **flow continuously** and create a **permanent magnetic field. The magnet in an MRI scanner is always "on."**

- Most scanners today have a **magnetic field strength** between **0.5 and 3 Tesla (T). Open MRI scanners,** those that do not completely encircle the patient in the scanning circle, have **lower field strengths of 0.1 to 1.0 T, which frequently results in decreased image quality.** By comparison, the earth's magnetic field is only about **50 micro Tesla.**

Step 1 Protons randomly oriented without external magnetic field

Step 2 All protons become aligned parallel to the external magnetic field (M) of the magnet along the longitudinal plane

Step 3 RF pulse is applied to the aligned protons

Step 4 Protons become excited by the RF pulse and flip from the longitudinal plane (dashed arrow) into the transverse plane (solid arrow)

Step 5 RF pulse ends and protons recover to longitudinal plane (solid arrow) =T1 relaxation, with accompanying decay of transverse magnetization (dashed arrow) =T2 relaxation

Fig. 21.1 A Relaxing Job. This graphic explains the various steps in the excitation and relaxation of the hydrogen protons in producing the T1 and T2 relaxation times.

Coils

- The **coils** within the magnet comprise an important part of the MRI scanner. These coils are responsible for either **transmitting** the **radiofrequency (RF) pulses (transmitter coils)** that excite the protons, or **receiving** the signal (or **echo**) given off by these excited protons (**receiver coils**) (Fig. 21.2).
- These coils are subjected to strong electrical currents and exist within a strong magnetic field that produces the repetitive "knocking" sound during an MRI scan.

Computer

- A computer dedicated to the MRI scanner processes the radiofrequency signals obtained by the receiver coils and converts them into an image.

WHAT HAPPENS ONCE SCANNING BEGINS

- When the patient is placed in the scanner magnet, the **transmitter coils** send a short (measured in milliseconds) electromagnetic pulse called a **radiofrequency (RF) pulse.** Remember that the spinning protons in the patient have already **aligned** with the external magnetic field of the magnet.
- This radiofrequency pulse is sent at a particular frequency that changes the orientation of the protons.
- When the **RF pulse is turned off,** the displaced protons **relax and realign** with the main magnetic field, and **energy** subsequently **released** in the **form of radiofrequency signals (the echo)** is **detected** by the **receiver coils.**

Fig. 21.2 Scanner Schematic. The **main magnet** produces the intense and stable magnetic field around the patient. **Shim coils** help make the magnetic field more homogeneous. The **gradient coils** are lower strength than the main magnetic field and produce a variable field adjusted to different body parts. **Radiofrequency coils** direct a pulse toward the area to be examined and are also adjusted for different body parts. The **scanner bore** is the horizontal tube in which the patient rests. The actual magnets reside inside the gantry housing.

Labels on figure: Scanner bore; Main magnet; Shim coils; Gradient coils; Radiofrequency coils

▶▶ IMPORTANT POINTS

- The times it takes for this **recovery** and **decay** to occur and the **echo** to be generated are **called *T1* and *T2*.**

- **T1 relaxation (or recovery)** is the time it takes for the tissue to recover to its **longitudinal state** (parallel to the magnetic field) (i.e., the time before the RF pulse was administered (see Fig. 21.1).
- **T2 relaxation (or decay)** is the time it takes for the tissue to regain its **transverse orientation** (perpendicular to the magnetic field) before the RF pulse was administered.
- **In summary,** as soon as the RF pulse stops, relaxation begins, and the spinning nuclei release energy that is subsequently detected by the receiver coil and ultimately used to produce an image.

Pulse Sequences

- **Pulse sequences** consist of a set of **imaging parameters** determined in advance by protocols for **specific diseases and body parts** and then preselected by the MRI technologist at the computer. A particular **imaging protocol** (e.g., a routine MRI brain protocol) **consists of a series of multiple pulse sequences** that determine the way different tissues will appear. A pulse sequence can last between 20 seconds and 15 minutes.

▶▶ IMPORTANT POINTS

- The **two main pulse sequences are spin echo (SE)** and **gradient recalled echo (GRE).** Spin echo sequences have a higher signal-to-noise ratio, but gradient recalled echo sequences are faster sequences preferred for rapid imaging techniques. **All of the pulse sequences used in MRI scanning are based on these two pulse sequences.**

- **TR and TE**
  - These parameters, which are set by the MRI operator at the console prior to scanning, determine how the image is **"weighted."**
  - **TR** is the **repetition time between two RF pulses,** and it influences the amount of **T1 weighting.**
    - Pulse sequences that feature a **short TR** (meaning a short amount of time between the RF pulses) will create what is called a **T1-weighted image.**
  - **TE,** which is the **echo time between a pulse and its resultant echo,** influences the amount of **T2 weighting.**
    - Pulse sequences that feature a **long TE** (meaning a long amount of time between the RF pulse and the echo) will create what is called a **T2-weighted image.**

HOW CAN YOU IDENTIFY A T1-WEIGHTED OR T2-WEIGHTED IMAGE?

- Different tissues have different T1 (recovery) and T2 (decay) values, which is why fat, muscle, and bone, for example, will appear differently not only from each other but also with different pulse sequences.

- **Tissues** that have a **short T1** will be **bright.**
- **Tissues** with a **long T2** will be **bright.**
- **Bright** translates into **whiter** or having **increased signal intensity** on MRI scans. **Dark** translates into **blacker** or having **decreased signal intensity** on MRI.

> ### ►► IMPORTANT POINTS
>
> - A key point is that **water** will be **dark** on **T1-weighted images** and **bright** on **T2-weighted images. Water is T1-dark and T2-bright.**
>   - A "**bright**" way to remember this fact is that the number "**2**" is both in **H_2O (water)** and **T2-weighted image.**
>   - Therefore, when looking at any MR image, **first try to find something you know is fluid (water),** such as the cerebrospinal fluid (**CSF**) **in the ventricles** and **spinal canal** or **urine** in the **bladder,** for example.
>   - If the fluid is **dark,** then you are probably looking at a **T1-weighted sequence** (Fig. 21.3A).
>   - If the fluid is **bright,** then chances are you are looking at a **T2-weighted image** (Fig. 21.3B).

- Certain tissues and structures are typically **bright on T1-weighted images.**
  - **Fat:** subcutaneous and intraabdominal fat, fat within yellow bone marrow, fat-containing tumors (see Fig. 21.3A)
  - **Hemorrhage:** although this varies depending on the **age** of the hemorrhage (Figs. 21.4)

- **Proteinaceous fluid:** proteinaceous fluid in renal or hepatic cysts, cystic neoplasms
  - However, a simple cyst containing water will be dark on T1 (and bright on T2), because remember that water is T1-dark (Fig. 21.5).
- **Melanin** (e.g., melanoma) (Fig. 21.6)
- **Gadolinium and other paramagnetic substances (manganese, copper)**
- Certain tissues and structures are typically **bright on T2-weighted images.**
  - **Fat:** subcutaneous and intraabdominal fat, fat within yellow bone marrow, fat-containing tumors (see Fig. 21.3B)
  - **Water, edema,** (Figs. 21.7 and 21.8) **inflammation, infection, cysts** (see Fig. 21.5)
  - **Hemorrhage:** although this varies depending on the **age** of the hemorrhage (see Fig. 21.4).
- Notice that **both fat and hemorrhage can be T1-bright and T2-bright.**
- **Suppression**
  - A useful feature of MRI is the ability to **cancel out** or **suppress** the signal from certain tissues selectively, thus making that tissue look **dark** on the image, and making other structures and pathology more conspicuous.
  - One body tissue that is **often suppressed** is **fat.**

Fig. 21.3 Normal T1-Weighted and T2-Weighted Axial Images of the Abdomen. Because cerebrospinal fluid is similar to water, it appears dark on the T1-weighted image (A) (*solid white arrow*) and bright on the T2-weighted image (B) (*open white arrow*). Subcutaneous fat (*dotted white arrows*) and intraabdominal fat (*dotted black arrows*) are bright on both T1- and T2-weighted images.

Fig. 21.4 Subcapsular Hematoma of the Kidney. (A) Axial T1-weighted, fat-suppressed image demonstrates a bright subcapsular hematoma (*solid white arrows*) involving the left kidney laterally. We can tell that this is a T1-weighted image because cerebrospinal fluid (CSF) in the spinal canal is dark (*open white arrow*). (B) Axial T2-weighted, fat-suppressed image again demonstrates a slightly bright left subcapsular hematoma, but also with a dark rim of hemosiderin (*dotted white arrows*) indicating surrounding older blood. There is a small amount of adjacent left perinephric fluid (*solid white arrow*). The bright signal of the CSF helps us to recognize this image as a T2-weighted image (*open white arrow*).

Fig. 21.5 Simple Left Ovarian Cyst. (A) Axial T2-weighted image demonstrates an ovoid, homogeneously bright lesion in the left ovary (*solid white arrows*) adjacent to a fibroid uterus (*dotted white arrows*). Note that urine in the bladder (*open white arrow*) and CSF in the spinal canal (*solid black arrow*) are both bright, which helps us identify this image as a T2-weighted image. (B) Axial, T1-weighted image shows that this left ovarian lesion is dark (*solid white arrows*) and therefore consistent with simple fluid. Urine in the bladder (*open white arrow*) and CSF in the spinal canal (*solid black arrow*) are also dark.

Fig. 21.6 Metastatic Melanoma. Sagittal T1-weighted image of the brain demonstrates a bright mass (*solid white arrow*) in the frontal lobe representing metastatic melanoma. Notice that both the yellow bone marrow within the skull (*solid black arrow*) and the overlying subcutaneous fat (*dotted white arrow*) are bright. We can tell that this is a T1-weighted image because the CSF in the lateral ventricles is dark (*open white arrow*).

Fig. 21.7 Glioblastoma Multiforme With Surrounding Edema. Axial T2-weighted image demonstrates bright vasogenic-type edema (*solid white arrows*) surrounding a large, lobulated frontal lobe mass (*dotted white arrows*) representing glioblastoma multiforme, an aggressive brain tumor. A few bright areas of cystic degeneration (*dotted black arrows*) appear within this mass. The frontal horns of the lateral ventricles are compressed (*solid black arrows*).

Fig. 21.8. Bone Marrow Edema Caused by Transient Lateral Patellar Dislocation. Axial proton-density, fat-saturated image (a T2-like sequence) demonstrates bright bone marrow edema involving the lateral (L) femoral (F) condyle (*dotted white arrows*) and medial aspect of the patella (P) (*solid black arrow*). This edema is due to recent lateral patellar dislocation with contusion of the patella as it struck the femur.

- **Fat** is normally bright on T1-weighted and T2-weighted images, but **will be dark on fat-suppressed images** (Fig. 21.9).
- This feature is useful when attempting to identify fat-containing lesions, such as **ovarian dermoid cysts, adrenal myelolipomas,** and **liposarcomas** (Fig. 21.10), as they will appear to change from **bright** on the **non–fat-suppressed** images to **dark** on the **fat-suppressed images.**
- Fat suppression is **also essential** for evaluation of tissues **after the administration of gadolinium contrast.**
- Many other pulse sequences besides T1-weighted and T2-weighted images typically comprise a particular MRI scan protocol, such as *diffusion-weighted images (DWI), proton density-weighted images,* and an entire alphabet soup of catchy acronyms such as **ADC, STIR, FLAIR, TOF,** *etc.*
- **Functional MRI (fMRI)** correlates the brain's changing **blood flow** requirements with changes in **neural activity** and translates them into differences in the MRI signal. It is being increasingly used to map neural activity in the brain, although it remains most commonly utilized in the research as opposed to the clinical setting.

MRI CONTRAST: GENERAL CONSIDERATIONS

> ### ⟫ IMPORTANT POINTS
>
> - **Gadolinium** is the most common intravenous contrast agent used in clinical MRI imaging.
>   - Gadolinium is a **rare-earth, heavy metal ion** that is chelated to different compounds to form MRI contrast agents. When chelated to an acid known as DOTA, it forms *gadoterate meglumine,* also known as the commonly used macrocyclic-structured contrast agent *Dotarem.*

Fig. 21.9 Normal T2-Weighted Fat-Suppressed Axial Image of the Abdomen. We can tell that this is a T2-weighted image because the cerebrospinal fluid in the spinal canal is bright (*open white arrow*). Note that the bile in the gallbladder (G) is also bright. It is a fat-suppressed image because the subcutaneous (*solid white arrow*) and intraabdominal (*dotted white arrow*) fat are dark. Fat is normally bright on a T2-weighted image without fat suppression.

- Gadolinium is **used in the same way that iodinated contrast media is used in CT.** It can be injected either by an intravascular or intraarticular route.
- After intravenous injection, gadolinium enters the blood pool, enhances organ parenchyma, and then is **excreted by the kidneys** via glomerular filtration.
  - Other special types of gadolinium-based contrast agents have a component of biliary excretion.
- **Gadolinium's effect is to shorten the T1 relaxation times** of hydrogen nuclei (and to a lesser extent also shorten T2). **T1 shortening will cause a brighter signal on T1-weighted images** than the same images without gadolinium and it is for this reason that **images obtained after gadolinium administration are usually T1-weighted** to take advantage of this effect.

Fig. 21.10 Fat in a Liposarcoma of the Right Spermatic Cord. (A) Axial T1-weighted image of the scrotum demonstrates a bright, heterogeneous right scrotal mass (*solid white arrows*). The left testis is unremarkable (*dotted white arrow*) and the right testis is not visualized. Note that subcutaneous fat is normally bright (*open white arrows*). (B) Axial T1-weighted, fat-suppressed, gadolinium-enhanced image demonstrates that the bright signal in the right scrotal mass is now dark, consistent with fat (*solid white arrows*). The subcutaneous fat is also dark on the fat-suppressed image (*open white arrows*). This was an unusual malignancy of the spermatic cord derived from fat cells.

- Fat is bright on T1 even before the administration of gadolinium. To increase detection of contrast enhancement in fat, the precontrast and postcontrast images are typically fat-suppressed (meaning darkened) to enhance the effect of the gadolinium (Fig. 21.11).

> **IMPORTANT POINTS**
>
> - Structures that become **bright on postgadolinium images are typically vascular** (e.g., tumors) (Fig. 21.12) **or are inflamed** tissues, and are described as **enhancing.**

Fig. 21.11 Fat Suppression and Normal Enhancement of the Abdomen Following the Administration of Intravenous Gadolinium. (A) T1-weighted image of a normal abdomen demonstrates normal bright subcutaneous and intraabdominal fat (*solid white arrows*). (B) T1-weighted, **fat-suppressed** image shows that the signal from the fat has been suppressed (*dotted white arrows*) and is now dark. Intraabdominal organs, such as the pancreas (P) and liver (L), now appear brighter relative to the adjacent suppressed fat. (C) T1-weighted, **fat-suppressed, early phase postgadolinium** image shows the normal enhancement of the aorta (*solid white arrow*), which enhances earlier than the inferior vena cava (I). The kidneys demonstrate normal corticomedullary phase enhancement (*dotted white arrows*), and the pancreas (P) enhances maximally during this phase. (D) T1-weighted, **fat-suppressed, later phase postgadolinium** image shows that the hepatic veins (*solid black arrow*) and inferior vena cava (I) are now well-enhanced. The kidneys (K) now demonstrate normal homogeneous enhancement, the optimal phase to detect renal masses.

Fig. 21.12 Right Parotid Pleomorphic Adenoma. (A) Axial T1-weighted image of the neck demonstrates a dark, ovoid mass with a slightly lobular contour (*solid black arrows*) located within the right parotid gland (*solid white arrows*). The left parotid gland is unremarkable (*dotted white arrows*). (B) Axial T1-weighted, fat-suppressed, postgadolinium-enhanced image demonstrates that the right parotid mass is very bright because of intense enhancement (*dotted white arrows*). Surgical resection of this mass yielded a pleomorphic adenoma, the most common benign tumor of the parotid gland. A clue that this image is a gadolinium-enhanced image is the presence of bright, enhancing vascular structures, such as the left retromandibular vein (*solid white arrow*).

MRI SAFETY ISSUES

Claustrophobia

- Compared with CT scans, the MRI bore is a narrower, more confined space than the CT gantry, and MRI examinations have a longer scan time. Patients can therefore occasionally suffer such extreme claustrophobia in the small confines of the MR scanner that **they will be unable to begin or complete** the study. Pretreatment with sedatives may help, in the appropriate clinical situation.
- Alternatively, the patient can be scanned in an **open magnet,** which is not as confining. The trade-off, however, is that open magnets, in general, have lower magnetic field strengths and poorer spatial resolution.

Ferromagnetic Objects

- Any ferromagnetic object inside the patient **can be moved** by the magnetic field of the MR scanner and potentially damage adjacent tissues. Such internal ferromagnetic objects also hold the potential to be **heated and cause burns** to surrounding tissues.

> ### ⟫ IMPORTANT POINTS
>
> - **Ferromagnetic objects inserted in a location where motion of the object may be harmful to the patient represent an absolute contraindication to MR imaging.** These objects include medically inserted items such as cerebral aneurysm repair clips, vascular clips, and surgical staples. Many vascular clips and staples are now manufactured to be MRI-compatible.

- Some **foreign bodies, such as bullets, shrapnel, and metal in the eyes** (as can sometimes be found in metal workers), can also be ferromagnetic.
  - Patients who may have a history of possible metallic foreign bodies in the eyes must have conventional orbital radiographs before undergoing an MRI and, if metal is present, an alternative means of imaging should be utilized.
- Ferromagnetic objects **outside** of the patient, such as **oxygen tanks, scissors, scalpels,** and **metallic tools,** also pose a risk to the patient as **they could become airborne** once they enter the magnetic field and for this reason are strictly forbidden in the MRI scanning room.
- The current terminology applied to identifying the safety of devices and whether they can enter an MRI environment is shown in Table 21.1.

Mechanical or Electrical Devices

- MRI cannot usually be performed in patients who have **pacemakers, pain stimulator implants, insulin pumps, other implantable drug infusion pumps,** and **cochlear implants.** An exception is a newer FDA-approved type of pacemaker that is specifically engineered to safely undergo MRI.

Pregnant Patients

- Although there are no known biological risks associated with MR imaging in adults, the effects of MRI on the fetus are not definitely known.

TABLE 21.1	**Is That Device MRI Compatible?**
Device Label	**Meaning**
MRI Safe	An item poses no known hazards in any MRI environment (e.g., plastic tubing)
MRI Conditional	The item is safe under predetermined conditions in some MRI environments (e.g., up to a certain field strength such as 3 Tesla)
MRI Unsafe	An item that is known to pose hazards in all MRI environments (e.g., a pair of scissors)

Source: American Society for Testing and Materials (ASTM) International, Designation: F2503-05. Standard Practice for Marking Medical Devices and Other Items for Safety in the Magnetic Resonance Environment. ASTM International, West Conshohocken, PA, 2005.

Fig. 21.13 MRI in Pregnancy. Coronal T2-weighted image demonstrates an intrauterine pregnancy. The maternal liver (*L*) and spleen (*S*) are partially imaged. The bright amniotic fluid (*A*) and fetal cerebrospinal fluid (*dotted white arrow*) help us to recognize this image as a T2-weighted image. The fetal body (*solid white arrow*) and leg (*dotted black arrow*) can be seen clearly. The umbilical cord (*solid black arrow*) is partially visualized.

- However, current data yield no evidence of definite harmful effects on the developing fetus using MRI with a field strength of 1.5 T. Therefore, the American College of Radiology states that pregnant patients **can** undergo MRI scans at any stage of pregnancy if it is decided that the risk-to-benefit ratio to the patient weighs in favor of performing the study (Fig. 21.13).

- **Gadolinium is not recommended in pregnant patients,** as gadolinium crosses the placenta, is subsequently excreted by the fetal kidneys, and has unknown effects on the fetus.

Nephrogenic Systemic Fibrosis

- In patients with renal insufficiency, gadolinium has been associated with a rare, painful, debilitating, and sometimes fatal disease called **nephrogenic systemic fibrosis (NSF).**
- NSF produces fibrosis of skin, eyes, joints, and internal organs resembling scleroderma.
- Patients with **end-stage or severe chronic kidney disease,** especially those on dialysis, were thought to be at the **greatest risk.**
    - However, the latest guidelines indicate that the now more-commonly used gadolinium-based contrast agents

have negligible if any risk of NSF, and can even be administered to patients with end-stage renal disease on dialysis.

- It has been discovered that gadolinium can deposit in brain tissue, particularly in patients who have received multiple doses of gadolinium-based contrast agents. The significance of this deposition is being actively investigated, but currently no known health risk or neurotoxicity has been associated with this phenomenon.

DIAGNOSTIC APPLICATIONS OF MRI

- Some of the many clinical uses of MRI are outlined in Table 21.2. The chapters in which some of the diseases are discussed in greater detail are indicated.

TABLE 21.2 Diagnostic Applications of MRI

System	Organ	Diseases
Musculoskeletal	Evaluate bone marrow, menisci, tendons, muscles	Meniscal tears; ligamentous and tendon injuries; contusions
	Bones	Occult or stress fractures
	Osteomyelitis	High negative predictive value if normal
	Spine **(see Chapter 23)**	Disc disease and marrow infiltration; differentiating scarring from prior surgery from new disease; evaluating spinal cord
Neurologic	Brain **(see Chapter 27)**	Ideal for studying brain, especially posterior fossa; tumor, infarction; multiple sclerosis
	Peripheral nerves	Impingement; injury
Gastrointestinal	Liver **(see Chapter 18)**	Characterize liver lesions; detect small lesions; cysts, hemangiomas; hepatocellular carcinoma; focal nodular hyperplasia; hemochromatosis; fatty infiltration
	Biliary system **(see Chapter 18)**	Magnetic resonance cholangiopancreatography for ductal dilatation, choledocholithiasis, strictures
	Small and large bowel	MR enterography; appendicitis in pregnant females
Endocrine/ reproductive	Adrenal glands	Adenomas; adrenal hemorrhage
	Female pelvis	Anatomy of uterus and ovaries; leiomyomas; adenomyosis; ovarian dermoid cysts; endometriosis; hydrosalpinx
	Male pelvis	Staging of rectal, bladder, and prostate carcinoma
Genitourinary	Kidneys	Renal masses; cysts versus masses

🏠 TAKE HOME POINTS

- MRI uses a very strong magnetic field to influence the electromagnetic activity of hydrogen nuclei, also called protons.
- **Protons** each have a charge and possess a spin. The constant movement of protons generates a small magnetic field causing the proton to behave like a mini-magnet. When the protons are placed in the much more powerful magnetic field of the MRI scanner, they all align with this external magnetic field.
- A **radiofrequency (RF) pulse,** transmitted by a transmitter coil, displaces the protons from their original alignment with the external magnetic field of the scanner.
- When the RF pulse is turned off, the displaced protons **relax and realign** with the main magnetic field, producing a radiofrequency signal (the echo) as they do so. Receiver coils receive this signal (or echo) given off by the excited protons. A computer reconstructs the information from the echo to generate an image.

- The main magnet in an MRI scanner is usually a **superconducting magnet** that is cooled to extremely low temperatures in order to carry the electrical current continuously.
- **Pulse sequences** consist of a set of imaging parameters that determine the way a particular tissue will appear. The two main pulse sequences on which all MRI pulse sequences are based are called **spin echo (SE)** and **gradient recalled echo (GRE).**
- **T1 and T2** are both time constants. T1 is called the **longitudinal** relaxation time, and T2 is called the **transverse** relaxation time.
- **TR** is the repetition time between two RF pulses. A short TR creates a T1-weighted image.
- **TE** is the echo time between a pulse and its resultant echo. A long TE creates a T2-weighted image.
- On T1-weighted images, fat, hemorrhage, proteinaceous fluid, melanin, and gadolinium are typically **bright (white).**

Continued

TAKE HOME POINTS—cont'd

- On T2-weighted images, fat, water, edema, inflammation, infection, cysts, and hemorrhage are typically **bright.**
- In summary, **fat is T1-bright and T2-bright. Water is T1-dark and T2-bright.**
- **Suppression** is a feature of MRI that will cancel out or eliminate signal from certain tissues and is most often used for fat. Although normally T1-bright, fat will be dark on T1-weighted, fat suppressed images. Fat suppression is particularly useful for tissue characterization after administration of gadolinium.
- **Gadolinium** is the most common intravenous contrast agent used in clinical MRI, and its effect is to **shorten the T1 relaxation time** of hydrogen nuclei yielding a **brighter signal.** Vascular structures, such as tumors and areas of

inflammation, enhance after gadolinium administration and become more conspicuous.
- **Ferromagnetic objects** must be kept outside of the MRI scanning room as they could become airborne when exposed to the magnetic field. Patients who may have metallic foreign bodies in their eyes must first have conventional orbital radiographs to determine if metal is present.
- In **pregnancy**, MRI is preferred in the second and third trimester, and gadolinium is contraindicated.
- **Nephrogenic systemic fibrosis** is a debilitating fibrotic disease that can occur in patients with renal insufficiency who receive intravenous gadolinium. Therefore, gadolinium is typically avoided in patients with severe renal disease.

More information on magnetic resonance imaging: understanding the principles and recognizing the basics is available to registered users online.

Recognizing Nontraumatic Abnormalities of the Appendicular Skeleton Including Arthritis

CONVENTIONAL RADIOGRAPHY, CT, AND MRI IN BONE IMAGING

- Most **examinations of bone start with conventional radiographs** obtained with at least **two views exposed at a 90-degree angle to each other** (called **orthogonal views**) so as to localize abnormalities better and to visualize as much of the bone as possible (Fig. 22.1).
- Still, conventional radiographs cannot visualize the entire circumference of a tubular bone and they are not particularly sensitive for demonstrating musculoskeletal soft-tissue abnormalities other than significant soft-tissue swelling.

- It is important to remember that, although the cortex completely surrounds the entire bone, on conventional radiographs it is best seen where it is viewed in profile (i.e., where the x-ray beam passes tangentially to the bone).
- CT and MRI are able to demonstrate the entire circumference and internal matrix of bone including, especially with MRI, the **surrounding soft tissues** not visible on conventional radiographs. This is accomplished by computer-aided reformatting and a superior ability to display more subtle differences in tissue densities (Fig. 22.2).
- **MRI** is an excellent means of studying the components of marrow, a fact that makes it so useful in the study of **marrow pathology.**

Fig. 22.1 Importance of Orthogonal Views. (A) On this frontal view of the knee, a bullet (*solid white arrow*) appears to lie within the distal femur. (B) The lateral view demonstrates that the bullet, in fact, is in the suprapatellar soft tissue (*dotted arrow*), not the femur. Conventional views of bone require two images at roughly 90 degrees to each other to help localize a finding.

Fig. 22.2 Normal Appearance of Bone. (A) This is an anteroposterior radiograph of the hip. When viewed in tangent, the cortex is seen as a smooth, white line, varying in thickness in different parts of the bone (*white arrows*). The **medullary cavity** lies within the **cortical shell** and contains an interlacing network of trabeculae (*white circle*). The **corticomedullary junction** is the interface between the inner margin of the cortex and the medullary cavity (*solid black arrow*). (B) An axial CT scan through the femoral shaft depicts the entire 360-degree circumference of the cortex (*dotted white arrow*) surrounding the less-dense medullary cavity containing both bony trabeculae and fat (*white circle*). This image is optimized to display bone, which is why the muscles and subcutaneous fat are less-well seen.

Whereas the cortex is the part of the bone most easily visualized on conventional radiographs, **cortical bone has a very low signal intensity on conventional MRI** sequences (Fig. 22.3).

NORMAL BONE AND JOINT ANATOMY

* On conventional radiographs, long bones are visualized as having a dense **cortex** of **compact bone** that completely envelopes a less-dense **medullary cavity** containing **cancellous bone** arranged as **trabeculae,** separated primarily by blood vessels, hematopoietic cells, and fat. The shaft of the bone is the **diaphysis**, capped on each end by the **epiphyses**. Where the diaphysis and epiphysis join (i.e., the **metaphysis**) is the site of the **epiphysial growth plate** in children.
* The proportions of cortical versus trabecular bone vary in different skeletal sites and even at different locations in the same bone (i.e., the **cortex is naturally thicker in some places than in others**) (see Fig. 22.2A).
* Fig. 22.4 contains a diagram of a typical synovial joint and compares the structures visualized on conventional radiographs and MRI.

DISEASES THAT AFFECT BONE DENSITY

The Effect of Bone Physiology on Bone Anatomy

* Bones reflect the general metabolic status of the individual. Their composition requires a **protein-containing, collagenous**

Fig. 22.3 Normal MRI of Knee. A sagittal view of the knee demonstrates the superior display of the internal matrix of bone and the surrounding soft tissues seen on MRI. There is fatty marrow in the distal femur (F), proximal tibia (T), and patella (P). The quadriceps (*solid black arrow*) and patellar (*dotted white arrow*) tendons are shown. The anterior cruciate ligament (*solid white arrow*) is visible. There is high signal fat in the infrapatellar fat pad (FP). Notice how the bone's cortex has a very weak signal, appearing dark (*dotted black arrow*).

Fig. 22.4 Diagram, Radiograph, and MRI Image of a True Joint. (A) A representation of a synovial joint shows the **articular cortex** that corresponds to the thin white line within the **joint capsule** that is usually capped by hyaline **articular cartilage**. The bone immediately beneath the articular cortex is called **subchondral bone**. Within the joint capsule is the **synovial membrane** and **synovial fluid**. (B) On conventional radiographs, the articular cortex (*solid white arrow*) and subchondral bone (*solid black arrows*) are visible, but the cartilage and synovial fluid are not (*dotted white arrow*). (C) A T1-weighted, coronal MRI of the knee shows the medial (MM) and lateral (LM) menisci, anterior (ACL) and posterior (PCL) cruciate ligaments, articular cartilage (*dotted black arrow*), joint capsule (*dotted white arrow*), synovial fluid (*solid white arrow*), and marrow in the subchondral bone (SC). The cortex of the bone (*solid black arrow*) produces little signal and is dark.

matrix (**osteoid**) upon which **bone mineral**, principally **calcium phosphate**, is transformed into cartilage and bone.

- Bones are continuously undergoing remodeling processes that include **resorption of old or diseased bone by osteoclasts** and **formation of new bone by osteoblasts.** Osteoblasts are responsible for bone matrix production, whereas osteoclasts resorb both the matrix and mineral.
- Both osteoclastic and osteoblastic activity depend on the presence of a **viable blood supply** to bring those cells to the bone.
- Bones also **respond to mechanical forces;** for example, the contractions of muscles and tendons, the process of bearing weight, constant use, or prolonged disuse, which help to form and/or maintain the shape as well as the content of each bone.
- In this section, we arbitrarily divide abnormalities of **bone density** into two major categories based primarily on their appearance on conventional radiographs: those that produce a pattern of either **increased** or **decreased** bone density (Table 22.1).

TABLE 22.1	**Changes in Bone Density**	
Density	**Extent**	**Examples Used in this Chapter**
Increased density	Diffuse	Diffuse osteoblastic metastases
	Focal	Localized osteoblastic metastases
		Avascular necrosis of bone
		Paget disease
Decreased density	Diffuse	Osteoporosis
		Hyperparathyroidism
	Focal	Localized osteolytic metastases
		Multiple myeloma
		Osteomyelitis

Fig. 22.5 Corticomedullary Junction: Normal and Abnormal. (A) The cortex normally projects as a smooth white line of varying thickness at the periphery of bone on conventional radiographs (*solid white arrows*), distinguishable from the less-dense medullary cavity (*asterisks*). (B) Diseases that cause a generalized increase in bone density "fill-in" the medullary cavity (*asterisks*) and make it as dense as the cortex (*dotted white arrows*). This obliterates the corticomedullary interface seen in normal bones. This patient had diffuse, osteoblastic metastatic prostate carcinoma.

DISEASES THAT INCREASE BONE DENSITY

Recognizing an Increase in Bone Density

- On conventional radiographs and CT, there is an **overall whiteness (sclerosis)** to all or most of the bones and a loss of the distinction between **the normal cortico-medullary junction** because of the abnormally increased density of the medullary cavity relative to the cortex (Fig. 22.5).
- Examples of diseases that cause increased bone density include metastatic disease, avascular necrosis of bone, and Paget disease.

Osteoblastic Metastatic Disease

- Diffuse, blood-borne, metastatic disease from **carcinoma of the prostate** is the **prototype for a generalized increase in bone density.** Osteoblastic metastatic disease, like that from the prostate, can also produce **focal areas** of increased bone density as well. These osteoblastic lesions are **most often** seen in the **vertebrae, ribs, pelvis, humeri,** and **femora** (Fig. 22.6). Osteoblastic activity occurs beyond the control of normal physiologic constraints.
- **Focal sclerotic lesions** can affect either the cortex, the medullary cavity, or both. Those that affect the **cortex** will usually produce **periosteal new-bone formation** *(periosteal reaction),* which leads to an appearance of **thickening of the cortex.** Those that affect the **medullary cavity** will result in **punctate,**

Fig. 22.6 Diffuse Metastatic Disease From Carcinoma of the Prostate. The bones are diffusely sclerotic from osteoblastic activity. You can no longer see the normal trabeculae nor the junction between the medullary cavity and the cortex. Contrast this picture with that of Paget disease of the pelvis (see Fig. 22.13).

amorphous, sclerotic lesions surrounded by the normal medullary cavity (Fig. 22.7).

- Metastatic disease to bone is found in a **significant percentage of autopsied patients with carcinoma of the prostate.** **Multiple** bone **metastases** from carcinoma of the prostate occur much **more frequently** than do **solitary bone lesions,** which are discussed later in this chapter (Box 22.1).

》 IMPORTANT POINTS

- The **radionuclide bone scan is currently the study of choice for detecting skeletal metastases**, regardless of the suspected primary (Box 22.2). With diffuse bone metastases, a so-called **superscan** may be seen on radionuclide bone scan. The superscan demonstrates high radiotracer uptake throughout the skeleton, with poor or absent renal excretion of the radiotracer (Fig. 22.8).

Fig. 22.7 Focal Sclerotic Metastases From Carcinoma of the Breast. Sclerotic lesions are seen in the L4 and S1 vertebral bodies (*white arrows*). Also present are multiple sclerotic lesions in the right ilium (*white circle*) and scattered throughout the pelvis. Metastatic breast carcinoma can be both osteolytic and osteoblastic.

Fig. 22.8 Metastatic Disease on Radionuclide Bone Scan. Anteroposterior and posteroanterior views of the axial and appendicular skeleton show the distribution of bone radiotracer uptake throughout the skeleton. This is the picture of the so-called **superscan** produced by osteoblastic metastatic disease involving every bone, leading to very high uptake throughout the skeleton and very little renal excretion of the radiotracer (*white arrows* point to the **absence** of excretion by the kidneys, a characteristic of a superscan).

BOX 22.1   Metastatic Disease to Bone

- **Metastases** to bone are far more common than primary bone tumors.
- Metastases to bone fall into two major categories: those that stimulate the production of new bone are called **osteoblastic** and those that destroy bone are called **osteolytic**; some metastases include lesions in which **both** osteoblastic and osteolytic changes are present.
- Metastatic bone lesions from any source are very uncommon distal to the elbow or the knee; when present in these locations, they are usually widespread and caused by lung or breast cancer.

Avascular Necrosis of Bone

- **Avascular necrosis (AVN)** of bone (also called **ischemic necrosis, aseptic necrosis, osteonecrosis**) results from cellular death and eventually leads to the collapse of the affected bone. It usually involves those bones that have a relatively **poor collateral blood supply** (e.g., scaphoid in the wrist, femoral head) and tends to affect the hematopoietic elements of marrow earliest so that **MRI is the most sensitive modality for detecting AVN.**

BOX 22.2   Finding Metastases to Bone: Bone Scan

- A radionuclide bone scan requires the intravenous administration of a minute amount of **technetium 99M MDP**, a radioactively tagged tracer that affixes to the surface of bone.
- Technetium 99M is the **radionuclide** used to tag methylene diphosphonate (MDP), the portion that **directs** the tracer to bone.
- Uptake of the radionuclide in bone depends, in part, on the bone's blood supply and rate of bone turnover: processes with extremely high or extremely low bone turnover may produce false–negative scans.
- **Osteoblastic lesions** almost always show increased activity (uptake of radiotracer). Even **osteolytic metastases** usually show increased uptake because of the repair that occurs in most, but not all, osteolytic processes.
- The bone scan is much **less sensitive** in detecting **multiple myeloma**, so conventional radiographic surveys of the skeleton are the initial study of choice when searching for myeloma lesions.
- Bone scans are **highly sensitive, but not very specific;** a positive scan almost always requires another imaging procedure (conventional radiographs, CT, or MRI) to rule out nonmalignant causes of a positive bone scan (e.g., fractures or osteomyelitis).

- There are a myriad of causes of avascular necrosis. Some of the more common are shown in Table 22.2.
- On conventional radiographs, the devascularized bone becomes **denser** and therefore appears more sclerotic than the remainder of the bone. This especially occurs in the **femoral head** (Fig. 22.9) and **humeral head** (Fig. 22.10).

- On **MRI,** there is usually a **decrease from the normal high signal** produced by fatty marrow (Fig. 22.11).
- On conventional radiographs, **old medullary bone infarcts** are recognized as dense, amorphous deposits of bone within the medullary cavities of long bones, frequently marginated by a thin, sclerotic membrane (Fig. 22.12).

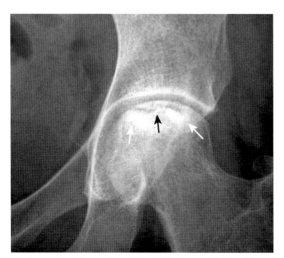

Fig. 22.9 Avascular Necrosis of the Left Femoral Head in a Patient on Long-Term Steroids for Systemic Lupus Erythematosus. A close-up view of the left femoral head shows a zone of increased sclerosis in the superior aspect of the femoral head (*white arrows*), a characteristic finding of avascular necrosis of the head. The linear, subcortical lucency (*black arrow*) represents subchondral fractures seen with this disease, called the **crescent sign**. Notice that the disease is isolated to the femoral head and involves neither the joint space nor the acetabulum (i.e., this it is not an arthritis).

TABLE 22.2	Some Causes of Avascular Necrosis of Bone	
Location	**Example of Disease**
Intravascular	Sickle-cell disease Polycythemia vera
Vascular	Vasculitis (Lupus and radiation-induced)
Extravascular	Trauma (fractures)
Idiopathic	Exogenous steroids and Cushing disease Legg-Calve-Perthes disease

Fig. 22.11 Avascular Necrosis: MRI. A T1-weighted coronal view of both hips demonstrates normal high signal from the fatty marrow in the right femur (*dotted white arrow*), but decreased signal in the left femoral head extending to the subchondral bone of the left hip joint (*solid white arrow*). The joint space is preserved. MRI is the most sensitive method of detecting avascular necrosis of the hip.

Fig. 22.10 Avascular Necrosis of Humeral Head. There is increased density seen at the very top of the humeral head (*black arrow*) in this patient with sickle-cell disease. Because the white cap on the bone was thought to resemble snow on a mountain-top, this sign of avascular necrosis has been called **snow-capping**. Avascular necrosis in sickle-cell disease does not usually manifest until young adulthood and, with the sensitivity of MRI, is more prevalent than originally had been thought using plain films alone.

Fig. 22.12 Old Medullary Bone Infarct. An amorphous calcification is seen in the medullary cavity of the proximal femur (*white arrows*). In general, the differential diagnosis for such an intramedullary calcification includes bone infarct or enchondroma. The characteristic sclerotic membrane surrounding this lesion suggests it is more likely an old bone infarct. This patient had been on long-term steroids for asthma.

Paget Disease

- Paget disease is a **chronic disease of bone**, most often occurring in older men, now believed to be caused by chronic paramyxoviral infection. It is **characterized by varying degrees of increased bone resorption and increased bone formation** with the latter predominating in those cases seen in more progressive forms of the disease.
- The end result is almost always a **denser bone** that, despite its density, is **mechanically inferior** to normal bone and thus **susceptible to pathologic fractures** or bone-softening deformities such as **bowing**. The **pelvis** is **most frequently involved**, followed by the **lumbar spine, thoracic spine, proximal femur,** and **calvarium.**

> **》 IMPORTANT POINTS**
>
> - Paget disease is usually diagnosed with conventional radiography. **The imaging hallmarks of Paget disease are:**
>   - **Thickening of the cortex.**
>   - **Coarsening and thickening of the trabecular pattern** (Fig. 22.13).
>   - **Increase in the size of the bone involved.** The "classical" history for Paget disease, rendered less useful since fashions have changed, was a gradual increase in a man's hat size as the calvarium increased in size from this disease.

DISEASES THAT DECREASE BONE DENSITY

Recognizing a Decrease in Bone Density

- As bones decrease in radiographic density, there may be a **diffuse loss of the normal network of bony trabeculae in the medullary cavity** because of the decreased number and thinning of many of the smaller trabecular structures.
- **Accentuation of the cortex** may be present, in which the cortex, although thinner than normal, **stands out more strikingly** because of the lower density of the medullary cavity (Fig. 22.14).

Fig. 22.13 Paget Disease of the Pelvis: Two Patients. (A) Frontal view of the pelvis shows an **increase in bony density** in the left hemipelvis, **accentuation** and coarsening of the **trabeculae** and **thickening** of the cortex (*white circle*), the hallmarks of Paget disease of bone. Compare the left hemipelvis with the normal right hemipelvis. (B) Axial CT scan of the pelvis of another patient with Paget disease demonstrates thickening of the cortex and accentuation of the trabeculae in the right ilium (*solid white arrow*). Compare it with the normal left side (*dotted white arrow*).

Fig. 22.14 Normal and Osteoporotic Foot. (A) Normal frontal view of the foot to contrast with (B) in the same patient some weeks later after prolonged immobilization. (B) There is overall decreased density of the bone and thinning of the cortices (*white arrows*) secondary to disuse osteoporosis. Conventional radiographs are subject to technical variations that can mimic osteoporosis even in a healthy individual.

- **Compression of vertebral bodies** (see Chapter 23).
- **Pathologic fractures** in the hip, pelvis, or vertebral bodies (see Chapter 24).
- Examples of diseases that cause a diffuse decrease in bone density include osteoporosis and hyperparathyroidism.

Osteoporosis

- **Osteoporosis** is defined as a systemic skeletal disorder **characterized by low bone mineral density** (BMD) and generally divided into **postmenopausal** and **age-related bone loss.**
  - **Postmenopausal osteoporosis** is characterized by **increased bone resorption** due to osteoclastic activity. **Age-related bone loss** begins around age 45 to 55 and is characterized by a **loss of total bone mass.**
- Additional factors that **increase the risk of osteoporosis** include exogenous steroid administration, Cushing disease, estrogen deficiency, inadequate physical activity, and alcoholism.
- Osteoporosis **predisposes to pathologic fractures** in the femoral neck, compression fractures of the vertebral bodies, and fractures of the distal radius (Colles fractures).
- **Conventional radiographs** are relatively **insensitive for detecting osteoporosis.** Almost **50% of the bone mass must be lost** before it is **recognizable** on conventional radiographs. Findings on conventional radiographs include **overall decreased density of bone, thinning of the cortex, and decrease in the visible number of trabeculae in the medullary cavity** (see Fig. 22.14B).
- Currently, **DEXA** (*Dual-energy X-ray Absorptiometry*) **scans are the most accurate** and widely recommended method for bone mineral density measurements.
  - DEXA scans are obtained by using a filtered x-ray source that produces two distinct energies that are differentially absorbed by bone and soft tissue, respectively. This allows for the more accurate calculation of bone density by subtracting the error introduced by varying amounts of overlying soft tissue. The x-ray dose is very low and the spine or hip are generally used for density measurements.

Hyperparathyroidism

- **Hyperparathyroidism** is a condition caused by excessive secretion of **parathormone (PTH)** by the parathyroid glands. Parathormone exerts its effects on bones, the kidneys, and the gastrointestinal tract. Its **effect on bones is to increase resorption** by stimulating osteoclastic activity. Calcium is removed from the bone and deposited in the bloodstream.
- There are **three forms** of hyperparathyroidism, which are listed in Table 22.3.
- The **diagnosis of hyperparathyroidism is based on clinical and laboratory findings,** but there are numerous findings of the disease on conventional radiographs and there are other imaging studies utilized to aid in surgery on the glands, if indicated. Imaging studies of the parathyroid glands themselves may include ultrasound, nuclear medicine parathyroid scans, and MRI scans.

TABLE 22.3 Forms of Hyperparathyroidism

Type	Remarks
Primary	Usually caused by a single adenoma in most patients (80% to 90%) and almost always results in hypercalcemia
Secondary	Results from hyperplasia of the glands secondary to imbalances in calcium and phosphorous levels, seen mostly with chronic renal disease
Tertiary	Occurs in patients with long-standing secondary hyperparathyroidism in whom autonomous hypersecretion of parathyroid hormone develops, leading to hypercalcemia

IMPORTANT POINTS

- Some of the **findings of hyperparathyroidism on conventional radiographs** include:
  - Overall **decrease in bony density.**
  - **Subperiosteal bone resorption,** especially on the radial side of the middle phalanges of the index and middle fingers (Fig. 22.15).
  - **Erosion of the distal clavicles** (Fig. 22.16).
  - **Well-circumscribed lytic lesions** in the long bones called **Brown tumors** (Fig. 22.17)

Focal Decreases in Bone Density

- Examples of diseases that cause a **focal decrease** in bone density include osteolytic metastatic disease, multiple myeloma, and osteomyelitis.

Osteolytic Metastatic Disease

- **Osteolytic metastatic disease** can produce focal destruction of bone (see Box 22.1). These lesions are most often produced by **focal infiltration of bone by cells other than osteocytes.**
- The **medullary cavity is almost always involved,** from which the disease may erode into and destroy the cortex as well. When the medullary cavity alone is involved, there must be almost a 50% reduction in mass in order for the lesion to be recognizable on **conventional radiographs** when viewed *en face.*
- MRI, on the other hand, is **excellent** at demonstrating the status of the medullary cavity and so is much more sensitive to the presence of metastatic disease than conventional radiography (Fig. 22.18).
- In **some cases, only the cortex is involved.** Cortical metastases may be easier to visualize on conventional radiographs because relatively less cortical destruction is needed for them to become apparent, especially if the lesions happen to be viewed in tangent.

Fig. 22.15 Subperiosteal Resorption in Hyperparathyroidism. Characteristic subperiosteal bone resorption is seen especially well on the radial aspect of the middle phalanges of the index and middle fingers (*solid white arrows*). Here the cortex appears shaggy and irregular, compared with the cortices on the opposite sides of the same bones, which are well defined. This patient also displays two other findings of hyperparathyroidism: a small **brown tumor** (*black arrow*) and resorption of the terminal phalanges **(acroosteolysis)** (*dotted white arrows*).

Fig. 22.17 Brown Tumor. There is a geographic lytic lesion in the midshaft of the tibia (*black arrows*). Brown tumors (also called **osteoclastomas**) are benign lesions that represent the osteoclastic resorption of a localized area of (usually) cortical bone and its replacement with fibrous tissue and blood. Their high hemosiderin content gives them a characteristic brown color; they were not named after a "Dr. Brown." These bone lesions can mimic osteolytic metastases or multiple myeloma, so that the clinical history of hyperparathyroidism is key. They can be seen with both primary and secondary hyperparathyroidism.

Fig. 22.16 Erosion of Distal Clavicle in Hyperparathyroidism. Another relatively common site of bone resorption in hyperparathyroidism is the distal end of the clavicle. Here the distal clavicle (*solid white arrow*), which should normally articulate with the acromion (*dotted white arrow*) has been resorbed, increasing the distance between it and the acromion. Other sites of bone resorption in hyperparathyroidism might include the lamina dura of the teeth, and the medial aspects of the tibia, humerus, and femur.

Fig. 22.18 Metastases to Lumbar Spine: MRI. (A) There is normal signal in the lumbar vertebral bodies on this T1-weighted sagittal view of the lumbar spine (*dotted white arrow*). (B) In another patient with a primary breast carcinoma, multiple metastatic deposits are replacing the normal marrow in the lumbar spine and sacrum (*black arrows*). The body of L4 is completely replaced by tumor (*solid white arrow*).

Fig. 22.19 Three Patterns of Lytic Bone Lesions. (A) This is a solitary **geographic** bone lesion with a gradual zone of transition between it and surrounding normal bone along with complete destruction of the cortex (*white arrow*). (B) This is a close-up of the femur in another patient that demonstrates several ill-defined lytic lesions (*dotted white arrows*) with indistinct margins implying a more aggressive malignancy. This appearance is called a **moth-eaten pattern**. (C) Another close-up of the femur in a different patient shows innumerable, small irregular holes in the bone (*white circle*) called a **permeative pattern**. Permeative lesions are called **round cell lesions** for the shape of the cells that produce them. Such diseases include Ewing's sarcoma, myeloma, and leukemia.

>> **IMPORTANT POINTS**

- On conventional radiographs, the **classical findings of osteolytic metastases** include:
  - **Irregularly shaped, lucent bone lesions,** which can be single or multiple.
    - These lytic lesions are frequently characterized as belonging to one (or sometimes more) of three patterns: **geographic, mottled, or permeative**, in order of decreasing size of the most discrete lesion visible (Fig. 22.19).
  - Osteolytic metastases typically **incite little or no reactive bone formation** around them. They can be **expansile** and **soap-bubbly** (i.e., contain bony septations), especially in renal and thyroid carcinoma (Fig. 22.20).
  - In the spine, they may preferentially **destroy the pedicles,** because of their blood supply (the **pedicle sign**), which can help to differentiate metastases from multiple myeloma (see below) that tends to spare the pedicle early in the disease (Fig. 22.21).

- The most common causes of osteoblastic and osteolytic bone metastases are listed in Table 22.4.

TABLE 22.4 Causes of Osteoblastic and Osteolytic Bone Metastases

Osteoblastic	Osteolytic
Prostate carcinoma (most common in older men)	Lung cancer (most common osteolytic lesion in male patients)
Breast carcinoma is usually osteolytic, but can be osteoblastic, especially if treated	Breast cancer (most common osteolytic lesion in female patients)
Lymphoma	Renal cell carcinoma
Carcinoid tumors (rare)	Thyroid carcinoma

Fig. 22.20 Expansile Renal Cell Carcinoma Metastasis. This is a very **aggressive** and **expansile** osteolytic metastasis in the humerus from a primary renal cell carcinoma. Notice that the cortex has been destroyed in several areas (*dotted white arrows*) and the lesion has a characteristic **soap-bubbly** appearance produced by fine septae (*solid white arrow*). Thyroid carcinoma and a solitary plasmacytoma could also produce these findings.

Myeloma

- **Myeloma,** the most common primary malignancy of bone in adults, can occur in a **solitary form,** often seen as a soap-bubbly, expansile lesion in the spine or pelvis (called a **solitary plasmacytoma**), or a **disseminated form** with multiple,

punched-out lytic lesions throughout the axial and proximal appendicular skeleton.

>> **IMPORTANT POINTS**

- **Findings of multiple myeloma on conventional radiographs:**
  - The most common early manifestation is **diffuse and usually severe osteoporosis.**
  - **Plasmacytomas** appear as **expansile, septated lesions, frequently with associated soft-tissue masses** (Fig. 22.22).
  - Later, in its disseminated form, **multiple, small, sharply-circumscribed** (described as **punched-out**) lytic lesions of approximately the same **size** are present, usually without any accompanying sclerotic reaction around them (Fig. 22.23).

- Classically, **conventional radiographs are more sensitive in detecting the lesions of multiple myeloma than radionuclide bone scans** that tend to underestimate the number and extent of lesions because of the absence of reactive bone formation.

Osteomyelitis

- **Osteomyelitis** refers to the **focal destruction of bone,** most often by a blood-borne **infectious agent,** the most common of which is *Staphylococcus aureus.*
- **In children,** the osteolytic lesion **tends to occur at the metaphysis** because of its rich blood supply.

>> **IMPORTANT POINTS**

- **Findings of acute osteomyelitis on conventional radiographs:**
  - **Focal cortical bone destruction** (Fig. 22.24)
  - **Periosteal new bone formation**
  - Inflammatory changes accompanying the infection may produce **soft-tissue swelling** and **focal osteoporosis** from hyperemia

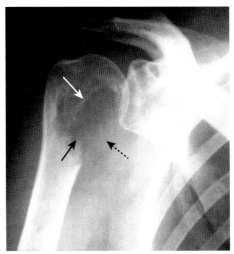

Fig. 22.22 Solitary Plasmacytoma: Shoulder. A large lytic lesion in the proximal humerus (*solid black arrow*), which has destroyed the cortex (*dotted black arrow*), contains multiple septations (*solid white arrow*). Solitary plasmacytomas can be a precursor to the more disseminated form of multiple myeloma. Renal cell and thyroid carcinoma can also produce such a picture (see Fig. 22.20).

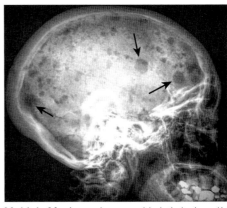

Fig. 22.23 Multiple Myeloma. Innumerable lytic lesions (*black arrows*) are seen in this lateral view of the skull. They are small, uniform in size, and have well-marginated edges, the so called **punched-out** lytic defects characteristic of multiple myeloma. Metastases to the skull can produce a similar picture, but tend to be fewer in number and less well-defined.

Fig. 22.21 Pedicle Sign. Each vertebral body should normally have two oval-shaped pedicles, one on each side, visible on the frontal radiograph of the spine (*solid white arrows*). The right pedicle of T10 (*dotted white arrow*) is missing because it has been destroyed by tumor. This is called the **pedicle sign**. Most metastatic lesions to the spine will also involve the vertebral body.

Fig. 22.24 Osteomyelitis: Middle Finger. Close-up view of the hand shows a lytic lesion in the terminal phalanx of the middle finger with destruction of a part of the cortex (*solid white arrows*). The soft tissue of the finger was edematous and the patient had a history of a penetrating injury to the finger weeks earlier.

- In **adults**, the **infection** tends to **involve the joint space more** often than it does in **children,** producing not only osteomyelitis but also **septic arthritis.**
- **Conventional radiographs can take up to 10 days to display the first findings of osteomyelitis** so that other imaging modalities, such as MRI and nuclear medicine studies, are frequently used for earlier diagnosis.
- A variety of radionuclide bone scans can demonstrate osteomyelitis, the most specific of which is currently a **tagged, white-cell scan** in which a sample of the patient's white blood cells is removed, tagged with a radioactive isotope (frequently indium), and injected back into the patient who is then imaged with a camera specific for nuclear studies to detect a site of abnormally increased radioactive tracer uptake.

DISEASES OF THE JOINTS: AN APPROACH TO ARTHRITIS

- Imaging studies play a key role in the diagnosis and management of arthritis and are the method by which many arthritides are first diagnosed. Other arthritides are initially diagnosed on clinical and laboratory grounds and imaging is used to document the severity, extent, and course of the disease (Table 22.5).
- **Conventional radiographs remain the study of first choice** in evaluating for the presence of arthritis. Conventional radiographs will demonstrate abnormalities of the **articular cortex** and the **subchondral bone** and will provide late, indirect evidence of the integrity of the articular cartilage. MRI is more sensitive in directly visualizing the soft tissues in and around a joint.

Classification of Arthritis

- An **arthritis is a disease that affects a joint and usually the bones on either side of the joint,** almost always accompanied by **joint space narrowing** (Fig. 22.25).
- We divide arthritides into **three main categories** (Table 22.6):
  - **Hypertrophic arthritis** is characterized, in general, by **bone formation** at the site of the involved joint(s). The bone formation may occur within the confines of the parent bone (**subchondral sclerosis**) or protrude from the parent bone (**osteophyte**) (Fig. 22.26A).
  - **Erosive arthritis** indicates underlying inflammation and is characterized by tiny, marginal, irregularly shaped lytic lesions in or around the joint surfaces called **erosions** (Fig. 22.26B).
  - **Infectious arthritis** is characterized by joint swelling, osteopenia, and **destruction of long, contiguous segments of the articular cortex** (Fig. 22.26C).

TABLE 22.5	Arthritis: Who Makes the Diagnosis?
Usually Diagnosed Clinically	**Frequently Diagnosed Radiologically**
Septic (pyogenic) arthritis	Osteoarthritis
Psoriatic arthritis	Early rheumatoid arthritis
Gout	Calcium pyrophosphate deposition disease
Hemophilia	Ankylosing spondylitis
	Septic (TB)
	Charcot (neuropathic) joint—late

Fig. 22.25 Arthritis or Not? (A) There is narrowing of the hip joint and both the femoral head and the acetabulum are abnormal (*white arrow*). This meets the criteria for an arthritis and represents osteoarthritis of the hip. (B) There is sclerosis of the femoral head (*dotted black arrow*), but the joint space remains normal as is the acetabulum (*solid black arrow*). This is avascular necrosis of the femoral head, not an arthritis.

TABLE 22.6   Classification of Arthritis

Category	Hallmarks	Types	Remarks
Hypertrophic arthritis	Bone formation Osteophytes	Primary osteoarthritis	Most common; mechanical stress; hands, hips, and knees most common
		Secondary osteoarthritis	Degenerative joint disease (DJD) secondary to prior trauma, or avascular necrosis
		Charcot arthropathy	Fragmentation; joint destruction; sclerosis; most often secondary diabetes
		CPPD	Chondrocalcinosis; DJD in unusual sites
Erosive arthritis	Erosions	Rheumatoid	Carpals, metacarpal-phalangeal joints, proximal interphalangeal joints of hands; osteoporosis; soft-tissue swelling
		Gout	Juxtaarticular erosions with over-hanging edges; long-latency; metatarsal-phalangeal joint of big toe; no osteoporosis
		Psoriatic	Juxtaarticular erosions of distal interphalangeal joints of hands; pencil-in-cup deformity; enthesophytes
		Hemophilia	Remodeling from hemarthroses and hyperemia; same changes in knee in female patients—think of juvenile rheumatoid arthritis
		Ankylosing spondylitis	HLA antigen B27 positive; bilateral sacroiliac (SI) joints; syndesmophytes
		Seronegative spondyloarthropathies	Rheumatoid factor negative; HLA antigen B27 positive; SI joints; syndesmophytes; reactive arthritis; psoriasis
Infectious arthritis	Osteopenia and soft-tissue swelling; early and marked destruction of most or all of the articular cortex	Pyogenic Tuberculosis	Early destruction of articular cortex; osteoporosis; gradual and late destruction of articular cortex; marked osteoporosis

CPPD, Calcium pyrophosphate deposition.

Fig. 22.26 The Imaging Hallmarks of the Three Major Categories of Arthritis. (A) **Hypertrophic arthritis** features subchondral sclerosis (*black arrows*) and marginal osteophyte production (*white arrow*). (B) **Erosive (inflammatory) arthritis** features characteristic marginal, lytic erosions (*white and black arrows*). (C) **Infectious arthritis** features destruction of the articular cortex (*dotted white arrow*).

- Within each of these three main categories, we will look at a few of the more common types of arthritis that also have characteristic imaging findings.

Hypertrophic Arthritis

- **Hypertrophic arthritis is characterized by bone formation,** either **subchondral sclerosis** or **osteophytes.**
- **Hypertrophic** arthritides are classified in Table 22.6.

Primary Osteoarthritis

- Primary osteoarthritis, also known as **primary degenerative arthritis** or **degenerative joint disease (DJD)**, is the **most common form of arthritis**, estimated to affect over 20 million Americans. It results from **intrinsic degeneration** of the **articular cartilage**, mostly from the mechanical stress of **excessive wear and tear** in weight-bearing joints.

• It mostly involves the **hips, knees,** and **hands** and increases in prevalence with increasing age.

>> **IMPORTANT POINTS**

- **The imaging findings of primary osteoarthritis** (Fig. 22.27):
  - **Marginal osteophyte formation. A hallmark of hypertrophic arthritis,** osseous transformation of cartilaginous excrescences and metaplasia of synovial lining cells leads to the production of these **bony protrusions at or near the joint.**
  - **Subchondral sclerosis.** This is a reaction of the bone to the mechanical stress to which it is subjected when its protective cartilage has been destroyed.
  - **Subchondral cysts.** As a result of chronic impaction, necrosis of bone, and/or imposition of synovial fluid into the subchondral bone, cysts of varying sizes form in the subchondral bone.
  - **Narrowing of the joint space.** Seen in all forms of arthritis.

>> **IMPORTANT POINTS**

- The radiographic findings of **secondary osteoarthritis** are the same as those for the primary form with several special clues to help suggest secondary osteoarthritis:
  - It **occurs at an atypical age** for primary osteoarthritis (e.g., a 30-year-old with osteoarthritis) (Box 22.3).
  - It has an **atypical appearance for primary osteoarthritis** (e.g., primary osteoarthritis is usually bilateral and often symmetric; severe osteoarthritic changes of one hip while the opposite appears perfectly normal point to the possibility of secondary osteoarthritis).
  - It may **appear in an unusual location** for primary arthritis, (e.g., the elbow joint) (Fig. 22.30).
- **Eventually any arthritis that affects the articular cartilage, no matter what the etiology, can lead to the changes of secondary osteoarthritis.**

• **What joints are involved?**
  • In osteoarthritis, destruction of the cartilaginous buffer between the apposing bones of a joint leads to narrowing of the joint space, most often on the **weight-bearing** side of the joint (i.e., **hip [superior and lateral] and knee [medial]**) (Fig. 22.28).
  • In most patients with osteoarthritis of the interphalangeal joints of the hands, the first carpometacarpal joint (**base of thumb) is also affected** (Fig. 22.29A). It is also common for osteoarthritis to affect the **distal interphalangeal joints,** especially in older women (Fig. 22.29B).

Secondary Osteoarthritis (Secondary Degenerative Arthritis)

• Secondary osteoarthritis is a form of degenerative arthritis of synovial joints that occurs because of an underlying, predisposing condition, **most frequently trauma,** that damages or leads to damage of the articular cartilage.

Fig. 22.27 Osteoarthritis. The hallmarks of osteoarthritis are demonstrated in this patient's right hip. There is **marginal osteophyte formation** (*solid white arrow*), **subchondral sclerosis** (*solid black arrows*), and **subchondral cyst formation** (*dotted black arrow*).

Fig. 22.28 Osteoarthritis of Hip (A) and Knee (B). (A) In the hip, the superior and lateral surface (*white arrow*) is the weight-bearing aspect and is most affected by osteoarthritis, whereas in the knee (B), the medial compartment bears the most weight and is more affected (*black arrow*).

Fig. 22.29 Osteoarthritis of the Hands. (A) There are osteophytes at the distal and proximal interphalangeal joints and the joint spaces are narrowed (*solid white arrows*). Subchondral sclerosis is also present at the carpal-metacarpal joint of the thumb (*black arrow*). (B) Large osteophytes are seen at the distal interphalangeal joints of the fingers (*dotted white arrows*) in another patient, an 87-year-old woman with joint pain.

Fig. 22.30 Secondary Osteoarthritis: Right Hip. There is a marked discrepancy in the appearance of each hip with advanced osteoarthritis and fusion of the right hip joint (*white circle*), but a normal left hip (*white arrow*). Many times, the severity of the findings in secondary arthritis leave little clue as to the original inciting cause. This patient had hip trauma on the right as a child.

Fig. 22.31 Erosive Osteoarthritis. This 56-year-old female patient had marked swelling, redness, and tenderness of the proximal and distal interphalangeal joints. There is a combination of erosions and osteophytes (*white and black arrows*) that produces a pattern called a **gull-wing deformity**, consistent with erosive osteoarthritis.

BOX 22.3 Some Causes of Secondary Osteoarthritis

- Trauma
- Infection
- Avascular necrosis
- Calcium pyrophosphate deposition disease
- Rheumatoid arthritis

Erosive Osteoarthritis

- Erosive osteoarthritis is a **type of primary osteoarthritis** characterized by more **severe inflammation** and by the development of **erosive joint changes**. It occurs most often in **perimenopausal women**.

- Erosive osteoarthritis may feature bilaterally symmetric changes like the osteophytes of primary osteoarthritis but with **marked inflammation (swelling and tenderness)** and **erosions** at the affected joints.
  - The **erosions are typically centrally located within the joint** and, combined with the small osteophytes associated with the disease, may produce the so-called *gull-wing deformity* (Fig. 22.31).
  - Erosive osteoarthritis most commonly occurs at the **proximal and distal interphalangeal joints of the fingers, first carpal-metacarpal, and the interphalangeal joint of the thumb.**
  - **Bony ankylosis may occur**, an uncommon finding in primary osteoarthritis.

Charcot Arthropathy (Neuropathic Joint)

- Charcot arthropathy develops from a **disturbance in sensation** that leads to **multiple microfractures** as well as an autonomic imbalance that leads to hyperemia, **bone resorption, and fragmentation of bone.**
- Even though the joint lacks sensory feedback, almost three of four patients with a Charcot joint **complain of some degree of pain**, although it is usually far less than would be expected for the degree of joint destruction present.
- **Soft-tissue swelling is a prominent feature.**
- The **most common cause** of a Charcot joint today is **diabetes** and most Charcot joints are found in the **lower extremities,** particularly in the **feet and ankles.**
- Causes of Charcot joints by location:
  - **Shoulders:** syrinx, spinal tumor, and syphilis
  - **Hips:** tertiary syphilis, diabetes
  - **Ankles and feet:** diabetes (common) and syphilis (uncommon)

Fig. 22.32 Charcot Arthropathy of Knees. A Charcot joint is a form of hypertrophic arthritis. The hallmark findings of a Charcot joint are fragmentation of the bones surrounding the joint (*white arrows*) as well as marked joint space destruction (*black arrows*). The most common cause of a Charcot joint of the knee is now diabetes.

▶ IMPORTANT POINTS

- **Radiographic findings of Charcot arthropathy:**
  - As a hypertrophic arthritis, a Charcot joint will demonstrate **extensive subchondral sclerosis.**
  - The **hallmark findings of a Charcot joint,** however, are:
    - **Fragmentation** of the bones surrounding the joint, which produces numerous small, bony densities within the joint capsule. Sometimes, **many—if not all—of the fragments may be resorbed** and no longer be visible (Fig. 22.32).
    - Eventual **destruction of the joint.** Charcot neuropathy is responsible for some of the **most dramatic examples of total joint destruction of any arthritis** (Fig. 22.33).
  - A Charcot joint shares findings with osteomyelitis and the two diseases may mimic each other in that they both produce **bone destruction** and **periosteal reaction (from fracture healing).** A radioisotope-tagged white-cell bone scan can help to differentiate infection from Charcot joint.

Calcium Pyrophosphate Deposition Disease (Pyrophosphate Arthropathy)

- Calcium pyrophosphate deposition disease is an arthropathy resulting from the deposition of **calcium pyrophosphate dihydrate (CPPD)** crystals in and around joints, **mostly in hyaline cartilage and fibrocartilage.** This is especially common in the **triangular fibrocartilage of the wrist** and the **menisci of the knee.**
- The terminology associated with describing this disease can be confusing.
  - **Chondrocalcinosis** refers only to **calcification** of the articular cartilage or fibrocartilage and is seen in about 50% of adults over the age of 85, most of whom are **asymptomatic.** Chondrocalcinosis can occur in other diseases besides CPPD, such as hyperparathyroidism or hemochromatosis (Fig. 22.34).
  - **Pseudogout** is a **clinical syndrome** consisting of an **acute, monoarticular arthropathy** characterized by **redness, pain,**

Fig. 22.33 Charcot Arthropathy of Foot. This patient had previously undergone an amputation of the phalanges of the second toe (*solid white arrow*) for diabetic gangrene, but the destruction and marked fragmentation of the remaining portion of the great toe (*solid black arrow*) and tarsal bones (*dotted white arrow*) are manifestations of Charcot neuropathy. Initially, a Charcot foot may manifest only inflammatory changes and be normal radiographically. Eventually, the hallmark deformity of this condition is collapse of the midfoot, called a **rocker-bottom** foot.

Fig. 22.34 Chondrocalcinosis. Calcification of the articular cartilage (*white arrows*) is common with advanced age and may be present without symptoms. If this same patient presented with inflammatory signs and symptoms, as well as crystals of calcium pyrophosphate dihydrate in the joint, it would be called **pseudogout.** Changes of pyrophosphate arthropathy are shown in Fig. 22.35.

and swelling of the affected joint (most commonly the knee) from which **calcium pyrophosphate dihydrate** crystals can be aspirated.

- **Pyrophosphate arthropathy** is a radiologic diagnosis and the most common form of CPPD.

>> **IMPORTANT POINTS**

- **Pyrophosphate arthropathy** may be indistinguishable from secondary osteoarthritis, but it does differ from it in several important respects:
  - CPPD affects joints not **usually affected by primary osteoarthritis** such as the **patellofemoral joint space of the knee,** the **radiocarpal joint,** the **metacarpophalangeal joints of the hands,** and the joints of the **wrist.**
  - **Chondrocalcinosis is usually present** in pyrophosphate arthropathy, but is not required for the diagnosis.
  - **Subchondral cysts** are **more common, larger, more numerous,** and more widespread than in primary osteoarthritis.
  - **Hook-shaped bony excrescences** along the second and third metacarpal heads are a common finding in this form of CPPD (Fig. 22.35A).
  - **In the wrist,** characteristic findings include **calcification of the triangular fibrocartilage,** narrowing of the radiocarpal joint, separation of the scaphoid and the lunate by more than 3 mm **(scapholunate dissociation),** and collapse of the distal carpal row toward the radius **(scapholunate advanced collapse)** (Fig. 22.35B).

Fig. 22.35 Pyrophosphate Arthropathy. (A) Hook-shaped bony excrescences along the second and third metacarpal heads are a common finding of pyrophosphate arthropathy (*white arrows*). The radiocarpal joint is narrowed (*black arrow*). (B) In the wrist, characteristic findings include calcification of the triangular fibrocartilage (*white arrow*), separation of the scaphoid (S) and the lunate (L) **(scapholunate dissociation)** and collapse of the capitate (C) toward the radius (*black arrow*) called **scapholunate advanced collapse (SLAC).**

Erosive Arthritis

- **Erosive arthritis** is composed of a large number of arthritides, all of which are associated with some degree of **inflammation** and **synovial proliferation** (**pannus formation**) that participates in the production of **lytic lesions in or near the joint** called **erosions,** especially in the small joints of the hands and feet.
- **Pannus** acts like a mass of growing and enlarging synovial tissue that leads to **marginal erosions** of the **articular cartilage and underlying bone.**
- Box 22.4 lists some of the many causes of erosive arthritis. We discuss four of the more common, which are **bolded** in the box.

Rheumatoid arthritis (RA)

- Rheumatoid arthritis is **more common in female patients,** frequently involving the **proximal joints of the hands and wrists.** It is **usually bilateral** and **symmetric.**
- Conventional radiographs remain the study of first choice in imaging RA.

> ### ▶▶ IMPORTANT POINTS
>
> - The **earliest** radiographic changes are **soft-tissue swelling** of the affected joints and osteoporosis, which tends to be most severe on both sides of the joint space (**periarticular osteoporosis or periarticular demineralization).**

- **In the hand,** the **erosions tend to involve the proximal joints:** the carpal-metacarpal joints, metacarpal-phalangeal, and proximal interphalangeal joints (Fig. 22.36).
  - **Late findings in the hands** include deformities such as **ulnar deviation of the fingers at the metacarpophalangeal (MCP) joints, subluxation of the MCP joints,** and

ligamentous laxity leading to deformities of the fingers (**swan-neck** and **boutonnière deformities).**

- In the **wrist,** erosions of the **carpals, ulnar styloid,** and **narrowing of the radio-carpal joint** space are frequently seen.
- Elsewhere in the body, the **larger joints usually show no erosions,** but there may be **marked uniform narrowing of the joint space with little or no subchondral sclerosis** (Fig. 22.37).
- In the spine, RA tends to involve the **cervical spine** by producing **ligamentous laxity,** which can lead to forward subluxation of C1 on C2 (**atlantoaxial subluxation**). Atlantoaxial subluxation can produce cord compression if severe (Fig. 22.38).
  - **RA may also cause narrowing, sclerosis, and eventual fusion of the facet joints in the cervical spine.**

Gout

- Gouty arthritis represents the **inflammatory changes incited by the deposition of calcium urate crystals** in the joint. There is characteristically an **extremely long latent period (5 to 7 years)** between the onset of symptoms and the visualization

> ### BOX 22.4   Some Causes of Erosive Arthritis
>
> - **Rheumatoid arthritis**
> - **Gout**
> - **Psoriatic arthritis**
> - **Ankylosing spondylitis (spine)**
> - Rheumatoid variants
> - Reactive arthritis
> - Sarcoid
> - Hemophilia

Fig. 22.36 Rheumatoid Arthritis, Hand (A) and Wrist (B). (A) The carpal-metacarpal joints (not shown), metacarpophalangeal (MCP) (*solid white arrows*), and proximal interphalangeal joints tend to be those most involved in the hand. There is also evidence of ulnar deviation of the fingers at the MCP joints (*white line*) and subluxation of the MCP joints (*dotted white arrow*). (B) In another patient's wrist with RA, erosions of the carpals (*dotted white arrow*), ulnar styloid (*solid white arrow*), and narrowing of the radio-carpal joint space (*dotted black arrow*) are seen.

of bone changes, so **gout is usually a clinical and not a radiologic diagnosis** (see Table 22.5).

- Gout tends to be **monoarticular** at its onset and **asymmetric later** in its course.
- It is **more common in male patients** and **most commonly affects the metatarsal-phalangeal joint of the great toe** at the time of symptom onset.

Fig. 22.37 Rheumatoid Arthritis of the Hip. There is marked uniform narrowing of the hip joint with little or no subchondral sclerosis (*black arrows*). Erosions are not present. If this were primary osteoarthritis, you should expect far more subchondral sclerosis and osteophyte production for this degree of joint space narrowing.

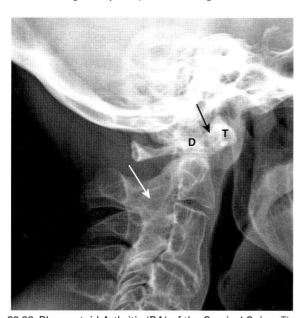

Fig. 22.38 Rheumatoid Arthritis (RA) of the Cervical Spine. The distance between the anterior border of the dens (D) and the posterior border of the anterior tubercle of C1 (T) is called the **predentate space** and is normally no more than 3 mm. This patient's predentate space measured 8 mm (*black arrow*) because of laxity of the atlantoaxial ligaments leading to **atlantoaxial subluxation.** RA may also cause fusion of the facet joints of the cervical spine (*white arrow*).

> **» IMPORTANT POINTS**
>
> - **Imaging findings of gout:**
>   - As an erosive arthritis, the hallmark of gout is the **sharply marginated, juxtaarticular erosion that tends to have a sclerotic border.** The appearance of the overhanging edges of gouty erosions have been called **rat-bites.**
>   - **Joint space narrowing may be a late finding** in the disease and there is **characteristically little or no periarticular osteoporosis** (Fig. 22.39).
>   - **Tophi**, collections of urate crystals in the soft tissues, are a late finding in gout and, when present, **rarely calcify.**
>   - **Olecranon bursitis is common** (Fig. 22.40).

Fig. 22.39 Gout. Gout, an erosive arthritis, displays sharply marginated, juxtaarticular erosions, which may have a sclerotic border (called **rat-bites**) (*white arrows*). As expected in gout, the metatarsophalangeal joint space is not particularly narrowed and there is no periarticular osteoporosis.

Fig. 22.40 Olecranon Bursitis in Gout. Olecranon bursitis is a relatively common manifestation of gout (large soft-tissue mass around elbow shown by *white arrows*) and its presence alone should alert you to the possibility of underlying gout. This patient also displays erosions adjacent to the elbow joint (*black arrow*).

Psoriatic arthritis

- **Most patients** with psoriatic arthritis **also have skin and nail changes of psoriasis** for many years, although for some, the joint manifestations may be the initial presentation of the disease. About 25% of patients with long-standing psoriasis develop psoriatic arthritis. It is **usually polyarticular.**
- Psoriatic arthritis typically involves the **small joints of the hands, especially the distal interphalangeal (DIP) joints.**

> **》 IMPORTANT POINTS**
>
> - The imaging hallmarks of psoriatic arthritis:
>   - **Juxtaarticular erosions,** especially of the **DIP joints** of the hands
>   - **Bony proliferation at the sites of tendon insertions (enthesophytes)**
>   - **Periosteal reaction along the shafts of the bone (not common)**
>   - **Resorption of the terminal phalanges** or the DIP joints with telescoping of one phalanx into another **(pencil-in-cup deformity)** (Fig. 22.41).
>   - **Absence of osteoporosis**

- In the **sacroiliac joints,** psoriasis can produce **bilateral, but asymmetric, sacroiliitis. The sacroiliac joints do not usually completely fuse as they do in ankylosing spondylitis** (see Chapter 23).

Fig. 22.41 Psoriatic Arthritis, Hand (A) and Foot (B). (A) The distal interphalangeal (DIP) joints (*white arrows*) are narrowed and eroded leading to telescoping of one phalanx into another **(pencil-in-cup deformity)**. (B) In the foot of another patient with psoriasis, there is ankylosis (fusion) of the second toe (*solid black arrow*) and more pencil-in-cup deformities (*dotted white arrows*).

Infectious arthritis

- **Infectious arthritis** (also called septic arthritis) usually occurs as a result of **hematogenous seeding of the synovial membrane from an infected source elsewhere in the body,** such as a wound infection or **from direct, contiguous extension from osteomyelitis** adjacent to the joint.
- It is usually subdivided into **pyogenic (septic) arthritis,** mostly caused by *Staphylococcal* and *Gonococcal* organisms, and **nonpyogenic arthritis,** due mostly to infection with *Mycobacterium tuberculosis.*
- **Risk factors** include intravenous drug use, steroids either injected or orally administered, joint prostheses, and recent joint trauma, including joint surgery.
- **In children and adults,** the **knee is frequently affected; in children,** the **hip is** another **common** site of infection. Hands may be infected from human bites and the feet from diabetes.
- Although **conventional radiographs** are obtained as the initial study, they are **relatively insensitive** to the early findings of the disease except for soft-tissue swelling and osteopenia.

> **》 IMPORTANT POINTS**
>
> - The **hallmark of infectious arthritis,** especially the pyogenic form, **is destruction of the articular cartilage and long contiguous segments of the adjacent articular cortex** from proteolytic enzymes released by the inflamed synovium.
> - This **destruction,** unlike other arthritides, **is usually relatively rapid.**
> - Infectious arthritis tends to be **monoarticular** and is associated with **soft-tissue swelling** and **osteopenia** from the hyperemia of inflammation (Fig. 22.42).

Fig. 22.42 Septic Arthritis and Osteomyelitis: Little Toe. This patient has septic arthritis (the metatarsal-phalangeal joint is destroyed) that has extended to the adjacent bone as osteomyelitis and destroyed either side of the joint space as well (*dotted white arrows*). Note the **normal** thin, white line that represents the articular cortex of the head of the fourth metatarsal (*black arrow*) as opposed to the destruction of the articular cortex in the affected toe. A large soft-tissue ulcer is overlying the lateral aspect of the left foot (*solid white arrow*). This patient was a diabetic.

- If septic arthritis is strongly suspected, aspiration of the joint will usually confirm the diagnosis.
- Because of its sensitivity, MRI is now used extensively in diagnosing septic joints. **Enhancement of the synovium** and the **presence of a joint effusion** have the best correlation with the clinical diagnosis of a septic joint.
- **Nonpyogenic infectious arthritis** is most often caused by *M. tuberculosis*, which **spreads via the bloodstream from lung.**
  - Unlike pyogenic arthritis, **tuberculous arthritis** has an **indolent and protracted course,** resulting in **gradual loss of the joint space** and **late destruction of the articular cortex.**
- Nonpyogenic infectious arthritis is **usually monarticular. Severe osteoporosis is a common finding.** In children, the spine is most often affected; in adults, the knee.
- Healing with fibrous and bony ankylosis occurs in both pyogenic and nonpyogenic infectious arthritis.

TAKE HOME POINTS

- Long bones consist of a **cortex** of compact bone surrounding a **medullary cavity** containing cancellous bone arranged as trabeculae, separated by blood vessels, hematopoietic cells, and fat.
- Conventional radiography relies on two views taken 90 degrees from each other to help localize findings **(orthogonal views).**
- On conventional radiographs, the cortex is best seen in tangent. On CT, the entire cortex is visualized. MRI is particularly sensitive to assessment of the marrow. Both CT and MRI are superior to conventional radiographs in evaluating soft tissues.
- Bone is undergoing continuous change from a combination of biochemical and mechanical forces.
- Abnormalities in bone density can arbitrarily be divided into those that **increase density** and those that **decrease density,** either **focally** or **diffusely.**
- **Osteoblastic metastases,** especially from carcinoma of the prostate and breast, can produce focal or generalized increases in bony density.
- The **radionuclide bone scan** is the modality of choice in screening for skeletal metastases. MRI is used primarily to solve specific questions related to a lesion's composition and extent.
- Other diseases that can increase bone density include avascular necrosis of bone and Paget disease.
- **Avascular necrosis** of bone usually involves bones with poor collateral blood supply, such as the femoral head, and is most readily detected by MRI.
- Hallmarks of **Paget disease** include thickening of the cortex, accentuation of the trabecular pattern, and enlargement and increased density of the affected bone.
- Examples of diseases that can cause a **generalized decrease in bone density** include osteoporosis and hyperparathyroidism.
- **Osteoporosis** is characterized by low bone mineral density and is most often either postmenopausal or age-related. Osteoporosis predisposes to pathologic fractures.
- **Hyperparathyroidism** is caused by excessive parathormone secretion, which leads to increased stimulation of osteoclastic activity. Its diagnosis is based on clinical and laboratory findings.
- **Osteolytic metastases,** especially from lung, renal, thyroid, and breast cancer, can produce focal areas of decreased bone density as can solitary plasmacytomas. **Plasmacytomas** are considered to be a precursor to multiple myeloma, the most common primary tumor of bone.
- **Osteomyelitis** is frequently caused by *Staphylococcus aureus* and more often spreads to an adjacent joint space in adults rather than in children.

- An **arthritis** is a disease of a joint that invariably leads to joint space narrowing and changes to the bones on both sides of the joint.
- Arthritides can be roughly divided into hypertrophic, erosive (inflammatory), and infectious categories.
- **Hypertrophic arthritis** features subchondral sclerosis, marginal osteophyte production, and subchondral cyst formation.
- **Primary osteoarthritis,** the most common form of arthritis, is a type of hypertrophic arthritis. It typically occurs on weight-bearing surfaces of the hip and knee as well as the distal interphalangeal joints of the fingers.
- Other hypertrophic arthritides include erosive osteoarthritis, Charcot joints, and CPPD. **Secondary osteoarthritis** may occur from either prior trauma or avascular necrosis or be superimposed on another underlying arthritis.
- **Erosive osteoarthritis** has findings similar to primary osteoarthritis, but tends to feature more inflammatory changes. The erosions are typically centrally located within the joint.
- **Charcot or neuropathic joints** feature fragmentation, sclerosis, and soft-tissue swelling. Diabetes is the most frequent cause of a Charcot joint today.
- **Pyrophosphate arthropathy** occurs with the deposition of calcium pyrophosphate crystals (chondrocalcinosis). It can produce large and multiple subchondral cysts, narrowing of the patellofemoral joint space, metacarpal "hooks," and proximal migration of the distal carpal row.
- **Erosive (or inflammatory) arthritis,** which is associated with inflammation and synovial proliferation (pannus formation), produces lytic lesions called **erosions** in or near the joint.
- Rheumatoid arthritis, gout, and psoriasis are three examples of erosive arthritis; the site of involvement is helpful in differentiating among the causes of erosive arthritides.
- **Rheumatoid arthritis** affects the carpals and proximal joints of the hand; it can widen the predentate space in the cervical spine and can lead to fusion of the posterior elements in the cervical spine.
- **Gout** most often affects the metatarsal-phalangeal joint of the great toe with juxtaarticular erosions and little or no osteoporosis. Tophi, which are late manifestations of the disease, usually do not calcify.
- **Psoriatic arthritis** usually occurs in patients with known skin changes of psoriasis; it affects the distal joints, primarily in the hands, and produces characteristic erosions that resemble a pencil-in-cup.
- **Infectious arthritis** features soft-tissue swelling and osteopenia and, in the case of pyogenic arthritis, relatively early and marked destruction of most or all of the articular cortex. It is mostly caused by *Staphylococcal* and *Gonococcal* organisms.

More information on recognizing nontraumatic abnormalities of the appendicular skeleton including arthritis is available to registered users online.

Recognizing Nontraumatic Abnormalities of the Spine

- **Magnetic resonance imaging,** with its superior soft-tissue differentiation, is the **study of choice** for most diseases of the spine because of its ability to visualize and detect abnormalities in **soft tissues,** such as bone marrow, the spinal cord, and the intervertebral disks; its ability to display images in **any plane;** and the **lack of exposure to radiation.**
- But MRI has its limitations. The study **remains relatively expensive** and its **availability is not as widespread** as CT or conventional radiographs, **patients with pacemakers** and certain internal ferromagnetic materials (e.g., certain aneurysm clips) **are not able to be scanned,** the procedure **takes more time** to complete and some patients cannot tolerate the **claustrophobia** they experience in some of the high-field-strength MRI scanners **(see Chapter 21).**

THE NORMAL SPINE (FIG. 23.1)

Vertebral Body

- Almost every vertebra has a **body** composed of inner cancellous bone and marrow and **posterior elements** made of compact dense bone consisting of the pedicles, laminae, facets, transverse processes, and a spinous process (Fig. 23.2A).
- From the level of **C3 through the level of L5** the vertebral bodies are more or less **rectangular in shape** and of about equal height posteriorly as anteriorly.
- The **endplates of contiguous vertebral bodies** are roughly **parallel** to each other.
- The **articular facets** of the **superior** and **inferior articular processes** are lined with cartilage and these facet joints are **true synovial joints.**
- In the frontal projection, each vertebral body displays **two ovoid pedicles** visible on each side of the vertebral body. The pedicles of L5 are frequently difficult to visualize, even in normal individuals, because of the lordosis of the lumbar spine (Fig. 23.2B).
- On conventional radiographs of the **lumbar spine** performed in the oblique projection, the anatomic structures normally superimpose to produce a shadow that resembles the front end of a Scottish terrier, the **Scottie dog** sign (Fig. 23.3).

Intervertebral Disks

- The intervertebral disks have a central gelatinous **nucleus pulposus** surrounded by an outer **annulus fibrosus** that is, in turn, made up of inner fibrocartilaginous fibers and outer cartilaginous fibers **(Sharpey's fibers).** The nucleus pulposus is located near the posterior aspect of the disk (Fig. 23.4).

> ▶ **IMPORTANT POINTS**
>
> - The **relative height of the disk space varies in each part of the spine.**
>   - In the **cervical spine,** the disk spaces are about **equal** to each other in height.
>   - In the **thoracic spine,** they are usually slightly **decreased** in size **from the cervical spine,** but **equal** in height to each other.
>   - In the **lumbar spine,** the disk spaces **progressively increase** in height with each successive interspace, **except for L5-S1,** which can be equal to or slightly less than the height of L4-L5 on conventional radiographs.

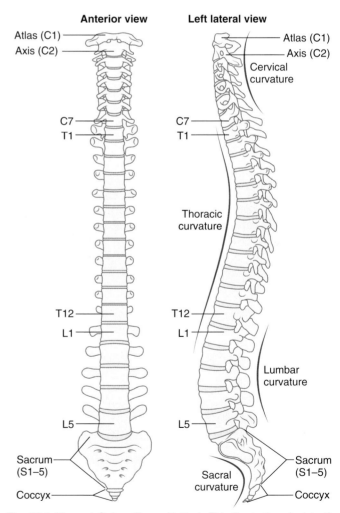

Fig. 23.1 Normal Spine (From Netter). This illustration depicts the entire spine consisting of 7 cervical vertebra, 12 thoracic vertebra—all of which normally bear ribs—5 lumbar vertebra, and 5 fused sacral vertebrae. The curvature of the cervical and lumbar spines is called lordotic and the curvature of the thoracic spine is kyphotic.

Fig. 23.2 Normal Spine: Axial CT (A) and Frontal Conventional Radiograph (B). (A) In this CT scan of a "typical" vertebral body, we see the body (B), pedicles (*solid white arrows*), laminae (*dotted white arrows*), transverse processes (T), spinal canal (C), and spinous process (S). (B) Each vertebral body has two pedicles that project as small ovals on either side of the vertebral body (*solid white arrows*). The spinous process (*dotted white arrow*) may be visualized slightly above the body to which it is attached. The facet joint is seen here *en face* (*solid black arrow*).

Fig. 23.3 Normal Scottie Dog. This is a left posterior oblique view of the lumbar spine (the patient is turned about halfway toward her own left). The **Scottie dog** is made up of the following: the **ear** (*solid black arrow*) is the superior articular facet, the **leg** (*solid white arrow*) is the inferior articular facet, the **nose** (*dotted black arrow*) is the transverse process, the **eye** (P) is the pedicle, and the **neck** (*dotted white arrow*) is the pars interarticularis. All these structures are paired: an identical set should be visible on the patient's right side.

Spinal Ligaments

- Several ligaments traverse the spine (Table 23.1) (see Fig. 23.4).

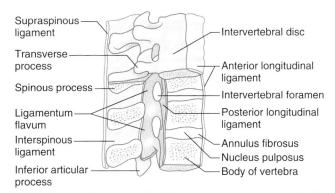

Fig. 23.4 Normal Spine and Soft Tissues. A partial cross-section illustration of the spine depicts the normal bony and ligamentous structures.

Spinal Cord and Spinal Nerves

- The spinal cord extends from the medulla oblongata to the level of L1-L2, ending as the **conus medullaris.** The **cauda equina** extends inferiorly from that point as a collection of nerve roots with each root exiting **below** its respectively numbered vertebral body.
- Each of the paired **neural foramina** of the spine contains a **spinal nerve, blood vessels,** and **fat.**
- **Spinal nerves** are named and numbered **according to the site they exit** from the spinal canal. **From C1-C7,** nerves exit **above**

their respective vertebrae. The **C8** nerve exits **between the seventh cervical and first thoracic** vertebrae. The **remaining nerves exit below** their respectively numbered vertebrae.

NORMAL MRI APPEARANCE OF THE SPINE

> ### » IMPORTANT POINTS
>
> - On **T1-weighted** sagittal MRI images of the spine, the **vertebral bodies,** containing bone marrow, will normally be of **high signal intensity (bright);** the **disks** will be **lower in signal intensity** and **cerebrospinal fluid (CSF)** in the thecal sac will have a **low signal intensity** (dark) (Fig. 23.5A).
> - On conventional **T2-weighted images,** the **vertebral body** will be slightly **lower in signal** intensity than the disks, whereas the **CSF will appear bright** (the reverse of T1) (Fig. 23.5B).
> - Cortical bone is **dark** (has a low signal) on all sequences.

TABLE 23.1	**Ligaments of the Spine**
Ligament	**Connects**
Anterior longitudinal ligament	Anterior surfaces of vertebral bodies
Posterior longitudinal ligament	Posterior surfaces of vertebral bodies
Ligamentum flavum	Laminae of adjacent vertebral bodies; lies in posterior portion of spinal canal
Interspinous ligament	Between spinous processes
Supraspinous ligament	Tips of spinous processes

BACK PAIN

- It has been estimated that **almost 80% of all Americans will have some episode of back pain** during their lifetime. The causes of back pain are numerous and the anatomic and physiologic interrelationships that produce it are still not known in many cases.
- Some causes of back pain are:
  - **Herniation of an intervertebral disk**
  - **Degeneration of an intervertebral disk**
  - **Arthritis involving the synovial joints of the spine**
  - **Diffuse idiopathic skeletal hyperostosis**
  - **Compression fractures,** usually from osteoporosis
  - **Spinal stenosis**
  - **Malignancy involving the spine**
  - **Infection of the spine**
  - **Ankylosing spondylitis**
  - Trauma to the spine
  - Muscle and ligament strain
- In this chapter we discuss all of these except muscle and ligament strains. Spinal trauma appears in **Chapter 24.**

Herniated Disks

- Only about 2% of patients with acute low back pain have a herniated disk. In the **lumbar region,** disk herniation may lead to **back pain** and **sciatica,** whereas herniation of a **cervical disk** may produce **radiculopathy** and **myelopathy. MRI is the study of choice for evaluating herniated disks.**

Fig. 23.5 Normal MRI Lumbar Spine: T1- and T2-Weighted Images. (A) Sagittal T1-weighted image demonstrates the normal dark appearance of the disk (D) relative to the vertebral body (V). The cerebrospinal spinal fluid (C) in the spinal canal is dark and the subcutaneous fat of the back (F) is bright. Cortical bone has a low signal (*white arrow*). (B) sagittal T2-weighted image demonstrates the normal appearance of the disk (D), which is slightly higher intensity (brighter) than the vertebral bodies. The CSF (C) in the spinal canal is now bright, and the subcutaneous fat (F) of the back remains bright.

Fig. 23.6 Herniated Disk: MRI. The spinal cord is dark (C) relative to the high intensity (whiter) signal surrounding it, which is the CSF in the spinal canal. A herniated disk (*solid white arrow*) extends posteriorly from the C4-C5 disk space and compresses the cord.

Fig. 23.7 Disk Herniation: L5-S1. Sagittal T2-weighted image of the lower lumbar spine demonstrates disk material (*solid white arrow*) beyond the confines of the L5-S1 intervertebral disk space, which represents a disk herniation extending inferiorly. Notice that degeneration and desiccation of the other disks has led them to become darker than normal on this T2-weighted image (*dotted white arrows*).

- In the **cervical spine,** disk herniations occur most frequently at **C4-C5, C5-C6,** and **C6-C7** (Fig. 23.6).
- Compared with the cervical and lumbar spine, **thoracic disks are very stable,** in part because they are protected by the rib cage that surrounds them.

>> **IMPORTANT POINTS**

- The majority of **disk herniations occur at** the lower three lumbar disk levels, **L3-L4, L4-L5 (most common), and L5-S1.** More than 60% of disk herniations occur **posterolaterally,** the location of the herniation determining the clinical presentation depending on which nerve roots are compressed.

- **Degeneration** of the outer annular fibers of the disk or **trauma** can lead to an interruption in those fibers and allow the disk material to **bulge,** which may or may not be associated with back pain.
- When the annular fibers rupture, the **nucleus pulposus** may **herniate** (usually posterolaterally) **through a weakened area of the posterior longitudinal ligament.**
- The herniated material may **protrude,** but remain in contact with the parent disk from which it originated, or it may be completely **extruded** into the spinal canal.
- Symptoms are caused by acute **compression** of the **nerve root.**

- Disk herniations can be visualized on both **CT** and **MRI.** CT demonstrates disk material compressing nerve roots or the thecal sac. On MRI, the herniated disk material is usually a **focal, asymmetric protrusion of hypointense disk material** that extends beyond the confines of the annulus fibrosus (Fig. 23.7).
- **Postlaminectomy syndrome** (also called **failed back surgery syndrome**) is persistent pain in the back or legs following spine surgery. In some studies, it has been estimated to occur in 40% of postoperative patients. Gadolinium-enhanced MRI studies of the spine are useful in differentiating persistent or recurrent **disk herniation** from **scar formation** as a cause of the pain.

Degenerative Disk Disease (DDD)

- With increasing age, the normally gelatinous nucleus pulposus becomes dehydrated and degenerates. This gradually leads to **progressive loss of the height of the intervertebral disk space.** At times, desiccation of the disk leads to **release of nitrogen** from tissues surrounding the disk resulting in the appearance of **air density in the disk space,** which is called a **vacuum-disk phenomenon.** A vacuum-disk represents a **late sign of a degenerated disk** (Fig. 23.8).

Fig. 23.8 Degenerative Disk Disease. The endplates of contiguous vertebral bodies have become sclerotic (*solid black arrow*), small osteophytes are produced at the margins of the vertebral bodies (*solid white arrow*), and there is desiccation of the disk with a **vacuum-disk phenomenon** (gas in the disk space), which is recognizable by the air density in place of the disk seen at L5-S1 (*dotted black arrow*).

- **Degenerative disk disease on MRI**
  - The decrease in water content of the nucleus pulposus results in a lower signal intensity of the disk on T2-weighted images (see Fig. 23.7).
- **Degenerative disk disease on conventional radiographs**
  - There is **disk space narrowing** and also changes in the vertebral bodies themselves.
  - The **endplates** of contiguous vertebral bodies become **eburnated** or **sclerotic. Small osteophytes** are produced at the margins of the vertebral bodies at each disk space (see Fig. 23.8).
  - At the same time, there is typically degeneration of the outer annulus fibrosus. This leads to the production of **larger marginal osteophytes** at the endplates than those seen with degeneration of the nuclear material.
- It should be noted that osteophytes are an **extremely common** finding, increasing in prevalence with increasing age, and that most patients with osteophytes of the spine are **asymptomatic.**

Osteoarthritis of the Facet Joints

- The **facet joints** (also known as the **apophyseal joints**) are **true joints** in that they have cartilage, a synovial lining, and

synovial fluid. As such, they are subject to an arthritis, such as **osteoarthritis,** similar to true joints in the appendicular skeleton.
- Some consider the small joint-like structures at the lateral edges of C3 to T1, called the **uncovertebral joints** or the **joints of Luschka,** to be true joints, whereas others do not.
  - In either case, the uncovertebral joints are frequent sites of osteophyte formation. **Osteophytes** at the **uncovertebral joints** are **frequently associated with** both **degenerative disk disease** and **osteophytes of the facet joints.**

> ### » IMPORTANT POINTS
>
> - In the **cervical spine, osteophytes that develop** at the **uncovertebral joints** can produce **protrusions of bone into** the normally oval-shaped **neural foramina,** which can be visualized on conventional radiographs taken in the oblique projection (Fig. 23.9A).

- There is usually a **complex interrelationship between degenerative disk disease and facet arthritis** such that the two frequently occur together. The osteophytes formed by osteoarthritis of the facet joints may also encroach on the neural foramina and produce radicular pain.
- In the **lumbar spine,** facet osteoarthritis may cause **narrowing** and **sclerosis of the facet joints,** best seen on oblique views of the spine (Fig. 23.9B). Facet arthritis is easier to visualize on CT scans of the spine than on conventional radiographs and actual nerve compression is easier to visualize on MRI of the spine.

Diffuse Idiopathic Skeletal Hyperostosis (DISH)

- DISH is a common disorder characterized by bone or calcium excrescences at the sites of ligamentous insertions. The excrescences are called **enthesophytes** and the conditions in which they form (of which DISH is only one) are called **enthesopathies.**
- DISH usually affects **men** over the age of **50;** it can occur anywhere in the spine, but **most often** affects the **lower thoracic and/or lower cervical spine.**
- Frequently patients with DISH complain of back stiffness, but may have **no pain** or **mild back pain.**
- **Conventional radiographs** of the spine are **sufficient** to make the diagnosis of DISH.

> ### » IMPORTANT POINTS
>
> - DISH is manifest by **thick bridging or flowing calcification/ossification** of the **anterior** or, sometimes, **posterior longitudinal ligaments.**
> - This ossification is visualized along the anterior or anterolateral aspects of at least **four contiguous vertebral bodies.** Unlike degenerative disk disease, the **disk spaces** and (usually) the **facet joints** are **preserved.** The flowing ossification seen in DISH is **separated slightly from the vertebral body** (Fig. 23.10A).

- Unlike ankylosing spondylitis, which may radiographically resemble DISH in the spine, the **sacroiliac joints are normal in DISH.**

Fig. 23.9 Uncovertebral Osteophytes and Facet Arthritis. (A) In the cervical spine, osteophytes may develop at the uncovertebral joints (*solid black arrow*) producing bony protrusions into the normally oval-shaped neural foramina (N) in this radiograph taken in the oblique projection. Osteophytes at the uncovertebral joints are frequently associated with both degenerative disk disease (*dotted white arrow*) and osteophytes of the facet joints (*solid white arrow*). (B) There is sclerosis and osteophyte formation involving the lower facet joints of the lumbar spine (*solid black arrows*).

Fig. 23.10 Diffuse Idiopathic Skeletal Hyperostosis (DISH) and Ossification of the Posterior Longitudinal Ligament (OPLL). (A) DISH is manifest by thick, bridging, or flowing calcification/ossification of the anterior longitudinal ligaments (*white arrow*). This ossification is visualized along the anterior or anterolateral aspects of at least four contiguous vertebral bodies. (B) OPPL (*white and black arrows*) can be associated with DISH and may contribute to the production of spinal stenosis.

- **Ossification of the posterior longitudinal ligament (OPLL)**, which is often present with DISH, is better visualized on CT and MRI than on conventional radiographs. It may cause compression of the spinal cord, especially in the cervical spine, because of narrowing of the spinal canal (Fig. 23.10B).

Compression Fractures of the Spine

- Vertebral compression fractures are **common**, affecting **women more than men**, and typically occur secondary to **osteoporosis**. They may be **asymptomatic** or they may produce **pain** in the mid-thoracic or upper lumbar area that typically disappears in 4 to 6 weeks. Sometimes they are first noticed because of increasing **kyphosis** or **loss of overall body height.**

- **Conventional spine radiographs are usually the study of first choice.** MRI can be utilized for differentiating **osteoporotic** compression fractures from compression fractures caused by **malignancy.** Both MRI and nuclear bone scans can help in establishing the **age** of a compression abnormality, which might be impossible on conventional radiographs alone.

- **Usually no neurologic deficit** is associated with an osteoporotic compression fracture because the fracture involves the anterior part of the vertebral body, away from the spinal cord.

» **IMPORTANT POINTS**

- **Osteoporotic compression fractures** usually involve the **anterior and superior** aspects of the vertebral body, **sparing the posterior body.** This will lead to a difference in the height between the **anterior and posterior** aspects of the same vertebral body **in excess of 3 mm.** Alternatively, the compressed body is typically more than 20% shorter than the body above or below it.
  - This compression pattern produces a **wedge-shaped deformity** that leads to accentuation of the normal kyphosis in the thoracic spine (the so-called **Dowager's hump**) and increases the **lordosis** in the lumbar spine (Fig. 23.11).

Spinal Stenosis

- Spinal stenosis refers to **narrowing of the spinal canal** or the neural foramina secondary to **soft-tissue or bony abnormalities,** either on an **acquired or congenital** basis. **Acquired etiologies,** such as those from **degenerative changes,** are more common than congenital causes.

- **Soft-tissue abnormalities** that can lead to **spinal stenosis** include hypertrophy of the ligamentum flavum, bulging disk(s), and OPLL.

- **Bony abnormalities** that can lead to **spinal stenosis** include a congenitally narrow spinal canal, osteophytes, facet osteoarthritis, or spondylolisthesis. A spinal canal that was borderline normal in size may become stenotic when any of these processes superimpose to further narrow the canal.

» **IMPORTANT POINTS**

- Spinal stenosis is **most common in the cervical and lumbar areas;** it can lead to radicular pain, myelopathy, or, in the lumbar region, neurogenic claudication. **Neurogenic claudication** is intermittent pain and paresthesias radiating down the leg worsened by standing or walking and relieved by flexing the spine by lying supine or squatting.

- **Conventional radiographs are usually obtained first** in evaluating for spinal stenosis, but **MRI is the study of choice** because the bony dimensions alone do not account for the soft tissues that can produce stenosis.

- **Conventional radiographic** findings may include an **anteroposterior diameter of the spinal canal of 10 mm or less,** **facet joint arthritis,** and **spondylolisthesis.**

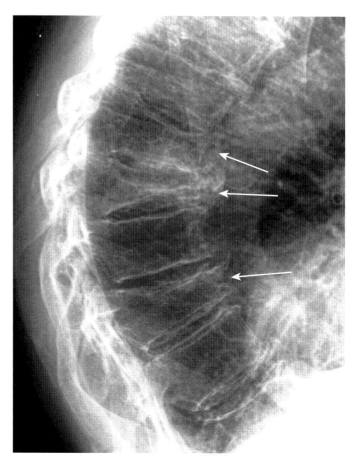

Fig. 23.11 Compression Fractures Secondary to Osteoporosis. The anterior and superior aspects of the vertebral body are most often involved (*white arrows*), sparing the posterior aspect. Progressive loss of overall body height is a common finding with compression fractures in the elderly.

- **CT** provides an excellent method of demonstrating bony abnormalities, but **MRI is the imaging modality of choice for detecting lumbar spinal stenosis** (Fig. 23.12).

Malignancy Involving the Spine

» **IMPORTANT POINTS**

- **Metastases** to bone are 25 times more common than **primary** bone tumors. Metastases usually occur where **red marrow** is found, with 80% of metastatic bone lesions occurring in the **axial skeleton** (i.e., spine, pelvis, skull, and ribs) because this is where, with normal aging, the red marrow exists.

- Because of the **rich blood supply** in the posterior portion of vertebral bodies, hematogenous **metastatic deposits to that part of the spine are common,** especially from **lung** and **breast** carcinoma.

- In the spine, metastases may lead to **compression fractures.** Metastases tend to **destroy the vertebral body,** including and especially the posterior aspect and the pedicles, which is different from **osteoporotic compression fractures** in which **the posterior vertebral body and pedicles remain intact** (see Fig. 23.11).

Fig. 23.12 Spinal Stenosis: CT. (A) On this CT myelogram, at the level of L2-L3, there are osteo-phytes (*solid white arrow*) that narrow the canal (C). A protruding disk (*dotted white arrow*) at L4-L5 reduces the size of the spinal canal at this level. (B) The canal (C) is narrowed by thickening of the lig-amenta flava (*white arrows*) and by bony overgrowth (*black arrows*) from osteoarthritis of the facet joints (F).

- As discussed in **Chapter 22, metastatic disease** can either be mostly bone-producing (i.e., **osteoblastic**) or mostly bone-destroying (i.e., **osteolytic**). Metastases that contain both osteolytic and osteoblastic processes occurring simultaneously are called **mixed metastatic lesions.**
- **Prostate cancer** is the prototype example of a primary malig-nancy that produces **osteoblastic metastases**; the prototype primary malignancy for the origin of osteoblastic metastatic disease in a **female** patient is **breast cancer.** The most common causes of primary malignancies that produce **osteolytic** meta-static lesions are **lung** and **breast** cancer. **Thyroid** and **renal** carcinomas may produce **osteolytic** lesions that are also expansile (see Fig. 22.20).
- The spine is also a frequent site of **multiple myeloma,** the most common primary malignancy of bone. Multiple myeloma is known for its tendency to produce almost **totally lytic lesions.** One of the hallmarks of multiple myeloma is osteo-porosis, so that myeloma may be associated with **diffuse spinal osteoporosis** and **multiple compression fractures** (Fig. 23.13).

▶ IMPORTANT POINTS

- The current **screening study of choice** for the detection of spinal metas-tases is a **technetium-99m (Tc-99m) bone scintiscan** (radionuclide bone scan). The technetium radioisotope is most commonly bound to **methylene diphosphonate (MDP)** that transports the Tc-99m to bone. A radionuclide bone scan is relatively inexpensive, widely available, and screens the entire body. Although bone scans are **highly sensitive** to the presence of meta-static deposits, they are **not very specific.** In many cases a confirmatory study, usually a conventional radiograph, is needed to exclude other causes of abnormal radio-tracer uptake, such as fractures, infection, and arthritis (Fig. 23.14).

Fig. 23.13 Multiple Myeloma of the Spine. There are multiple com-pression fractures of the vertebral bodies (L1-L5) from the osteopo-rosis (*white arrows*) produced by multiple myeloma. Notice how the posterior aspects of the vertebral bodies remain essentially normal in height in osteoporotic fractures, whereas the central and anterior aspects collapse.

Fig. 23.14 Metastases, Radionuclide Bone Scan, and CT. (A) A technetium-99m methylene diphosphonate (MDP) bone scan demonstrates abnormal tracer uptake in numerous areas, including the spine (*solid white arrows*) and pelvis (*dashed white arrow*). Because of the nonspecific nature of positive bone scans, a confirmatory study, usually conventional radiography, is obtained as well. In this case the patient had undergone a CT scan and the coronal reformatted image (B) shows numerous osteoblastic lesions in the spine (*dotted white arrows*) and the pelvis (*solid black arrow*) corresponding to the lesions seen on bone scan. This patient had known breast carcinoma.

MRI in Metastatic Spine Disease

- MRI can detect changes of some spinal metastases even **earlier than a radionuclide scan** and techniques are being described that may allow for a rapid, **whole-body screening** utilizing MRI, similar to radionuclide bone scanning.

> ### » IMPORTANT POINTS
>
> - With neoplastic infiltration of the bone marrow, there is a **decrease** in the normally high signal of the vertebra on **T1-weighted images** and there is usually a **high signal on T2-weighted** images (Fig. 23.15).

- Unlike osteoporotic compression fractures which tend to spare the posterior aspects of the bodies while the central and anterior portions collapse, **spinal metastases** will more often **affect the entire body** including the posterior portion.

Diskitis/Osteomyelitis of the Spine

- **Infection of the disk (diskitis)** is almost always associated with **osteomyelitis** of the adjacent **vertebrae** and it almost always spreads **hematogenously** from infection in another organ (e.g., urinary tract or soft tissues). The **lumbar region** is most commonly involved, and *Staphylococcus aureus* is most often the pathogen. **Back pain** and **tenderness** are presenting symptoms.

- Because of the blood supply, children are more likely to start with diskitis, which then spreads to the adjacent vertebrae, whereas adults more frequently develop vertebral osteomyelitis that spreads to the disk.

> ### » IMPORTANT POINTS
>
> - **Diskitis/osteomyelitis** should be considered any time there are abnormalities of a disk space **(narrowing, irregularity)** and **destruction of the adjacent vertebral body endplates**. Findings on conventional radiographs may take weeks or months to manifest. CT is more sensitive and can also detect extra-spinal disease, such as an abscess. MRI is most sensitive (Fig. 23.16).

- Treatment is antibiotics, sometimes along with surgery.

Ankylosing Spondylitis

- Ankylosing spondylitis is a chronic and progressive arthritis characterized by **inflammation** and eventual **fusion of the**

Fig. 23.15 Metastases to the Spine: MRI. (A) T1-weighted sagittal MRI of the thoracic spine demonstrates marrow replacement in the T8 vertebral body (*solid white arrow*). The signal is decreased compared with the normal bodies above and below it. (B) T2-weighted sagittal MRI shows abnormally high signal in the compressed vertebral body (*dotted white arrow*). The patient had primary breast carcinoma.

Fig. 23.16 Diskitis/Osteomyelitis. (A) There is destruction of the anterior, superior portion of the endplate of L4 (*solid black arrow*) with narrowing of the disk space at L4-L5 (*dotted black arrow*). (B) Sagittal CT in another patient shows narrowing of the disk space at L4-L5 (*dotted white arrow*) with destruction of large portions of the endplates of the adjacent two vertebral bodies (*solid white arrows*), a combination of findings highly suggestive of diskitis with osteomyelitis.

sacroiliac joints along with the spinal facet joints and involvement of the paravertebral soft tissues.

- More **common in young males**, the disease characteristically **ascends the spine starting in the sacroiliac joints** and moves to the lumbar, thoracic, and finally cervical spine.

- Almost all patients with ankylosing spondylitis test **positive** for the **human leukocyte antigen B27 (HLA-B27)** as opposed to only about 5% to10% of the general population.

- Conventional radiographs of the affected areas are the usual study performed for diagnosis and follow-up of patients with ankylosing spondylitis.

- Like DISH, ankylosing spondylitis is an **enthesopathy**. There is inflammation, with subsequent **calcification** and **ossification** at and around the **entheses**, the insertion **sites of tendons, ligaments,** and **joint capsules.**

> ## IMPORTANT POINTS
>
> - **Sacroiliitis** is the hallmark of ankylosing spondylitis. It is usually **bilaterally symmetric** and **eventually leads to bony fusion** or **ankylosis** of these joints until they appear either as a thin white line (instead of a joint space) or they disappear altogether (Fig. 23.17).

- In the spine, there is **ossification of the outer fibers of the annulus fibrosis** producing **thin bony bridges** joining the

corners of one vertebra to another, called **syndesmophytes.** Progressive syndesmophyte production connecting adjacent vertebral bodies produces a **bamboo-spine** appearance (Fig. 23.18).

Fig. 23.17 Ankylosing Spondylitis. Bony overgrowth is seen at the ischial tuberosity, the insertion point of the hamstring muscles (*solid white arrow*). Bilaterally symmetric sacroiliitis eventually leads to bony fusion or ankylosis of the sacroiliac joints until they disappear as joints altogether (*solid black arrows*). The symphysis pubis is also ankylosed (*dotted black arrow*).

Fig. 23.18 Ankylosing Spondylitis: Frontal (A) and Lateral (B) Spine. There are flowing syndesmophytes (*solid white arrows* in [A] and *dotted white arrows* in [B]). Progressive ossification connecting adjacent vertebral bodies produces the **bamboo-spine** appearance seen here, which is characteristic of ankylosing spondylitis.

TAKE HOME POINTS

- Conventional radiographs, CT, and MRI are all used to evaluate the spine, but MRI is the study of choice for most diseases of the spine because of its superior ability to display soft tissues.
- Normal features of the vertebral bodies, intervertebral disks, the spinal cord, spinal nerves, and spinal ligaments are described.
- Some of the more **common causes of back pain** are muscle and ligament strain, herniation of an intervertebral disk, degeneration of an intervertebral disk, arthritis involving the synovial joints of the spine, diffuse idiopathic skeletal hyperostosis, and spinal stenosis.
- Most **herniated disks** occur posterolaterally in the lower cervical or lower lumbar spine and are best evaluated with MRI.
- **Postlaminectomy syndrome** is persistent pain in the back or legs following spine surgery. Gadolinium-enhanced MRI can be very helpful in its detection.
- With increasing age, the nucleus pulposus becomes dehydrated and degenerates, leading to changes of **degenerative disk disease,** such as progressive loss of the height of the disk space, marginal osteophyte production, sclerosis of the endplates of the vertebral bodies, and, occasionally, the appearance of a vacuum disk.
- The facet joints are true joints and so are subject to changes of osteoarthritis; **facet osteoarthritis,** which is frequently associated with degenerative disk disease, can lead to radicular pain.
- **Diffuse idiopathic skeletal hyperostosis** is manifest by thick, bridging, or flowing calcification/ossification of the anterior longitudinal ligaments, usually occurring in men over the age of 50. The disk spaces and the facet joints are most often preserved.
- **Compression fractures** of the spine, which are most often secondary to osteoporosis, are seen more commonly in women. They can be seen on conventional radiographs and, because they usually disproportionately involve the anterior portion of the body, can produce an exaggerated kyphosis in the thoracic spine.
- **Spinal stenosis** is a narrowing of the spinal canal or the neural foramina secondary to soft-tissue or bony abnormalities, either on an acquired (more common) or congenital basis; it is most common in the cervical and lumbar regions.
- **Metastatic lesions to the spine** occur mostly in the blood-rich, posterior aspect of the vertebral body, including the pedicles; lung (mixed), breast (mixed), and prostate (osteoblastic) metastases are the most common.
- **Multiple myeloma** also frequently involves the spine, with either severe osteoporosis which can produce compression fractures, or lytic destruction of the vertebral body.
- **Ankylosing spondylitis** is a chronic and progressive arthritis characterized by symmetric fusion of the SI joints and ascending involvement of the spine eventually producing a bamboo-spine appearance.

 More information on recognizing nontraumatic abnormalities of the spine is available to registered users online.

Recognizing Trauma to the Bony Skeleton

RECOGNIZING AN ACUTE FRACTURE

- It seems like everyone is fascinated by an x-ray of a broken bone. Fractures are a favorite among those learning radiology, perhaps because of how common and seemingly straightforward they are. In this chapter we tell you how to recognize a fracture, describe it, name it, and avoid overlooking it.
- A fracture is described as a **disruption in the continuity of all or part of the cortex of a bone.**
  - If the **cortex** is **broken through and through,** the fracture is called **complete.**
  - If only a **part of the cortex** is fractured, it is called **incomplete.** Incomplete fractures tend to occur in bones that are "softer" than normal, such as those in children or in adults with bone-softening diseases, such as Paget disease (see Chapter 22).
  - Examples of **incomplete** fractures in children are the **greenstick fracture,** which involves only one part of, but not the entire cortex, and the **torus fracture (buckle fracture),** which represents compression of the cortex (Fig. 24.1).

>> **IMPORTANT POINTS**

- **Radiologic features of acute fractures** (Box 24.1)
  - **Fracture lines**, when viewed in the optimum orientation, **tend to be "blacker" (more lucent)** than other lines normally found in bones, such as **nutrient canals** (Fig. 24.2A).
  - There may be an **abrupt discontinuity of the cortex**, sometimes associated with **acute angulation** of the normally smooth contour of bone (Fig. 24.2B).
  - Fracture lines tend to be **straighter** in their course yet **more acute in their angulation** than any naturally occurring lines (such as **epiphyseal plates**) (Fig. 24.3).
  - The **edges** of a fracture may be **jagged** or **irregular.**

BOX 24.1 Characteristics of an Acute Fracture

- Abrupt disruption of all or part of the cortex
- Acute changes in the smooth contour of a normal bone
- Fracture lines are black and linear
- Where fracture lines change their course, they tend to be sharply angulated
- Fracture fragments are jagged and not smoothly corticated

Fig. 24.1 Greenstick and Buckle (Torus) Fractures. (A) There is a greenstick fracture (*dotted white arrow*) that involves only one part of, but not the entire, cortex (*solid white arrow*). (B) The buckle fracture is characterized by bulging of the cortex (*black arrows*).

Fig. 24.2 Nutrient Canal Versus Fracture. (A) This is a normal nutrient canal (*white arrows*). Notice how the nutrient canal has a sclerotic (whiter) margin and is confined to the cortex. (B) This is a true fracture (*dotted black arrows*) seen in another patient. Fracture lines are blacker and traverse the cortex and medullary cavity. The edges of a fracture tend to be jagged and rough.

Fig. 24.3 Fracture Versus Epiphyseal Plate. Fracture lines (*black arrow*) tend to be straighter in their course and more acute in their angulation than any naturally occurring lines, such as the **epiphyseal plate** in the proximal humerus (*white arrows*). Because the top of the humeral metaphysis has irregular hills and valleys, the epiphyseal plate has an undulating course that allows you to see it on both the anterior and posterior margins of the humeral head, leading to the appearance that there is more than one epiphyseal plate.

⚠ DIAGNOSTIC PITFALLS

- **Sesamoids, accessory ossicles, and unhealed fractures** (Table 24.1)
  - **Sesamoids** are bones that normally form in a tendon as it passes over a joint. The **patella** is the largest and most famous sesamoid bone.
  - **Accessory ossicles** are accessory epiphyseal or apophyseal ossification centers that fail to fuse with their parent bone.
  - **Old, unhealed fracture fragments** can sometimes mimic acute fractures (Fig. 24.4A).
  - Unlike fractures, these small bones are **corticated** (i.e., there is a white line that completely surrounds the bony fragment) and their edges are usually **smooth**.
  - In the case of **sesamoids** and **accessory ossicles**, they are **usually bilaterally symmetric** so that a view of the opposite extremity will usually demonstrate the same bone in the same location. They also **occur at anatomically predictable sites.**
    - There are almost always sesamoids present in the thumb, the posterolateral aspect of the knee **(fabella)**, and the great toe (Fig. 24.4B).
    - Accessory ossicles are most common in the foot (Fig. 24.4C).

RECOGNIZING DISLOCATIONS AND SUBLUXATIONS

- In a **dislocation,** the bones that originally formed the two components of a joint are no longer in apposition to each other. Dislocations can only occur at joints (Fig. 24.5A).
- In a **subluxation,** the bones that originally formed the two components of a joint are in **partial contact** with each other. Subluxations also occur only at joints (Fig. 24.5B).
- Some characteristics of common dislocations of the shoulder and hip are shown in Table 24.2.

DESCRIBING FRACTURES

- There is a common lexicon used in describing fractures to facilitate a reproducible description and to assure reliable and accurate communication.

TABLE 24.1 Differentiating Fractures, Ossicles, and Sesamoids

Feature	Acute Fracture	Sesamoids and Accessory Ossicles[a]
Abrupt disruption of cortex	Yes	No
Bilaterally symmetric	Almost never	Almost always
"Fracture line"	Unsharp, jagged	Smooth
Bony fragment has a cortex completely around it	No	Yes

[a]Old, unhealed fractures will not be bilaterally symmetric.

TABLE 24.2 Dislocations of the Shoulder and Hip

Shoulder	Hip
Anterior, subcoracoid most common	Posterior and superior more common
Caused by a combination of abduction, external rotation, and extension	Frequently caused by knee striking dashboard transmitting force to hip
Associated with fractures of humeral head **(Hill-Sachs deformity)** and glenoid **(Bankart fracture)**	Associated with fractures of posterior rim of the acetabulum

Fig. 24.4 Pitfalls in Fracture Diagnosis. (A) Old, **unhealed fracture fragments** (*white arrow*), (B) **sesamoids** (bones that form in a tendon as it passes over a joint) (*dotted white arrows*), and (C) **accessory ossicles** (accessory epiphyseal or apophyseal ossification centers that do not fuse with the parent bone), such as this **os trigonum** (*white arrow*), can sometimes mimic acute fractures.

Fig. 24.5 Dislocation and Subluxation. (A) In a **dislocation,** the bones that originally formed the two components of the interphalangeal joint are no longer in apposition to each other (*white arrows*). The terminal phalanx of the little toe is dislocated laterally. (B) In a **subluxation,** the bones that originally formed the two components of a joint are in partial contact with each other. The humeral head (H) is subluxed inferiorly (*white arrow*) in the glenoid (G) because of a large hematoma in the joint secondary to a fracture of the surgical neck of the humerus (*black arrow*). The hematoma itself is not visible by conventional radiography.

Fig. 24.6 Segmental Fracture and Butterfly Fracture. (A) There is a **segmental fracture** in which a portion of the shaft exists as an isolated fragment. Notice how the fibula has a center segment (S) and two additional fragments, one on either side (*white arrows*). (B) A **butterfly fragment** is a comminuted fracture in which the central fragment has a triangular shape (*dotted white arrow*).

TABLE 24.3 **How Fractures Are Described**	
Parameter	**Terms Used**
Number of fracture fragments	Simple or comminuted
Direction of fracture line	Transverse, oblique (diagonal), spiral
Relationship of one fragment to another	Displacement, angulation, shortening, and rotation
Open to the atmosphere (outside)	Closed or open (compound)

- **Fractures are usually described using four major parameters** (Table 24.3):
  - The **number of fragments**
  - The **direction of the fracture line**
  - The **relationship of the fragments** to each other

- Whether the fracture communicates **with the outside atmosphere**

How Fractures Are Described—By the Number of Fracture Fragments

- If the fracture produces **two fragments,** it is called a **simple fracture.**
- If the fracture produces **more than two** fragments, it is called a **comminuted fracture.** Some comminuted fractures have special names.
  - A **segmental fracture** is a comminuted fracture in which a portion of the shaft exists as an isolated fragment (Fig. 24.6A).
  - A **butterfly fragment** is a comminuted fracture in which the central fragment has a triangular shape (Fig. 24.6B).

How Fractures Are Described—By the Direction of the Fracture Line (Table 24.4)

- In a **transverse fracture,** the fracture line is perpendicular to the long axis of the bone. Transverse fractures are caused by a force directed **perpendicular to the shaft** (Fig. 24.7A).
- In a **diagonal** or **oblique fracture,** the fracture line is diagonal in orientation relative to the long axis of the bone. Diagonal or oblique fractures are caused by a force usually applied along the **same direction as the long axis** of the affected bone (Fig. 24.7B).
- With a **spiral fracture,** a twisting force or torque produces a fracture like those that might be caused by planting the foot in a hole while running. Spiral fractures are usually **unstable** and often associated with soft-tissue injuries such as **tears** in **ligaments** or **tendons** (Fig. 24.7C).

TABLE 24.4   Direction of Fracture Line and Mechanism of Injury

Direction of Fracture Line	Mechanism
Transverse	Force applied perpendicular to long axis of bone; fracture occurs at point of impact
Diagonal (also known as oblique)	Force applied along the long axis of bone; fracture occurs somewhere along shaft
Spiral	Twisting or torque injury

How Fractures Are Described—By the Relationship of One Fracture Fragment to Another

> ### ▶▶ IMPORTANT POINTS
>
> - By convention, abnormalities of the position of bone fragments secondary to fractures describe **the altered relationship of the distal fracture fragment relative to the proximal fragment.** These descriptions are based on the expected position the distal fragment would have normally assumed had the bone not been fractured.

- There are four major parameters most commonly used to **describe the relationship** of **fracture fragments.** Some fractures display more than one of these abnormalities of position. The four parameters are:
  - **Displacement**
  - **Angulation**
  - **Shortening**
  - **Rotation**
- **Displacement** describes **the amount by which the distal fragment is off-set,** front-to-back and side-to-side, from the proximal fragment. Displacement is most often described either in terms of **percent** (For example, "*The distal fragment is displaced by 50% of the width of the shaft.*") or by **fractions** ("*The distal fragment is displaced ½ the width of the shaft of the proximal fragment.*") (Fig. 24.8A).
- **Angulation** describes **the angle between the distal and proximal fragments** as a function of the degree to which the distal fragment is deviated from the position it would have assumed were it in its normal position. Angulation is described in degrees and by position ("*The distal fragment*

Fig. 24.7 Transverse, Diagonal, and Spiral Fracture Lines. (A) In a **transverse fracture** (*black arrow*), the fracture line is perpendicular to the long axis of the bone. (B) Diagonal or **oblique fractures** (*black arrow*) are diagonal in orientation relative to the normal axis of the bone. (C) **Spiral fractures** (*white arrows*) are usually caused by twisting or torque injuries.

Fig. 24.8 Fracture Orientation Parameters. (A) **Displacement** describes the amount by which the distal fragment (*white arrow*) is off-set, front-to-back and side-to-side, from the proximal fragment (*black arrow*). (B) **Angulation** describes the angle between the distal and proximal fragments (*dotted black line*) as a function of the degree to which the distal fragment is deviated from its normal position (*solid white line*). (C) **Shortening** describes how much, if any, overlap occurs at the ends of the fracture fragments (*white and black arrows*). (D) The opposite term from shortening is **distraction,** which refers to the distance the bone fragments are separated from each other (*two white arrows* show pull of tendons on fracture fragments of patella; *black arrow* points to distraction of fracture). *D*, Distal; *P*, proximal.

is angulated 15° anteriorly relative to the proximal fragment.") (Fig. 24.8B).

- **Shortening** describes how much, if any, **overlap** there is of the **ends of the fracture fragments,** which translates into how much shorter the length of the fractured bone is than it would be had it not been fractured (Fig. 24.8C).
  - The opposite term from shortening is **distraction,** which refers **to the distance the bone fragments are separated from each other** (Fig. 24.8D).
  - Shortening (overlap) or distraction (lengthening) are usually described by a number of centimeters (*"There are 2 cm of shortening of the fracture fragments."*).
- **Rotation** is an unusual abnormality in fracture positioning almost always involving the **long bones,** such as the femur or humerus. Rotation describes the orientation of the joint at one end of the fractured bone relative to the orientation of the joint at the other end of the same bone.
  - Normally, for example, when the hip joint is pointing forward, the knee joint is also pointing forward. If there is **rotation** about a fracture of the femoral shaft, the hip joint could be pointing forward while the knee joint is oriented in another direction (Fig. 24.9). To appreciate rotation, both the joint above and the joint below a fracture should be visualized, preferably on the same radiograph.

How Fractures Are Described—By the Relationship of the Fracture to the Atmosphere

- A **closed fracture** is the **more common** type of fracture in which there is **no communication** between the fracture fragments and the outside air/atmosphere.

Fig. 24.9 Rotation. To appreciate rotation, which usually occurs in long bones, both the joint above and the joint below a fracture must be visualized, preferably on the same radiograph. In this patient, the proximal tibia (*black arrow*) is oriented in the frontal plane, whereas the distal tibia and ankle (*white arrow*) are rotated and oriented laterally.

Fig. 24.10 Open (Compound) Fracture: Fifth Metacarpal. Open or compound fractures (*black arrows*) have an open wound or break in the skin allowing the bone to communicate with the outside (*white arrow*). Whether a fracture is open or not is best evaluated clinically.

Fig. 24.11 Avulsion Fractures: Anterior Superior Iliac Spine and Lesser Trochanter. There is an avulsion of the **anterior superior iliac spine** (*solid white arrow*), which is the site of the insertion of the sartorius muscle. There is also an avulsion of a portion of the lesser trochanter, on which the iliopsoas muscle inserts (*dotted white arrow*). The patient had participated in track and field events a week prior to these injuries.

- In an **open or compound fracture,** there is **communication between the fracture and the outside** atmosphere (e.g., a fracture fragment penetrates the skin) (Fig. 24.10). Compound fractures have implications regarding the way in which they are treated in order to avoid the complication of **osteomyelitis.** Whether a fracture is open or not is best diagnosed **clinically.**

AVULSION FRACTURES

- Avulsion is a **common mechanism** of fracture production in which the fracture fragment (called the **avulsed fragment**) is pulled from its parent bone by **the pull of a tendon** or **ligament.**
- Although avulsion fractures can and do occur at any age, they are **particularly common in younger individuals** engaging in athletic endeavors; in fact, they derive many of their names from the **type** of athletic activity that produces them (e.g., **Dancer's fracture, Skier's fracture,** and **Sprinter's fracture**).
- They **occur in anatomically predictable locations** because tendons insert on bones in a known location (Table 24.5) and the avulsed fragment is **typically small** (Fig. 24.11).
- They sometimes **heal with such exuberant callus formation** that they can be mistaken for a bone tumor (Fig. 24.12).

TABLE 24.5 Avulsion Fractures Around the Pelvis

Avulsed Fragment	Muscle That Inserts on That Fragment
Anterior, superior iliac spine	Sartorius muscle
Anterior, inferior iliac spine	Rectus femoris muscle
Ischial tuberosity	Hamstring muscles
Lesser trochanter of femur	Iliopsoas muscle

SALTER-HARRIS FRACTURES: EPIPHYSEAL PLATE FRACTURES IN CHILDREN

- Salter-Harris fractures are discussed in **Chapter 28** on pediatrics.

CHILD ABUSE

- Child abuse is discussed in **Chapter 28** on pediatrics.

STRESS FRACTURES

- Stress fractures **occur as a result of numerous microfractures** in which bone is subjected to repeated stretching and compressive forces.

Fig. 24.12 Healing Avulsion Fracture of Ischial Tuberosity. There is a healing fracture (*black arrows*) of the ischial tuberosity, which had been caused by forceful contraction of the hamstring muscles. There is a large amount of external callus present called **exuberant callus** (*white arrow*).

> ## ▶▶ IMPORTANT POINTS
>
> - Although **conventional radiographs are usually the study first obtained**, they may **initially appear normal in as many as 85%** of stress fractures, so it is common for a patient to complain of pain yet have a normal-appearing radiograph at first.
> - The **fracture may not be diagnosable** until after periosteal new bone formation occurs or, in the case of a **healing** stress fracture of cancellous bone, **the appearance of a thin, dense zone of sclerosis across the medullary cavity** (Fig. 24.13).

- Radionuclide **bone scan will usually be positive much earlier** than conventional radiographs: **within 6 to 72 hours** after the injury.
- Some **common locations for stress fractures** are the **shafts of long bones,** such as the proximal femur or proximal tibia, as well as the calcaneus and the second and third metatarsals (the latter called **march fractures**).

COMMON FRACTURE EPONYMS

- There are almost as many fracture eponyms as there are types of fractures. If you harbored a desire to have a fracture named after you some day, then you are probably too late. We focus on six of the most commonly used eponyms.
- **Colles fracture** is a **fracture of the distal radius with dorsal angulation** of the distal radial fracture fragment caused by a **f**all **on** the **o**utstretched **h**and (sometimes abbreviated as

Fig. 24.13 Stress ("March") Fracture; Two Frontal Views Taken 3 Weeks Apart. (A) Although conventional radiographs are the study of first choice, they may initially appear normal, as in this patient one day after pain began. (B) The fracture may not be diagnosable until after periosteal new bone formation forms (*white arrow*) or after the appearance of a thin dense zone of sclerosis across the medullary cavity (*black arrow*). This radiograph was taken 3 weeks after the first.

Fig. 24.14 Colles Fracture: Frontal (A) and Lateral (B) Views. A Colles fracture is a fracture of the distal radius (*solid white arrows*) with dorsal angulation of the distal radial fracture fragment (*angled black arrow*) caused by a fall on the outstretched hand. There is frequently an associated fracture of the ulnar styloid (*dotted white arrow*).

FOOSH). There is frequently an associated fracture of the ulnar styloid (Fig. 24.14).

- **Smith fracture** is a fracture of the distal radius with palmar angulation of the distal radial fracture fragment (in effect, it is a **reverse** Colles fracture). It is caused by a fall on the back of the flexed hand (Fig. 24.15).

- **Jones fracture** is a transverse fracture of the fifth metatarsal about 1 to 2 cm from its base, caused by plantar flexion of the foot and inversion of the ankle. A Jones fracture may take longer to heal than the more common avulsion fracture of the base of the fifth metatarsal (Fig. 24.16).

- **Boxer's fracture** is a fracture of the neck of the fifth metacarpal (little finger) with palmar angulation of the distal fracture fragment. Sometimes the fourth metacarpal may be involved. It is most often the result of punching a person or wall (Fig. 24.17).

- **March fracture** is a type of **stress fracture** cause by repeated microfractures to the foot from trauma (such as marching) most often affecting the **shafts of the second and third metatarsals** (see Fig. 24.13).

- **Lisfranc fracture-dislocations** are relatively uncommon and most often result from either athletic injuries or motor vehicle collisions/industrial accidents. They may be obvious, as in the example shown (Fig. 24.18), or inapparent on conventional radiographs. CT or MRI may be needed to show the injury.

SOME SUBTLE FRACTURES OR DISLOCATIONS

- Look at these areas carefully when evaluating for a possible fracture; then look a second and third time.

Fig. 24.15 Smith Fracture. A Smith fracture is a fracture of the distal radius (*white arrow*) with palmar angulation of the distal radial fracture fragment (*angled black line*), the reverse of a Colles fracture. It is caused by a fall on the back of the flexed hand.

Fig. 24.16 Jones Fracture. A Jones fracture is a transverse fracture of the base of the 5th metatarsal (*white arrow*) that occurs about 1 to 2 cm from the tuberosity of the 5th metatarsal (*black arrow*). It is caused by plantar flexion of the foot and inversion of the ankle.

Fig. 24.17 Boxer's Fracture. A Boxer's fracture is a fracture of the neck of the 5th metacarpal with palmar angulation of the distal fracture fragment (*black arrow*). Despite its name, it is **not** a fracture commonly sustained by professional boxers whose second and third metacarpals and radius bear the brunt of the force.

Fig. 24.18 Lisfranc Fracture-Dislocation. (A) A close-up view of a **normal** right foot. Notice how the lateral border of the **1st MT** (*solid white arrow*) aligns with the lateral border (*dotted white arrow*) of the first or medial cuneiform (**1st C**) and the medial border of the **2nd MT** (*solid black arrow*) lines up with the medial border of the second or middle cuneiform (**2nd C**) (*dotted black arrow*). The Lisfranc ligament is depicted by the white bar that joins the 1st C with the base of the 2nd MT. (B) This is a Lisfranc fracture-dislocation. The lateral border of the **1st MT** (*solid white arrow*) no longer aligns with the lateral border of the **1st C** (*dotted white arrow*) and the medial border of the **2nd MT** (*solid black arrow*) no longer aligns with the **2nd C** (*dotted black arrow*). There is a fracture at the base of the **2nd MT** (*white circle*). All of the metatarsals are dislocated laterally (*curved arrow*), called a **homolateral** dislocation. *C,* Cuneiform; *MT,* metatarsal.

- **Scaphoid fractures**
  - Scaphoid (navicular) fractures are common injuries clinically suspected if there is tenderness in the **anatomic snuff box** after a fall on an outstretched hand. Look for **hairline-thin radiolucencies** on special angled views of the scaphoid (Fig. 24.19). Fractures across the **waist** of the scaphoid can lead to **avascular necrosis of the proximal pole** of that bone.
    - Because of peculiarities of vascularization, a fracture through the mid-portion (**waist**) **of the scaphoid interrupts blood supply to the proximal pole** while the remainder of the bones of the wrist continues to undergo the process of bone turnover. The result is an apparent relative **increase in the density** of the **devascularized part compared** with the **remainder of the bone** (Fig. 24.20).

- **Buckle fractures of radius and/or ulna in children**
  - These are common fractures in children. Look for **acute and sudden angulation of the cortex**, especially near the wrist (**see** Fig. 24.1B). These are impacted fractures and usually heal quickly with no deformity.
- **Radial head fracture**
  - A fracture of the radial head is the **most common fracture of the elbow in an adult.** Look for a crescentic lucency of fat along the posterior aspect of the distal humerus produced by normally invisible **intracapsular, extrasynovial fat** that is lifted away from the bone by swelling of the joint capsule due to a **traumatic hemarthrosis**—the **positive posterior fat-pad sign** (Fig. 24.21).

Fig. 24.19 Scaphoid Fracture. Look for linear fracture lines on special angled views of the scaphoid (*white arrow*). Fractures across the waist of the scaphoid can lead to avascular necrosis of proximal pole of that bone.

Fig. 24.20 Avascular Necrosis of the Proximal Pole of the Scaphoid. A close-up frontal view of the wrist demonstrates that the proximal pole of the scaphoid (*black arrow*) is denser than the distal pole (*solid white arrow*). There is a fracture through the waist of the scaphoid (*dotted white arrow*).

Fig. 24.21 Fracture of Radial Head with Joint Effusion: Frontal (A) and Lateral (B) Views. (A) Radial head fractures (*dotted black arrows*) are the most common fractures of the elbow in an adult. (B) There is a crescentic lucency along the dorsal aspect of the distal humerus (*solid black arrow*)—the **positive posterior fat-pad sign**. Virtually all studies of bones will include at least two views at 90-degree angles to each other called **orthogonal views**. Many protocols call for two additional oblique views that enable you to visualize more of the cortex in profile.

- **Supracondylar fracture of the distal humerus in children**
  - This is the **most common fracture of the elbow in a child.** Most of these fractures produce **posterior displacement** of the distal humerus and they can be quite subtle (Fig. 24.22).
- **Posterior dislocation of the shoulder (uncommon injury)**
  - In a posterior dislocation, the humeral head is fixed in internal rotation and looks like a "light bulb" in all views

of the shoulder. Look at a view like the **axillary** or **"Y"** view to see if the humeral head still lies within the glenoid fossa. On the "Y" view (an oblique view of the shoulder), the head will lie **lateral to the glenoid** in a posterior dislocation (Fig. 24.23).

- **Hip fractures in the elderly**
  - Hip fractures are common and frequently related to osteoporosis. If possible, conventional radiographs of the femoral

Fig. 24.22 Supracondylar Fracture. On a true lateral film, the **anterior humeral line** (a line drawn tangential to the anterior humeral cortex and shown here in *black*) should bisect the middle third of the ossification center of capitellum (C). When there is a supracondylar fracture, this line will pass more anteriorly, as it does here. There is a positive **posterior fat pad sign** present (*white arrow*).

Fig. 24.23 Posterior Dislocation; Anterior Dislocation. (A) In a posterior dislocation, look for the humeral head (H) to be persistently fixed in internal rotation and resemble a **light bulb** no matter how the patient turns the forearm. There is also an increased distance between the head and the glenoid (G) (*black arrow*). (B) On the angled "Y" view of the shoulder in a posterior dislocation, the head (H) will lie under the acromion (A), a posterior structure of the scapula. (C) In a Y view of an **anterior dislocation**, the humeral head (H) lies under the anterior coracoid process (C) of the scapula.

neck should be performed with the patient's leg in internal rotation so as to display the femoral neck in profile. Look for **angulation of the cortex** or zones of **increased density indicating impaction** (Fig. 24.24).

- Sometimes hip fractures may be very subtle and require an MRI or radionuclide bone scan for diagnosis.
- Look also for **indirect signs** indicating the possibility of an underlying fracture (Table 24.6).

Fig. 24.24 Impacted Subcapital Hip Fracture. Subcapital hip fractures occur at the junction between the femoral head and neck. Most hip fractures in the elderly (90%) occur as a result of a fall, frequently a minor fall such as from the standing position. Look for a step-off of the cortex (*white arrow*) and zones of increased density (*black arrows*) indicating impaction or overlying bone fragments.

TABLE 24.6 Indirect Signs of Possible Fracture

Sign	Remarks
Soft-tissue swelling	Frequently accompanies a fracture but, if present, does not necessarily mean that a fracture is present.
Disappearance of normal fat stripes	The **pronator quadratus fat stripe** on the volar aspect of the wrist, for example, may be displaced with a fracture of the distal radius (Fig. 24.25).
Joint effusion	The **positive posterior fat pad sign** seen on the dorsal aspect of the distal humerus from a traumatic joint effusion is an example (see Fig. 24.21B).
Periosteal reaction	Sometimes the healing of fractures will be the first manifestation that a fracture was present, especially with stress fractures of the foot.

FRACTURE HEALING

- Fracture healing is determined by many factors, including the **age of the patient,** the **fracture site,** the **position of the fracture fragments,** the degree of **immobilization,** and the **blood supply** to the fracture site (Table 24.7).
- Immediately following a fracture, there is hemorrhage into the fracture site.
- Over the next several weeks, osteoclasts act to remove the diseased bone. The fracture line may **minimally widen** at this time.
- Then, over the course of several more weeks, **new bone (callus)** begins to bridge the fracture gap (Fig. 24.26).

> ## ⟫ IMPORTANT POINTS
>
> - **Internal endosteal healing** is manifest by **indistinctness of the fracture line** leading to eventual obliteration of the fracture line, in most cases.
> - **External periosteal healing** is manifest by external callus formation eventually leading to **bridging of the fracture site.**

- **Remodeling** of bone **begins at about 8 to 12 weeks** postfracture as mechanical forces, in part, begin to adjust the bone to its original shape.
  - In **children, this occurs much more rapidly** and usually leads to a bone that will eventually appear normal. In **adults, this process may take years** and the healed fracture may never assume a completely normal shape.
- **Complications of the healing process.**
  - **Delayed union. The fracture does not heal in the expected time** for a fracture at that particular site (e.g., longer than 6 to 8 weeks for a fracture of the shaft of the radius). **Most** cases of **delayed union** will eventually **progress to complete healing** with further immobilization.
  - **Malunion.** Healing of the fracture fragments occurs in a **mechanically** or **cosmetically unacceptable position.**
  - **Nonunion.** This implies that **fracture healing will never occur.** It is characterized by **smooth** and **sclerotic fracture margins** with **distraction of the fracture fragments** (Fig. 24.27). A **pseudarthrosis,** complete with a synovial lining, may form at the fracture site.
    - **Motion at the fracture site** may be demonstrated under fluoroscopic manipulation or on stress views.

TABLE 24.7 Factors That Affect Fracture Healing

Accelerate Fracture Healing	Delay Fracture Healing
Youth	Old age
Early immobilization	Delayed immobilization
Adequate duration of immobilization	Too short a duration of immobilization
Good blood supply	Poor blood supply
Physical activity after adequate immobilization	Steroids
Adequate mineralization	Osteoporosis, osteomalacia

Fig. 24.25 Normal and Abnormal Pronator Quadratus Fat Plane. (A) This is an example of a normal fascial plane produced by the pronator quadratus (*white arrow* points to lucency) on the volar aspect of the wrist compared with the bulging fascial plane (*dotted white arrow*) in (B), which has occurred because of soft-tissue swelling accompanying a fracture of the distal radius (*black arrow*).

Fig. 24.26 Healing Humeral Fracture. Internal endosteal healing occurs several weeks after a fracture and is manifest by indistinctness of the fracture line (*black arrow*) eventually leading to obliteration of the fracture line. External, periosteal healing is manifest by external callus formation (*white arrows*) leading to bridging of the fracture site

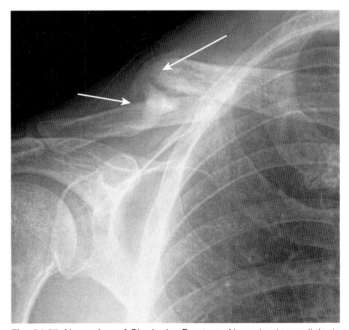

Fig. 24.27 Nonunion of Clavicular Fracture. Nonunion is a radiologic diagnosis that implies fracture healing is not likely to occur as the processes leading to the repair of bone have ceased. It is characterized by smooth and sclerotic fracture margins with distraction of the fracture fragments (*white arrows*). A **pseudarthrosis**, complete with a synovial lining, may form at the fracture site.

SPINAL TRAUMA

- Fractures of the spine are infrequent compared with fractures of other parts of the skeleton. When they occur, they have particular importance because of the implications for associated spinal cord injury.
- **CT**, with its ability to reformat images in different planes and provide additional information about the soft tissues, now supplements and, in many cases, **has replaced conventional radiography in the evaluation of spinal trauma.** CT is utilized to determine **the extent of the injury** in any patient in whom a traumatic spinal injury has already been demonstrated by conventional radiographs.
- CT is also utilized to **detect bony lesions not visible on conventional radiographs** and to **evaluate soft-tissue abnormalities** in patients who are unable to undergo an MRI examination.
- Most spinal fractures occur in the **thoracic** and **lumbar spines.** Cervical spine fractures account for the remaining spinal fractures. The **most commonly fractured vertebrae are L1, L2, and T12,** accounting for more than half of all thoracolumbar spine fractures. **Compression fractures** are the most common type of spinal fracture.
- **The three cervical lines** (Fig. 24.28).
  - Many trauma protocols include a **cross-table lateral view** of the cervical spine (the patient's neck is immobilized,

the patient remains on the stretcher or examining table, and the x-ray beam is directed **horizontally** so that the patient's **head is not moved**).
- This view enables a **quick assessment for spinal fracture/subluxation** before further studies that might involve motion of the patient's neck are performed.
- Three, parallel arcuate lines should be envisioned on the lateral spine radiograph. Deviation from the normal parallel curvature of these lines should suggest a subluxed and/or fractured vertebral body.

> ### ⟫ IMPORTANT POINTS
>
> - Some of the more common spinal fractures:
>   - **Compression fractures** are discussed in **Chapter 23.**
>   - **Jefferson fracture**
>   - **Hangman's fracture**
>   - **Burst fracture**
>   - **Chance fracture**

Jefferson Fracture

- A Jefferson fracture is a **fracture of C1** usually involving both the anterior and posterior arches. In its classical presentation, there are **bilateral fractures of both the anterior and posterior arches of C1,** producing four fractures in all.
- It is **caused by an axial loading injury** (e.g., diving into a swimming pool and hitting one's head on the bottom).

> ### ⟫ IMPORTANT POINTS
>
> - On **conventional radiographs,** the hallmark of a Jefferson fracture is **bilateral, *lateral* offset of the lateral masses of C1 relative to C2 as seen on the *open-mouth view* (atlantoaxial view)** of the cervical spine. The fracture is **confirmed utilizing CT** (Fig. 24.29).

- A Jefferson fracture is a **self-decompressing** fracture in that the spinal canal at the level of the fracture is usually wide enough to accommodate any swelling of the cord. There is typically **no neurologic deficit** associated with this type of fracture.

Hangman's Fracture

- A Hangman's fracture is a **fracture of the posterior elements of C2.** Hangman's fractures **result from a hyperextension-compression injury** typically occurring in an unrestrained occupant in a motor vehicle accident who strikes his or her forehead on the windshield with the neck extended.
- They are **best evaluated on the lateral view** of the cervical spine on conventional radiography and the **sagittal view** on CT.

Fig. 24.28 The Three Cervical Lines. Three parallel arcuate lines should smoothly join all of the **spinolaminar white lines** that occur first at the junctions between the laminae and the spinous processes (*dashed black line*); a second line should join all of the **posterior aspects of the vertebral bodies** (*solid black line*); and a third line should join all of the **anterior aspects of the vertebral bodies** (*dashed white line*).

> ### ⟫ IMPORTANT POINTS
>
> - The fracture effectively **separates** the **posterior aspect** of the **C2** vertebral body from the **anterior** aspect of **C2** allowing the anterior aspect of C2 to **sublux forward** on the body of C3 (Fig. 24.30).

Fig. 24.29 Normal Open-Mouth View; Jefferson Fracture, Open-Mouth View and CT. (A) A normal "open-mouth" view of C1 and C2 demonstrates that the lateral margins of C1 (1) line up with the lateral margins of C2 (2) (*solid white arrows*). (B) The hallmark of a Jefferson fracture is bilateral, lateral offset of the lateral masses of C1 (1) (*solid white arrows*) relative to C2 (2). (C) The fracture is confirmed utilizing CT, which shows fractures of both the right and left anterior arches (*solid white arrows*) and the right posterior arch of C1 (*dotted white arrow*). *1, lateral masses of C1; 2, C2.*

Fig. 24.30 Hangman's Fracture. The fracture (*dotted white arrow*) effectively separates the posterior aspect of the C2 vertebral body from the anterior aspect of C2 allowing the anterior aspect to sublux forward on the body of C3 (*solid white arrow*). Notice that the spinolaminar line of C2 (*solid black arrow*) lies abnormally posterior to the spinolaminar lines of the other vertebral bodies.

- Some Hangman's fractures have so little displacement that CT may be needed for their detection.
- Because Hangman's fractures lead to overall **widening** of the **spinal canal**, they are usually **not associated with neurologic deficits.** This is in contradistinction to the injury after which this fracture is named, the fracture incurred during a **judicial hanging** in which there was **hyperextension** leading to a fracture of C2 and **marked distraction** of C2 from C3 with distraction of the **spinal cord** itself.

Burst Fractures

- Burst fractures are most common in the **cervical spine, thoracic spine, and upper lumbar spine.**
- They are high-energy **axial-loading injuries,** typically secondary to motor vehicle accidents or falls, in which the disk above is driven into the vertebral body below and the vertebral body bursts. This in turn drives bony fragments **posteriorly** into the **spinal canal (retropulsed fragments),** whereas the anterior aspect of the vertebral body is displaced **forward.**

Fig. 24.31 Burst Fracture: Radiograph and CT. (A) Findings include a comminuted compression fracture of the vertebral body in which the anterior vertebral body is displaced forward (*dotted white arrow*), whereas the posterior aspect of the body is propelled dorsally toward the spinal canal (*black arrow*). Notice how the posterior aspects of the normal vertebral bodies are concave inward (*solid white arrows*). (B) Axial CT scan of the spine shows a fracture of the vertebral body (*black arrow*) and the retropulsed fragment (*white arrow*) protruding into the spinal canal (C).

- Because these fractures involve incursion on the spinal canal, the **majority of burst fractures** are **associated** with a **neurologic deficit.**

> ▶▶ **IMPORTANT POINTS**
>
> - Findings of burst fractures include a **comminuted compression fracture** of the **vertebral body** in which the **posterior aspect** of the **body** is **bowed backward toward** the **spinal canal.** **CT** is the **best imaging modality** for identifying **bony fragments** in the spinal canal (Fig. 24.31).

Chance Fracture

- Chance fractures (named after George Q. Chance, a British radiologist who first described them) are **transverse fractures** through the **entire vertebral body, pedicles, and spinous process,** frequently occurring as a result of a fall or motor vehicle accident in which the occupant was using only a lap seatbelt. They typically occur in the **upper lumbar-lower thoracic spine** and are associated with a relatively **high incidence** of **intraabdominal visceral injuries,** especially to the duodenum, pancreas, and mesentery.

> ▶▶ **IMPORTANT POINTS**
>
> - Radiographic findings include a **horizontal fracture** that shears through the vertebral body, pedicles, and spinous process. The vertebral body component may not be as obvious as the fractures through the posterior elements (eVideo 24.1).

Locked Facets

- Bilateral locking of the facets in the cervical spine can occur as a result of a **hyperflexion injury** in which the **inferior facets** of one **vertebral body slide over** and **in front** of the **superior facets** of the **body below.** In this position, the slipped facets cannot return to their normal position without medical intervention; thus, the term **locked.**
- Locked facets occur with **forward slippage** of the affected vertebral body on the body below it **by at least 50% of its anteroposterior diameter.**

> ▶▶ **IMPORTANT POINTS**
>
> - On **lateral (sagittal) imaging** of the cervical spine, the **inferior articular facet will lie in front of the superior facet** of the body below. This is the **reverse** of the **normal** anatomic relationship between adjacent facets (Fig. 24.32).
>   - Since the superior articular facet is no longer "covered" by the inferior facet above it, this appearance was described on CT as the **naked facet sign.**

- This injury virtually **always results in neurologic impairment.**

PATHOLOGIC FRACTURES

- Pathologic fractures are those that occur in **bone with a preexisting abnormality.** Pathologic fractures tend to occur with **minimum** or **no trauma.**

Fig. 24.32 Normal and Bilateral Locked Facets. (A) Normally the inferior articular facet of the body above (in this case C4—*white arrow*) covers and lies **posterior** to the superior articular facet of the body below (in this case C5—*black arrow*). (B) The inferior articulating facet of C4 (*dotted white arrow*) lies **anterior** to the superior articular facet of C5 (*dotted black arrow*), the reverse of normal. Locking of the facets in the cervical spine can occur as a result of a hyperflexion injury, which results in forward slippage of the affected vertebral body on the body below it by at least 50% of its anteroposterior diameter (*solid white arrow*).

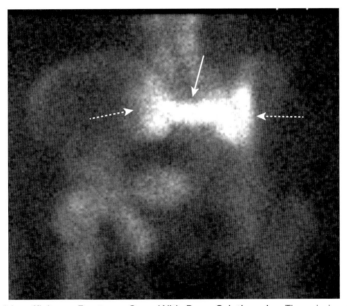

Fig. 24.33 Sacral Insufficiency Fractures Seen With Bone Scintigraphy. There is increased radiotracer uptake in vertical fractures through the sacral ala (*dotted white arrows*) and a horizontal fracture through the body of the sacrum (*solid white arrow*). This has been called the **Honda Sign** because it resembles the carmaker's insignia. The sacrum is a common site for such fractures from osteoporosis.

- **Insufficiency fractures** are a type of pathologic fracture (Box 24.2).
- Diseases that produce either an **increase** or a **decrease** in bone density tend to **weaken the normal architecture** of bone and predispose to pathologic fractures.
- Diseases that predispose to pathologic fractures may be **local** (e.g., metastasis) or **diffuse** (e.g., osteoporosis). In general, pathologic fractures occur more often in the **ribs, spine, and proximal appendicular skeleton** (especially, humerus and femur).

BOX 24.2 Insufficiency Fractures

- Insufficiency fractures are a type of pathologic fracture in which mechanically weakened bone fractures from a normal or physiologic stress.
- They are most common in postmenopausal women secondary to osteoporosis.
- Common sites include the pelvis, thoracic spine, sacrum, tibia, and calcaneus.
- Unlike other fractures that manifest themselves by a lucency in the bone, most insufficiency fractures display a sclerotic band (representing healing) on conventional radiographs.
- CT, MRI, or nuclear medicine bone scans are more sensitive than conventional radiographs in detecting insufficiency fractures (Fig. 24.33).

Fig. 24.34 Pathologic Fracture. In this patient with metastatic renal cell carcinoma to the humerus, there is a geographic lytic lesion seen in the distal humerus (*black arrows*) through which a transverse pathologic fracture has occurred (*white arrow*).

- **Recognizing pathologic fractures** (Fig. 24.34).
  - First, there has to be a fracture present.
  - The bone surrounding the fracture will demonstrate abnormal density or architecture.
  - **Delayed healing** is **common** in pathologic fractures.
- Attempts to predict "impending" fractures in diseased bone have, by and large, proved to be unreliable.
- The treatment of a pathologic fracture depends in part on successful treatment of the underlying condition that produced it.

🏠 TAKE HOME POINTS

- A **fracture** is described as a disruption in the continuity of all or part of the cortex of a bone.
- **Complete fractures** involve the entire cortex, are more common, and typically occur in adults; **incomplete fractures** involve only a part of the cortex and typically occur in bones that are softer, such as those of children; **torus** and **greenstick fractures** are incomplete fractures.
- **Fracture lines** tend to be blacker, more sharply angled, and more jagged than other lucencies in bones such as nutrient canals or epiphyseal plates.
- Sesamoids, accessory ossicles, and unhealed fractures may mimic acute fractures, but all will have smooth and corticated margins.
- **Dislocation** is present when two bones that originally formed a joint are no longer in contact with each other; **subluxation** is present when two bones that originally formed a joint are in partial contact with each other.
- Fractures are described in many ways, including the number of fracture fragments, direction of the fracture line, relationship of the fragments to each other, and whether or not they communicate with the outside atmosphere.
- **Simple fractures** have two fragments; **comminuted fractures** have more than two fragments; segmental and butterfly fractures describe two types of comminuted fracture.
- The direction of fracture lines is described as **transverse, diagonal, or spiral.**
- The relationships of the fragments of a fracture are described by four parameters: **displacement, angulation, shortening, and rotation.**
- **Closed fractures** are those in which there is no communication between the fracture and the outside atmosphere; they are much more common than **open or compound fractures** in which there is a communication with the outside atmosphere.
- **Avulsion fractures** are produced by the forceful pull of a tendon or ligament; they can occur at any age, but are particularly common in younger, athletic individuals.
- **Stress fractures**, such as march fractures in the metatarsals, occur as a result of numerous microfractures and frequently are not visible on conventional radiographs taken when the pain first begins; after some time, bony callus formation and/or a dense zone of sclerosis becomes visible.
- Some common, named fractures are **Colles fracture** (of the radius), **Smith fracture** (of the radius), **Jones fracture** (of the base of the fifth metatarsal), **Boxer's fracture** (of the head of the fifth metacarpal), **march fracture,** and the **Lisfranc fracture-dislocation** of the foot.
- Some fractures are more difficult to detect than others; the **more subtle fractures** include scaphoid fractures, buckle fractures of the radius and ulna, radial head fractures, supracondylar fractures, posterior dislocations of the shoulder (which are uncommon), and hip fractures.
- Soft-tissue swelling, the disappearance of normal fat stripes and fascial planes, joint effusions, and periosteal reaction are **indirect signs** that should alert you to the possibility of an underlying fracture.
- **Fractures heal** with a combination of endosteal callus, recognized by a progressive indistinctness of the fracture line, and external callus that bridges the fracture site; many factors affect fracture healing, including the age of the patient, the degree of mobility of the fracture, and its blood supply.
- **Delayed union** refers to a fracture that is taking longer to heal than is usually required for that site; **malunion** means the fracture is healing, but in a mechanically or cosmetically unacceptable way; **nonunion** is a radiologic diagnosis that implies there is little if any likelihood the fracture will heal.
- **Spinal fractures** are less common than fractures of the appendicular skeleton, but they have important implications because of the possibility of spinal cord injury. CT has replaced conventional radiography as the modality of imaging in many cases of spinal trauma.
- The findings in a Jefferson fracture, Hangman's fracture, burst fracture, Chance fracture, and locked facets are discussed; the first two are self-decompressing injuries that are usually not associated with neurologic deficit.
- **Pathologic fractures** are those that occur with minimal or no trauma in bones that had a preexisting abnormality.

More information on recognizing trauma to the bony skeleton is available to registered users online.

Recognizing the Imaging Findings of Trauma to the Chest

- Trauma is the leading cause of death, hospitalization, and disability in Americans from the age of 1 year through age 45. The major imaging findings of chest trauma will be discussed in this chapter. Table 25.1 summarizes some of the traumatic injuries that are discussed in other chapters.
- Trauma-related injuries can be divided by the two major mechanisms that produce them.
  - **Blunt trauma** is usually the result of motor vehicle accidents and is the more common of the two.
  - **Penetrating trauma** is usually the result of accidental or criminal stabbings and gunshot wounds.
  - Table 25.2 is an overview of the initial imaging work-up for penetrating injuries to various body parts.
- In this chapter, we discuss various manifestations of chest trauma, starting from the periphery (chest wall) and progressing centrally (aorta).

TABLE 25.1 Other Manifestations of Trauma

Injury	Discussed in
Pleural effusion/hemothorax	Chapter 8
Aspiration	Chapter 9
Fractures and dislocations	Chapter 24
Spinal trauma	Chapter 24
Abdominal and pelvic trauma	Chapter 26
Head trauma	Chapter 27

TABLE 25.2 Initial Imaging Workup of Penetrating Trauma

Body Part	Modality of Choice
Head	CT scan of the head without and then possibly with contrast.
Neck	Mostly CT first (plain films used less often) followed by CT-angiography if damage to the neck vessels is suspected.
Chest	Chest radiographs are obtained first; then a CT scan of the chest as a follow-up in almost all patients except those who are hemodynamically unstable.
Abdomen	Abdominal CT scanning is study of choice in identifying and assessing the severity of visceral organ injury.

CHEST TRAUMA

- Chest injuries in trauma patients are **very common** and are responsible for one of four of the trauma-related deaths. The overwhelming majority of chest trauma is the result of motor vehicle accidents.

CHEST WALL TRAUMA

Rib Fractures

- **Rib fractures are common** sequelae of blunt chest trauma and the associated morbidity and mortality from such trauma increases as the **number** of rib fractures increases. The severity of underlying visceral injury is usually more important than the rib fractures themselves, but their presence might provide clues to unsuspected pathology.

> ⟫ **IMPORTANT POINTS**
>
> - Fractures of the **first three ribs** are relatively **uncommon** and, if they occur following blunt trauma, **indicate a sufficient amount of force** to produce other internal injuries (Fig. 25.1).

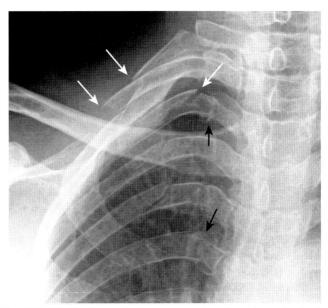

Fig. 25.1 Rib Fractures. Fractures present as linear lucencies in the ribs and are easier to detect when the fracture ends are displaced (*white arrows*). Do not mistake the normal costovertebral junctions (*black arrows*) near the spine for a fracture.

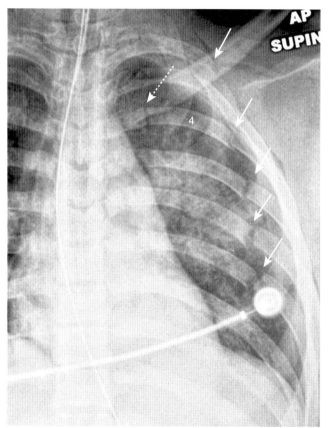

Fig. 25.2 Flail Chest. There are two or more fractures (*dotted white arrow* demonstrates second fracture in rib 4) present in more than three contiguous ribs (*solid white arrows*) in this patient struck by an automobile. The airspace disease in the left lung is an underlying pulmonary contusion, which almost always accompanies a flail chest.

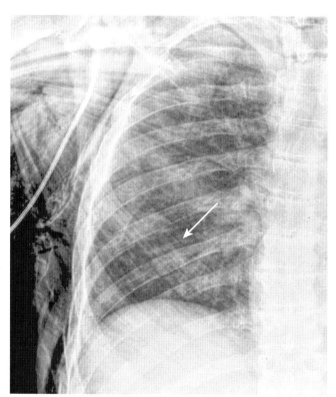

Fig. 25.3 Subcutaneous Emphysema. Air dissecting along muscle bundles produces this characteristic striated appearance (*white arrows*). Although dramatic radiographically, subcutaneous emphysema usually produces no serious clinical effects by itself.

- Fractures of **ribs 4 to 9 are common** and especially important if they are displaced (they can produce a pneumothorax) or if there are two fractures in each of three or more contiguous ribs (**flail chest**).
  - **Flail chest** is almost always accompanied by a pulmonary contusion (see later in this chapter). Because of the severity of the injuries with which it is usually associated, a flail chest has a significant mortality (Fig. 25.2).
- Fractures of **ribs 10 to 12** may indicate the presence of **underlying trauma** to the **liver** (right side) or the **spleen** (left side), especially if they are displaced (eVideo 25.1).
- In cases of minor trauma, it is **not unusual for rib fractures to be undetectable on the initial examination,** but to become visible in several weeks after callus begins to form.

Subcutaneous Emphysema

- **Air** can **extend into the soft tissues** of the **neck, chest, and abdominal walls** from the mediastinum or it can dissect in the subcutaneous tissues from a thoracotomy drainage tube or a penetrating injury to the chest wall.
- **Air dissecting along muscle bundles** produces a **characteristic comb-like, striated appearance** that superimposes on the underlying lung, often making it difficult to evaluate the lungs by conventional radiography (Fig. 25.3).

- Even though it may present a striking imaging appearance, **subcutaneous emphysema usually produces no serious clinical effects by itself.**
- Depending on the volume of subcutaneous air present, it may require **several days** to **a week** or longer for the air to reabsorb.

PLEURAL ABNORMALITIES: PNEUMOTHORAX

Causes of a Pneumothorax

- **Spontaneous**
  - **Spontaneous pneumothoraces** are common and often develop from **rupture of an apical, subpleural bleb** or bulla. They **characteristically occur in tall thin men between 20 and 40 years of age.** Trauma is not a prerequisite for a spontaneous pneumothorax.
- **Traumatic**
  - Trauma is the **most common cause** of a **pneumothorax, either accidental or iatrogenic.** The trauma may be:
    - Through the chest wall (e.g., stab wound)
    - Internal (e.g., rupture of a bronchus from a motor vehicle collision)
    - Iatrogenic (e.g., following an attempt at central venous catheter insertion)
- **Diseases that decrease lung compliance**
  - Chronic fibrotic disease (e.g., eosinophilic granuloma or diseases such as hyaline membrane disease in infants)
- **Rupture of an alveolus or bronchiole** (e.g., asthma)

Fig. 25.4 Simple Pneumothorax With No Shift. There is a large left-sided pneumothorax (*white arrows*) with no shift of the heart or trachea to the right. There is subcutaneous emphysema in the region of the left shoulder (*black arrow*). Can you detect why the patient had all of these findings? Yes, that is a bullet superimposed on the heart (but on CT it was actually posterior to the heart in the left lower lobe).

Fig. 25.5 Large Left-Sided Tension Pneumothorax. In this patient with a spontaneous pneumothorax, the left lung is almost totally collapsed (*solid white arrow*) and there is a shift of the trachea (*solid black arrow*) and heart to the right side. The left hemidiaphragm is depressed because of the elevated left intrathoracic pressure (*dotted white arrow*).

Types of Pneumothoraces

- Pneumothoraces can be categorized as **primary** (i.e., occurring in what appears to have been normal lung [**spontaneous pneumothorax** being an example]) or **secondary** (i.e., those that occur in diseased lung [as in **emphysema**]).
- Pneumothoraces have also been classified based on the presence or absence of a **"shift" of the mobile mediastinal structures, such as the heart and trachea.**
  - **Simple pneumothorax:** there is usually **no shift of the mediastinal structures** (Fig. 25.4).
  - **Tension pneumothorax:** there is a **shift of the mediastinal structures away from the side of the pneumothorax** frequently associated with cardiopulmonary compromise (Fig. 25.5).

Tension Pneumothorax

- Progressive loss of air into the pleural space through a one-way check-valve mechanism may cause a shift of the heart and mediastinal structures **away** from the side of the pneumothorax. The air may be entering through a rent in the parietal pleura or visceral pleura or from the tracheobronchial tree.
- The continuously **increasing intrathoracic pressure may lead to cardiopulmonary compromise** by **impairing venous return to the heart.**
- Besides a shift of the mobile mediastinal structures **away** from the side of the pneumothorax, there may be **inversion of the hemidiaphragm** (especially on the left side) and there may be **flattening of the heart contour on the side under tension.**

BOX 25.1 How Large Is the Pneumothorax?

- Size measurements of pneumothoraces on conventional radiographs correlate poorly with CT scans of their actual size.
- There is poor correlation between the size of the pneumothorax and the degree of clinical impairment.
- **The 2 cm rule:** If the distance between the lung margin and the chest wall at the apex is <2 cm, a chest tube is usually not needed; a distance >2 cm usually requires chest tube drainage.
- Assessment of the patient's clinical status is the most important determinant in deciding whether chest tube drainage is required.

- There should **never** be a shift of the heart or mediastinal structures **toward** the side of a pneumothorax.
- The question "**How large is the pneumothorax?**" is an oft-repeated question, but the actual issue is "Does this patient require a chest tube to drain the pneumothorax?" Box 25.1 summarizes the answer.

IMAGING MODALITIES USED TO DIAGNOSE A PNEUMOTHORAX

Pneumothorax: Conventional Radiographs

- A **pneumothorax occurs when air enters the pleural space.**
  - The negative pressure normally present in the pleural space rises higher than the intraalveolar pressure and the lung collapses.

- The parietal pleura remains on the inner surface of the chest wall, but the visceral pleura retracts toward the hilum attached to the collapsing lung.
  - The **visceral pleura becomes visible as a thin white line** outlined by air on both sides, marking the outer border of the lung and indicating the presence of the pneumothorax. The visible visceral pleura is called the **visceral pleural white line** or simply the **visceral pleural line.**

> ▶ **IMPORTANT POINTS**
>
> - You should be able to **identify the visceral pleural line** (Fig. 25.6) in order **to make the definitive diagnosis of a pneumothorax.**

- Even as the lung collapses, it tends to maintain its usual lung-like shape so that the curvature of **the visceral pleural line parallels the curvature of the chest wall**; that is, the visceral pleural line is **convex outward toward the chest wall** (Fig. 25.7).
  - Most other linear densities that **mimic** a pneumothorax do not demonstrate this spatial relationship with the chest wall.
- There is usually, but not always, an **absence of lung markings peripheral to the visceral pleural line.**

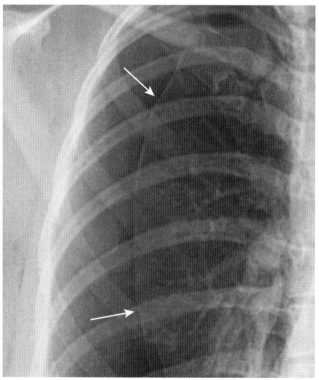

Fig. 25.6 Visceral Pleural Line in a Pneumothorax. You should see the visceral pleural line to make the definitive diagnosis of a pneumothorax (*white arrows*). The visceral and parietal pleurae are normally not visible, both normally lying adjacent to the chest wall.

> **!** **DIAGNOSTIC PITFALLS**
>
> - **Pleural adhesions** may keep part, but not all, of the visceral pleura adherent to the parietal pleura, even in the presence of a pneumothorax. On conventional radiographs, it may be possible to visualize lung markings in front or in back of the pneumothorax and to overlook the presence of a pneumothorax because lung markings appear to extend to the chest wall (Fig. 25.8).
> - **Absence** of lung markings **alone** is **not sufficient** for the **diagnosis of a pneumothorax,** nor is the **presence of lung markings distal** to the **visceral pleural line sufficient** to eliminate the possibility of a pneumothorax.

- The **presence of an air-fluid interface in the pleural space** is, by definition, an indication that there is a pneumothorax present (see Fig. 8.16).
  - For more about recognizing a **hydropneumothorax,** see **Chapter 8.**
- In the supine position, air in a relatively large pneumothorax may collect anteriorly and inferiorly in the thorax and manifest itself by **displacing the costophrenic sulcus inferiorly** while, at the same time, producing **increased lucency of that costophrenic sulcus.** This is called the **deep sulcus sign** and it is presumptive evidence for the presence of a pneumothorax on a supine chest radiograph (Fig. 25.9).
- The key signs for recognizing a pneumothorax are summarized in Box 25.2.

> **BOX 25.2   Recognizing a Pneumothorax: Signs to Look for**
>
> - Visualization of the **visceral pleural line**—a must for the diagnosis
> - Convex curve of the visceral pleural line paralleling the contour of the chest wall
> - Absence of lung markings distal to the visceral pleural line (most times)
> - The **deep sulcus sign** of an inferiorly displaced costophrenic sulcus seen on a supine chest
> - The presence of an air-fluid interface in the pleural space

Fig. 25.7 Pneumothorax Seen on CT. As the lung collapses, it tends to maintain its usual shape so that the curvature of the visceral pleural line (*solid white arrows*) parallels the curvature of the chest wall (*dotted white arrows*). This patient also has **subcutaneous emphysema**—air in the soft tissues—of the left lateral chest wall (*white stars*). The patient had been stabbed by a former friend.

Fig. 25.8 Pneumothorax With Pleural Adhesions. (A) There is a pneumothorax (*white arrows*) that is prevented from collapsing the lung by pleural adhesions (*black arrows*). (B) On a CT scan, the pleural adhesions (*black arrows*) are seen tethering the partially collapsed lung (*white arrows*) to the parietal pleura. Adhesions most frequently result from prior infection or blood in the pleural space.

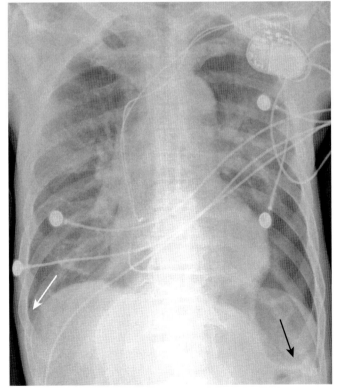

Fig. 25.9 Deep Sulcus Sign. In the supine position, air in a relatively large pneumothorax may collect anteriorly and inferiorly in the thorax, producing increased lucency of the lateral costophrenic sulcus (*black arrow*). This is called the **deep sulcus sign** and is a sign of a pneumothorax on a supine radiograph. Notice how much lower the left costophrenic sulcus appears than the right sulcus (*white arrow*).

Pitfalls in Misdiagnosing a Pneumothorax

- Several pitfalls can lead to the mistaken diagnosis of a pneumothorax.

⚠ DIAGNOSTIC PITFALLS

- **Pitfall 1: Absence of lung markings mistaken for a pneumothorax.**
  - The simple absence of lung markings is not sufficient to warrant the diagnosis of a pneumothorax as there are other diseases that produce such a finding.
  - These diseases include:
    - **Bullous disease of the lung** (Fig. 25.10)
    - **Large cysts in the lung**
    - **Pulmonary embolism,** which can lead to a lack of perfusion and hence a decrease in the number of vessels visible in a particular part of the lung **(Westermark sign of oligemia)**
  - In none of these diseases would the treatment ordinarily include the insertion of a chest tube and, in fact, insertion of a chest tube into a bulla might actually **produce** an intractable pneumothorax.
  - **Solution:** Look at the contour of the structure you believe is the visceral pleural line. Unlike the margin of a bulla, the **visceral pleural line** will be **convex outward** toward the chest wall and will **parallel the curve of the chest wall** (Fig. 25.11). If in doubt, consider CT of the chest.
- **Pitfall 2: Mistaking a skin fold for a pneumothorax**
  - When the patient lies directly on the radiographic cassette (as for a portable supine radiograph), a **crease of the patient's skin** may become trapped between the patient's back and the surface of the cassette. This is called a **skin fold.**
  - A skin fold can produce an **edge** in the expected position of the visceral pleural line that **may, in fact, parallel the chest wall** just as you would expect the visceral pleural line in a pneumothorax (Fig. 25.12).
  - **Solution:** Unlike the thin white line of the visceral pleura, **skin folds produce a relatively thick white band of density.**
- **Pitfall 3: Mistaking the medial border of the scapula for a pneumothorax**
  - Ordinarily the patient is positioned for an **upright** frontal chest radiograph in such a way that the scapulae are retracted lateral to the outer margin of the rib cage, thus preventing the medial border of the scapula from overlapping the lung fields.
  - Most trauma patients undergo supine chest radiographs. With **supine** radiographs, the **medial border of the scapulae may superimpose on the upper lobes** and **mimic the visceral pleural line** of a pneumothorax (Fig. 25.13).
  - **Solution:** Before diagnosing a pneumothorax, make sure you can **trace the outlines of the scapula** on the side in question and identify its medial border as being separate from the suspected pneumothorax.

Pneumothorax: CT of the Chest

- Today, CT of the chest has essentially replaced conventional radiography alone if there is a strong clinical suspicion of a pneumothorax that is not demonstrated on conventional

Fig. 25.10. Bullous Disease: Right Upper Lobe. There is a thin white line visible on this close-up of the right upper lobe (*solid white arrows*) and there are few lung markings peripheral to it. Unlike the visceral pleural line of a pneumothorax, this white line is convex **away** from the chest wall and does not parallel the curvature of the chest wall. This is the classical appearance of a **bulla** in a patient with emphysema. The walls of several other bullae are visible in this patient (*dotted white arrows*). On rare occasions, bullae can grow so large as to render the hemithorax seemingly devoid of visible lung tissue (**vanishing lung syndrome**).

Fig. 25.11 Bullous Disease on Right; Pneumothorax on Left. This axial section from a chest CT demonstrates the different appearances of bullous disease, seen on the right as a rounded, cystic lucency (*dotted white arrow*), and a pneumothorax seen here on the left with its border convex, paralleling the chest wall (*solid white arrow*). This patient also has subcutaneous emphysema on the left (*solid black arrow*).

A   B

Fig. 25.12 Skin Fold Mimicking a Pneumothorax and a True Pneumothorax. (A) When patients lie directly on the radiographic cassette as they might for a portable supine radiograph, a fold of the patient's skin may produce an **edge** (*dotted white arrow*) in the expected position of a pneumothorax and that edge may, in fact, parallel the chest wall just as you would expect a pneumothorax to appear. (B) While skin folds produce relatively thick white bands of density, this different patient demonstrates the thin white line of the visceral pleura (*solid white arrow*). A skin fold is an **edge;** the visceral pleura produces a **line.**

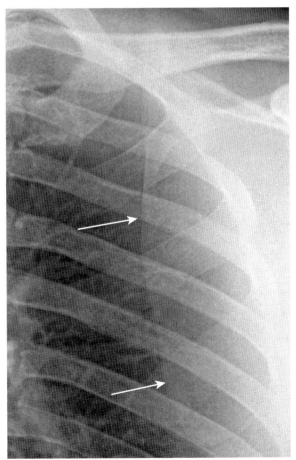

Fig. 25.13 Scapular Edge Mimicking a Pneumothorax. On supine radiographs, the medial border of the scapula (*white arrows*) will frequently superimpose on the upper lung field and may mimic the visceral pleural line of a pneumothorax. Before diagnosing a pneumothorax, make sure you can identify the medial border of the scapula as being separate from the suspected pneumothorax.

radiographs. **CT is able to detect extremely small amounts of air in the pleural space** (Fig. 25.14).

Pneumothorax: Other Imaging Techniques

- **Ultrasound** (see Chapter 20)
- **Decubitus chest x-rays**
  - Because air rises to the highest point in the body, lateral decubitus films of the chest with the affected side "up" and the x-ray beam directed horizontally (parallel to the floor) may detect a small pneumothorax not seen in the supine position. This method may be helpful in demonstrating a pneumothorax in an infant.
- **Delayed films** are sometimes obtained about **6 hours after a penetrating injury** to the chest in patients in whom no pneumothorax is visible on the initial examination because of the occasional appearance of a delayed traumatic pneumothorax.

TRAUMA-RELATED PARENCHYMAL LUNG ABNORMALITIES

Pulmonary Contusions

- Pulmonary contusions are the **most frequent** parenchymal complications of **blunt chest trauma.** They represent **hemorrhage into the lung**, usually at the point of impact.

> ### ▶▶ IMPORTANT POINTS
>
> - **Recognizing a pulmonary contusion:**
>   - The **history of trauma** is of **paramount importance** as contusions present as **airspace disease** that is **indistinguishable from other airspace diseases** such as pneumonia or aspiration.
>   - Contusions tend to be **peripherally placed** and **frequently occur at the point of maximum impact.** Air bronchograms are usually **not present** because blood fills the bronchi as well as the airspaces (Fig. 25.15).

Fig. 25.14 Pneumothorax Seen Only on CT. (A) Close-up view of the right lung demonstrates no evidence of a pneumothorax. (B) CT scan in the same patient shows air in the pleural space (*black arrow*) with the lung and visceral pleura retracted from the chest wall (*white arrow*) by a small pneumothorax. It is frequently impossible to obtain an upright chest radiograph in a traumatized patient. Smaller pneumothoraces may be visible only on CT scans of the chest.

Fig. 25.15 Pulmonary Contusions, Chest Radiograph and CT. (A) Pulmonary contusions tend to be peripherally placed and frequently at the point of maximum impact (*dotted white arrow*). They do not usually contain air bronchograms. (B) Another patient, who was an unrestrained passenger in an automobile accident, also has a large contusion (*solid white arrow*) associated with multiple rib fractures (*solid black arrows*).

- Classically, contusions **appear within 6 hours after the trauma** and, because blood in the airspaces tends to be reabsorbed quickly, **disappear within 72 hours**, frequently sooner.
- Airspace disease that **lingers more than 72 hours** should **raise suspicion** of another process, such as **aspiration, pneumonia,** or a **pulmonary laceration.**

Pulmonary Lacerations (Pulmonary Hematoma or Traumatic Pneumatocele)

- Pulmonary hematomas result from a **laceration of the lung parenchyma** and, as such, may accompany more severe **blunt trauma** or **penetrating chest trauma.**
- A pulmonary laceration is also called a **traumatic pneumatocele** or **hematoma.**
- They are sometimes masked by the airspace disease from a surrounding pulmonary contusion, at least for the first few days until the contusion resolves.

> ▶▶ **IMPORTANT POINTS**

- **Recognizing a pulmonary laceration:**
  - Their **appearance** will depend on **whether they contain blood** and, if so, **how much blood** fills the laceration.
    - If they are **completely filled with blood**, they will appear as a solid, usually **ovoid mass.**
    - If they are **partially filled with blood** and **partially filled with air**, they may contain a visible **air-fluid level** or demonstrate a **crescent sign** as the blood begins to form a clot and pull away from the wall of the laceration.
    - If they are **completely filled with air**, they will appear as an **air-containing, cyst-like structure** in the lung (Fig. 25.16).

- Unlike pulmonary contusions that clear rapidly, **pulmonary lacerations,** especially if they are blood filled, **may take weeks or months to clear completely.**

Pulmonary Interstitial Emphysema

- When the pressure or volume in the alveolus becomes sufficiently elevated, the **alveolus may rupture,** leading to extraalveolar air.
- This extraalveolar air may take one of two main paths:
  - If the alveolus is in close proximity to a pleural surface, the **air may burst outward into the pleural space and create a pneumothorax.**
  - Alternatively, the air can **track backward along the bronchovascular bundles in the lung to the mediastinum,** then into the neck and out to the subcutaneous tissues of the chest and abdominal wall. Occasionally the air can track downward into the abdomen as well as retroperitoneum.
  - It is also possible for air to dissect **both** into the **pleural space** and backward along the **bronchovascular sheaths** at the same time.
- The air that tracks backward toward the hilum does so along the **perivascular connective tissue of the lung,** forming **small cystic collections** of extraalveolar air that **dissect retrograde through the bronchovascular sheaths** to the hila. When the extraalveolar air is confined to the interstitial network of the lung, it is called **pulmonary interstitial emphysema** or **perivascular interstitial emphysema.**
- Presumably because of the looser connective tissue in the lungs of children and young adults, pulmonary interstitial emphysema is **more likely to occur** in those **under the age of 40.**

Fig. 25.16 Pulmonary Lacerations: Conventional Radiograph and CT. (A) If lacerations are completely filled with blood, they will appear as an ovoid mass (*dotted white arrow*). (B) If they are partially filled with blood and partially filled with air, they may contain a visible air-fluid level (*black arrow*). Unlike the neighboring pulmonary contusion (*solid white arrow*), pulmonary lacerations may take weeks or months to clear completely, especially if they are blood filled. The top of the left hemidiaphragm (D) is seen in this image.

Fig. 25.17 Pulmonary Interstitial Emphysema. This coronal reformatted CT scan of the chest demonstrates air (*solid white arrows*) surrounding the pulmonary arteries (white branching structures) in the lung. This air arose from a ruptured alveolus in a patient with asthma and is tracking back to the hilum where it also produced pneumomediastinum and subcutaneous emphysema. The patient also has bilateral basilar pneumothoraces (*dotted white arrows*).

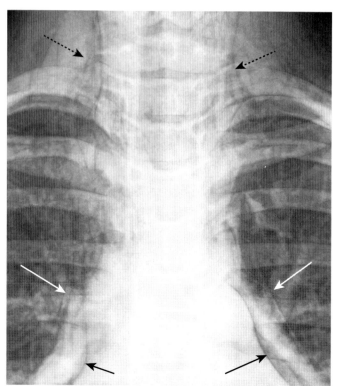

Fig. 25.18 Pneumomediastinum, Pneumopericardium, and Subcutaneous Emphysema. This patient with asthma developed spontaneous pneumomediastinum, most likely from rupture of an alveolus followed by formation of pulmonary interstitial emphysema. The air tracked back to the hila, then into the mediastinum where it produced streaky white linear densities (*solid white arrows*) extending to the neck. In the neck, there is subcutaneous emphysema (*dotted black arrows*). In adults, air does not usually enter the pericardium except by direct penetration, so it is somewhat unusual that this patient also developed pneumopericardium (*solid black arrows*).

- **Assisted mechanical ventilation increases the risk** of developing pulmonary interstitial emphysema and its formation **heralds a significant risk for the imminent appearance of a pneumothorax,** frequently within a matter of a few hours or days.
- Other causes of increased intraalveolar pressure and rupture include asthma and barotrauma.
- **Pulmonary interstitial emphysema may not be recognizable** on conventional radiographs because the air **collections are small** and because there is usually a **considerable amount of coexisting disease** in the lung that obscures it. It may, however, be more visible on CT scans of the chest (Fig. 25.17).

Pneumomediastinum

- About **one in three patients** with **pulmonary interstitial emphysema will develop pneumomediastinum** (more than three in four develop pneumothorax). Pneumomediastinum can occur in trauma because the air tracks backward along the bronchovascular bundles until it enters the mediastinum
- Pneumomediastinum may also develop **when there is perforation of an air-containing viscus that lies within the mediastinum,** such as the esophagus or tracheobronchial tree.
  - **Rupture of the distal esophagus,** usually the left posterolateral wall, can occur with increased intraesophageal pressure from retching or vomiting in **Boerhaave's syndrome.**

- **Rupture of the tracheobronchial tree** is most often **secondary to significant trauma,** either **iatrogenic,** such as during a traumatic **intubation,** or **accidental,** such as from a penetrating wound or severe blunt trauma.

> ## IMPORTANT POINTS

- **Radiographic findings of pneumomediastinum:**
  - **Linear, streak-like lucency** associated with a **thin white line paralleling the left heart border**
  - **Streaky air outlining the great vessels** (aorta, superior vena cava, carotid arteries)
  - Linear streaks of air **parallel to the spine** in the upper thorax extending into the neck and surrounding the esophagus and trachea (Fig. 25.18)
  - **Continuous diaphragm sign:** With pneumomediastinum, air can outline the central portion of the diaphragm beneath the heart, producing an unbroken superior surface of the diaphragm that extends from one lateral chest wall to the other (Fig. 25.19).

Pneumopericardium

- **Pneumopericardium is usually due to direct penetrating injuries** to the pericardium, caused either **iatrogenically**

Fig. 25.19 Continuous Diaphragm Sign of Pneumomediastinum. (A) The central portion of the diaphragm is usually not visible because it is obscured by the heart, which has the same soft-tissue density as the diaphragm on radiographs. When air enters the mediastinum, the entire diaphragm under the heart may become visible (*black arrow*). This is called the **continuous diaphragm sign**. (B) A coronal reformatted CT scan of the chest in another patient shows pneumomediastinum outlining the central portion of the diaphragm (*black arrow*) and the remainder of the pneumomediastinum extending superior to the great vessels (*white arrows*).

(during cardiac surgery) **or accidentally** (from penetrating trauma). Pneumopericardium is **more common in pediatric patients** than in adults and may develop in neonates with hyaline membrane disease.

- It is **rare for air in the pleural space to enter the pericardium,** except in those who have a pericardial defect, such as a surgical "window" incised in the pericardium that allows free exchange between the pleural and pericardial spaces.

> ## ▶▶ IMPORTANT POINTS
>
> - Pneumopericardium produces a **continuous** band of **lucency that encircles the heart** bound by the parietal pericardial layer **that extends no higher than the root of the great vessels** (corresponding to the level of the main pulmonary artery) (Fig. 25.20).
>   - **Pneumomediastinum,** in contrast, **does extend** above the root of the great vessels into the uppermost thorax.

- **CT is usually necessary to demonstrate the findings of pneumopericardium.**

AORTIC TRAUMA

- Trauma to the aorta is most frequently the result of **deceleration injuries in motor vehicle accidents.** Although the survival rates are improving, **most patients** with rupture of the thoracic aorta **die before reaching the hospital** and, of those who survive an aortic injury, the likelihood of death increases the longer the abnormality remains untreated. Only those with **incomplete** tears in which the **adventitial lining prevents exsanguination** (producing a **pseudoaneurysm**) survive to be imaged.

Fig. 25.20 Pneumopericardium. This patient sustained penetrating chest trauma. There is a pneumopericardium as shown by the visible parietal pericardium (*solid white arrows*) outlining air around the heart in the pericardial space. Notice how the air does not extend above the reflection of the aorta and main pulmonary artery (*dotted white arrow*) as it would in a pneumomediastinum. There is also a right-side hemo-pneumothorax as evidenced by the air-fluid level in the right hemithorax (*solid black arrow*).

> ## ▶▶ IMPORTANT POINTS
>
> - The most common site of injury is the **aortic isthmus**, which is the portion of the **aorta just distal to the origin of the left subclavian artery.** Seat-belt injuries may involve the abdominal aorta, but such injuries are far less common than the deceleration injuries to the thoracic aorta.

- Only emergency surgery will prevent approximately 50% of patients with blunt aortic injuries from dying within the first 24 hours if left untreated.

Recognizing Aortic Trauma

- **Findings seen on conventional radiographs of the chest** are the same as those discussed under **Aortic Dissection in Chapter 12.** A **completely normal chest radiograph** has a relatively **high negative predictive value** for aortic injury, but, if the **chest x-ray is in any way abnormal**, the abnormalities are usually so nonspecific that identifying aortic injuries requires additional imaging.
  - There may be **loss of the normal shadow of the aortic knob, a left apical pleural cap** of fluid or blood, a **left pleural effusion, or deviation of the trachea or esophagus to the right** (Fig. 25.21).
  - Under most circumstances, suspected aortic injuries are now studied using CT that allows for rapid image acquisition in one breath-hold and appropriately timed contrast delivery to the aorta (**CT-angiography**). Most experts agree that a negative CT-angiogram obviates the need for catheter angiography. The findings of aortic injury are **frequently subtle** and require experience to recognize because those patients with the more obvious findings may not have survived to be imaged.
- **Findings on contrast-enhanced CT scans of the chest** (Fig. 25.22):
  - **Aortic intimal flap.** A lucent defect in the contrast column of the aorta arising from a **tear** in the intima and media.
  - **Contour or caliber abnormalities.** Abrupt change in the smooth contour or size of the aorta at the point of injury.
  - **Periaortic hematoma.** Delineation of a **contrast-filled collection outside of the normal confines of the aorta** representing pseudoaneurysm or extravasation.

- **Mediastinal hematoma.** Increased attenuation in the mediastinum from an admixture of blood and normal fat. May be present in the absence of an aortic injury, presumably due to small vessel trauma.
- **Hemopericardium.** Fluid of high-attenuation (i.e., blood) in the pericardial sac indicates a significant injury to the aorta or heart itself.
- Patients with **equivocal** CT findings may need a catheter study of the aorta (**aortography**).

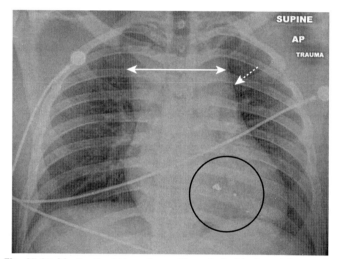

Fig. 25.21 Mediastinal Hematoma. There is "widening of the mediastinum" (*double white arrow*), an inexact finding on an anteroposterior supine portable chest radiograph. More importantly, the shadow of the aortic knob is obscured by something of soft-tissue density (*dotted white arrow*). Because the patient had been shot (bullet fragments in the *black circle*), these findings did lead to a request for a CT-angiogram that demonstrated a large mediastinal hematoma.

Fig. 25.22 Aortic Trauma: Three Different Patients. (A) There is a tear at the level of the aortic isthmus represented by the linear defect in the wall of the descending aorta (*solid white arrow*). A mediastinal hematoma is also present (*dotted white arrows*). (B) There is a large mediastinal hematoma (*solid white arrows*). (C) There are periaortic hematomas containing extravasated blood (*black arrows*) and a large mediastinal hematoma (*solid white arrows*). *AA,* Ascending aorta; *AR,* aortic arch; *DA,* descending aorta; *PA,* pulmonary artery.

TAKE HOME POINTS

- Trauma is generally divided into **blunt** and **penetrating** trauma. Most trauma-related injuries are due to blunt trauma, with motor vehicle accidents contributing the majority.
- **Rib fractures** may herald more serious internal injuries, such as lacerations of the liver or spleen or pneumothoraces. Most rib fractures occur in ribs 4 to 9.
- A **flail chest** is defined as one in which at least two fractures occur in each of three contiguous ribs. It is associated with significant morbidity and mortality.
- **Subcutaneous emphysema** may produce dramatic, but largely clinically insignificant, findings. It heralds the presence of an underlying abnormality, but usually does not require treatment itself.
- There is normally no air in the pleural space; air in the pleural space is called a **pneumothorax.** You must identify the visceral pleural white line to diagnose a pneumothorax.
- Beware of the pitfalls that resemble pneumothoraces: **bullae, skin folds,** and the medial border of the **scapula.**
- **Simple pneumothoraces** are those with no shift of the heart or mobile mediastinal structures; most pneumothoraces are simple.
- **Tension pneumothoraces** (usually associated with cardiorespiratory compromise) produce a shift of the heart and mediastinal structures **away** from the side of the pneumothorax by virtue of a check-valve mechanism that allows air to enter the pleural space but not leave.
- Most pneumothoraces are **traumatic** in etiology, either accidental or iatrogenic.
- Conventional chest radiographs are poor at estimating the size of a pneumothorax; CT is better; the most important assessment to be made is the clinical status of the patient.

- Besides the conventional upright chest radiograph, other ways to diagnose a pneumothorax include ultrasound, decubitus views, and delayed images. CT remains the mainstay for detecting small pneumothoraces.
- **Pulmonary contusions** are the most common manifestation of blunt chest trauma and represent hemorrhage into the lung, usually at the point of impact. They classically clear in a few days.
- **Pulmonary lacerations** are tears in the lung parenchyma that may be fluid or air-containing. Their presence may be hidden by a surrounding contusion and they typically take longer than a contusion to clear.
- **Pulmonary interstitial emphysema** results from an increase in the intraalveolar pressure that in turn, leads to rupture of an alveolus and dissection of air back toward the hila along the bronchovascular bundles; it is frequently difficult to visualize.
- **Pneumomediastinum** can occur when air tracks back to the mediastinum from a ruptured alveolus or from perforation of an air-containing viscus, such as the esophagus or trachea; it can produce the **continuous diaphragm sign** on a frontal chest radiograph.
- **Pneumopericardium** usually requires direct penetration of the pericardium to occur rather than dissection of air from a pneumomediastinum; it can be difficult to differentiate from a pneumomediastinum, but a key is that pneumopericardium does not extend above the roots of the great vessels, whereas pneumomediastinum does.
- **Aortic injuries** usually occur at the isthmus, require rapid recognition for optimum survival, and may appear on contrast-enhanced CT as intimal flaps, contour abnormalities, or hematomas.

 More information on imaging findings of chest trauma is available to registered users online.

Recognizing the Imaging Findings of Trauma to the Abdomen and Pelvis

ABDOMINAL TRAUMA

- The role of advanced imaging techniques deserves special mention in abdominal trauma. Radiology has made a significant impact on the lives of traumatized patients by distinguishing those patients who can be managed conservatively from those who need surgical or other interventions and by helping to direct the most appropriate intervention for those who need it.

▶▶ IMPORTANT POINTS

- **CT is the study of choice in abdominal trauma.**
  - **Intravenous contrast is always used** (unless contraindicated) to identify devascularized areas, hematomas, active extravasation of blood, or extraluminal urine (after contrast has passed through the kidneys) (Box 26.1).
    - If a **head CT is to be done** as well, it should be **done first** before contrast is injected for the abdomen.
  - **Oral contrast** is usually not administered. **Rectal contrast** is occasionally administered in penetrating trauma to search for a bowel laceration.
  - It is always best to consult with the radiologist so as to tailor the best study to fit the patient's needs.

- In some emergency settings, a quick abdominal ultrasound is used in unstable trauma patients to evaluate for hemoperitoneum (FAST Scan: see Chapter 20).
- The most commonly affected solid organs in **blunt** abdominal trauma (in order of decreasing frequency) are the **spleen, liver, kidney, and urinary bladder.** Traumatic injuries to each of them will be discussed under each organ.

Liver

- The liver is discussed first because it is actually the **most frequently injured organ** if **both penetrating and blunt trauma** are included together. The liver is the largest intraabdominal organ and is fixed in position, making it especially susceptible to injury. Injuries to the liver account for the **majority of deaths from abdominal trauma.**
- The posterior aspect of the right lobe is injured most frequently. Most hepatic injuries are associated with blood in the peritoneal cavity (**hemoperitoneum**).
- **Contrast-enhanced CT is the study of choice** and, because of its ability to demonstrate both the nature and extent of the trauma, the overwhelming majority of patients with liver trauma are now managed conservatively and do not require surgery.

BOX 26.1 Contrast Reactions and Renal Failure

- Intravenous contrast materials available today are nonionic low osmolar solutions containing a high concentration of iodine that circulate through the bloodstream, opacify those tissues and organs with high blood flow, are absorbed by x-ray (and therefore appear "whiter" on images), and are finally excreted in the urine by the kidneys.
- In some patients (e.g., those with diabetes, dehydration, multiple myeloma) who have compromised renal function evidenced by creatinine >1.5, iodinated contrast may produce a nephrotoxic effect resulting in **acute tubular necrosis**. Though usually reversible, in a small number of patients with underlying renal insufficiency, renal dysfunction may permanently worsen. This effect is dose-related.
- Iodinated contrast agents can sometimes produce mild side effects, including a feeling of warmth, nausea and vomiting, local irritation at the site of injection, and itching and hives; these side effects usually require no treatment. Occasional idiosyncratic, allergic-like reactions include itching, hives, and laryngeal irritation.
- Asthmatics and those with a history of severe allergies or prior reactions to IV contrast have a higher likelihood of contrast reactions (but still very low overall) and may benefit from steroids, Benadryl, and cimetidine administered prior and/or after injection. Prior shellfish allergy bears absolutely NO relationship to iodinated contrast reactions.
- In about 0.01% to 0.04% of all patients, severe and idiosyncratic reactions to contrast can occur that can produce intense bronchospasm, laryngeal edema, circulatory collapse and, very rarely, death (1 in 200,000 to 300,000).

▶▶ IMPORTANT POINTS

- **CT findings in hepatic trauma:**
  - **Subcapsular hematoma.** Lenticular fluid collections that conform to the shape of the outer contour of the liver but which frequently flatten the adjacent liver parenchyma. Most occur anterolaterally over the right hepatic lobe (Fig. 26.1A).
  - **Lacerations.** Most common finding. Irregularly marginated, low attenuation, linear, or branching defects, usually at the periphery. "Fracture" is a term that has been used to describe a laceration that avulses a section of the liver (Fig. 26.1B).
  - **Intrahepatic hematomas.** Focal high attenuation lesions first caused by blood; hematomas may progress to low attenuation, mass-like lesions filled with serous fluid (Fig. 26.1C).
  - **Wedge-shaped defects.** Devascularized sections of liver parenchyma that do not contrast-enhance.
  - **Contusions.** A term used to describe an area of minimal parenchymal hemorrhage; they are lower in attenuation than the surrounding liver and have indistinct margins.
  - **Pseudoaneurysms and acute hemorrhages.** Irregular collections of high attenuation, extravasated contrast that often require angiography with embolization and/or surgery.

Fig. 26.1 Hepatic Trauma: Three Different Patients. (A) There is a lenticular fluid collection involving the lateral portion of the right lobe of the liver that represents a **subcapsular hematoma** (*solid black arrow*). There is also a **laceration** of the right lobe (*dotted black arrow*). (B) There are multiple **lacerations** of the right lobe of the liver (*black circle*). (C) There is active **extravasation** of contrast-enhanced blood (*solid black arrow*) from a large intrahepatic laceration with **hematoma** (*dotted black arrow*) and both **subcapsular** blood and hemoperitoneum (*solid white arrow*).

Fig. 26.2 Splenic Trauma: Three Different Patients. (A) There is crescent-shaped collection of fluid in the subcapsular space, which compresses the normal splenic parenchyma, representing **subcapsular hematoma** (*solid white arrow*). (B) This patient has a splenic (*solid white arrow*) and hepatic (*solid black arrow*) **laceration** and a large **hepatic contusion** (*dotted black arrow*). There is also pneumoperitoneum (*dotted white arrow*). (C) This patient has active **extravasation** of contrast-enhanced blood (*solid black arrow*) and a large **intrasplenic hematoma** (*solid white arrow*).

Spleen

- Splenic trauma is usually caused by **deceleration injuries** in unrestrained occupants in motor vehicle collisions, by a fall from a height, or being struck by a motor vehicle as a pedestrian.
- Because the **spleen is the most highly vascular organ, hemorrhage** represents the most serious complication of trauma. Despite its vascular nature and the delayed presentation of many splenic injuries, **most splenic trauma is treated conservatively** (nonsurgically).

Fig. 26.3 Splenic Contusions. There are several low attenuation lesions in the spleen (*white and black arrows*) in this patient who fell from a ladder. The treatment for splenic contusions is usually conservative. *L,* Liver; *S,* stomach (containing oral contrast).

≫ IMPORTANT POINTS

- **CT is the study of choice for evaluating splenic trauma.** Findings include:
  - **Subcapsular hematoma.** Low attenuation, crescent-shaped collection of fluid in the subcapsular space that frequently compresses the normal splenic parenchyma (Fig. 26.2A).
  - **Laceration.** Irregular, low attenuation defect that typically transects the spleen (Fig. 26.2B).
  - **Intraparenchymal hematoma.** Lacerations filled with blood; they are intrasplenic, rounded areas of low attenuation that may have a mass effect and enlarge the spleen (Fig. 26.2C).
  - **Contusion.** Alterations in the normal homogeneous appearance of the spleen, including mottled areas of low attenuation (Fig. 26.3).
  - **Intraperitoneal fluid or blood.** Hemoperitoneum occurs with almost all splenic injuries, also producing small amounts of blood in the pelvis. Its presence does not necessarily indicate active hemorrhage.

Kidneys

- Motor vehicle accidents are the most common cause of blunt abdominal trauma to the kidneys in the United States. Almost all patients with renal trauma will have **hematuria.**

Fig. 26.4 Renal Trauma: Two Different Patients. (A) Coronal-reformatted, contrast-enhanced CT scan shows a low-attenuation linear defect representing a **renal laceration** (*black arrow*) and a **subcapsular hematoma** (*white arrow*). (B) Axial CT scan of another patient also shows a renal laceration (*solid black arrow*) and a **perinephric hematoma** (*dotted black arrow*).

- **Contrast-enhanced CT is the study of first choice** and has almost completely replaced the intravenous urogram and standard cystogram.

> **IMPORTANT POINTS**

- **CT findings in renal trauma:**
  - **Contusion.** Ill-defined, patchy low attenuation areas in the contrast-enhanced kidney.
  - **Subcapsular hematoma.** Crescentic or elliptic densities that compress the more dense underlying renal parenchyma (Fig. 26.4A).
  - **Perinephric hematoma.** Ill-defined fluid collection surrounding the kidney confined by Gerota's fascia (Fig. 26.4B).
  - **Laceration.** Low-attenuation linear or branching defects in the renal parenchyma. More severe lacerations may extend through the renal hilum into the collecting system, renal artery, or vein. "Fracture" is a term that may be used when the laceration connects the hilum with the cortex (see Fig. 26.4B).
  - **Vascular injuries.** If arterial, there may be no flow to the kidney and hence, no contrast enhancement. They may also produce wedge-shaped defects in the kidney.
  - **Injuries to the collecting system.** Extraluminal contrast arising from the renal pelvis or ureter (Fig. 26.5).

Fig. 26.5 Tear of Proximal Ureter. There is a tear of the ureter at the level of the left ureteropelvic junction demonstrated by extraluminal contrast (*white arrow*) representing contrast-containing urine that is leaking from the collecting system. The patient was an unrestrained driver in a motor vehicle accident.

Shock Bowel

- **Shock bowel** usually occurs with **blunt abdominal trauma** in which there is severe **hypovolemia** and profound **hypotension**, with complete reversibility of these findings following resuscitation.
- **Recognizing shock bowel on CT:**
  - Diffuse **thickening** of the **small bowel wall** with **increased enhancement.**
  - Fluid-filled and **dilated loops** of bowel (Fig. 26.6A).
- Other findings include a **small inferior vena cava** (<1 cm) **and aorta** (<6 mm) and decreased perfusion of the **spleen** (Fig. 26.6B).

PELVIC TRAUMA

Rupture of the Urinary Bladder

- About **70% of bladder ruptures** occur with **pelvic fractures** and about 10% of patients with pelvic fractures have an associated rupture of the bladder.
- They are best demonstrated by a **CT cystogram** in which contrast is infused under gravity through a Foley catheter into the bladder, but they can also be well-demonstrated by antegrade filling of the bladder from renal excretion of intravenously injected contrast.

Fig. 26.6 Shock Bowel. (A) There is marked enhancement of the bowel wall with multiple dilated and fluid-filled loops (*solid white arrow*). There is also peritoneal fluid present (*dotted white arrows*). (B) In another patient with shock bowel, the aorta (*solid black arrow*) and inferior vena cava (*dotted black arrow*) are diminutive in size. The bowel wall enhances (*solid white arrow*). Shock bowel usually occurs with severe hypovolemia and profound hypotension.

Fig. 26.7 Bladder Ruptures: Extraperitoneal and Intraperitoneal. (A) Contrast-containing urine (*white arrows*) has leaked into the **extraperitoneal** spaces from a perforated bladder following pelvic fractures. Iodinated contrast, the tip of a Foley catheter and air are seen inside of the partially filled urinary bladder (B). (B) **Intraperitoneal** bladder ruptures are less common and may occur with blunt trauma. The contrast flows freely away from the bladder (B) up the paracolic gutters (*solid white arrows*) and outlines loops of bowel (*dotted white arrow*).

⟫ IMPORTANT POINTS

- There are **two major types** of bladder rupture (Fig. 26.7):
  - **Extraperitoneal** bladder rupture is more common (80%) and usually the **result of a pelvic fracture** with **direct puncture** of the bladder. Extraluminal contrast **remains around the bladder**, especially the retropubic space.
  - **Intraperitoneal** bladder rupture is less common and usually the **result of a forceful blow to the pelvis with a distended bladder,** especially in children. Rupture usually occurs at the **dome** of the bladder adjacent to the peritoneal cavity. Contrast runs freely through the **peritoneal cavity, surrounds bowel, and extends into the paracolic gutters** (Fig. 26.8).

Fig. 26.8 Bladder Rupture: Intraperitoneal. Following a cystogram, iodinated contrast flows freely through a rent in the dome of the bladder (not shown) into the peritoneal cavity to outline the exterior of the bowel (*white arrows*).

Urethral Injuries

- Urethral injuries are associated with significant pelvic trauma in **males** and occur most often from **blunt trauma.**
- Urethral injuries should be investigated when there are **straddle fractures** of the pelvis or **penetrating injuries** in the region

of the **urethra.** Hematuria, blood at the urethral meatus, and inability to void are suggestive clinical findings.

- Imaging is done most often using **retrograde urethrography (RUG)** in which contrast is instilled retrograde at the urethral meatus and there is retrograde filling of the urethra. This is done before insertion of a Foley catheter into the bladder.

    - The **most common injury** is a rupture of the **posterior urethra** through the urogenital diaphragm into the proximal bulbous urethra. Extraluminal contrast can be seen outside of the urethra in the pelvis and perineum (Fig. 26.9).

LESS COMMON ABDOMINAL INJURIES

Diaphragm

- Diaphragmatic injuries are estimated to occur in up to 5% of trauma patients. The **left hemidiaphragm** is involved more than the right and the posterolateral portion of the diaphragm is affected most often.
- It is easier to visualize defects in the diaphragm on the left than the right. There may be **herniation** of abdominal contents into the thorax. The intraabdominal contents may be **constricted** where they pass through the diaphragmatic rent, producing the **collar sign** (Fig. 26.10).
- There may be **delayed presentation** of a ruptured diaphragm, either from **delayed rupture** of the diaphragm or **delayed detection** of a diaphragmatic rupture.

Pancreas

- Pancreatic injury is relatively uncommon but occurs more frequently with **penetrating trauma** than with blunt. It is almost always accompanied by injuries to other organs no matter what the cause.
- CT is the imaging study of choice. The CT findings may be subtle, including **peripancreatic fluid** and diffuse **enlargement** of the pancreas. The most obvious finding is a **fracture** through the pancreas (Fig. 26.11). Magnetic resonance cholangiopancreatography (MRCP) may be used to visualize the pancreatic duct.
- Complications can include pseudocysts, recurrent pancreatitis. or fistula formation.

Fig. 26.9 Urethral Trauma. Contrast that was instilled retrograde through the penile urethra (*white arrow*) is seen to leak from the posterior urethra secondary to a perforation (*dotted black arrow*) and collects outside of the urinary system in the perineum and extraperitoneal bladder spaces (*solid black arrows*). The patient had pelvic fractures secondary to a fall.

Fig. 26.10 Ruptured Diaphragm. (A) There is a rent in the right hemidiaphragm that allows a portion of the liver (HL) to extrude through the rupture. Where the organ passes through the rupture, a constricted zone is seen (*black arrows*) called the **collar sign.** (B) The sagittal view demonstrates the herniated portion of the liver (*dotted white arrow*). *HL,* Herniated portion of liver; *L,* liver.

Fig. 26.11 Pancreatic Laceration. There is a laceration (transection) of the tail of the pancreas (P) (*solid white arrows*) with an associated left renal injury (*dotted white arrow*). There is a high likelihood of damage to the pancreatic duct in such injuries, a finding that would increase morbidity and mortality. The patient had been stabbed in the abdomen.

 TAKE HOME POINTS

- CT has had a profound impact on traumatized patients by distinguishing those patients who can be managed conservatively from those who need surgical or other interventions.
- The most commonly affected solid organs in **blunt** abdominal trauma (in order of decreasing frequency) are the spleen, liver, kidney, and urinary bladder.
- The **liver** is commonly injured in **both blunt and penetrating trauma** and its injuries account for the majority of the deaths from abdominal trauma. The liver may demonstrate lacerations, hematomas, wedge-shaped defects, pseudoaneurysms, and acute hemorrhage.
- Because the **spleen** is highly vascular, hemorrhage is the most serious sequela of splenic trauma whose other findings include hematomas, lacerations, and contusions.
- Patients who have had **renal trauma** almost always have hematuria and may show contusions, lacerations, hematomas, or vascular pedicle injuries on CT.

- They may also demonstrate extraluminal contrast from an injury to the renal pelvis or ureter.
- **Shock bowel** is a consequence of profound hypotension and shows diffuse small bowel wall thickening with enhancement of dilated and fluid-filled loops on CT.
- **Bladder ruptures** may be either extraperitoneal (more common) or intraperitoneal, the former demonstrating extraluminal contrast surrounding the bladder and the latter showing contrast that flows freely in the peritoneal cavity.
- **Urethral injuries** occur almost exclusively in males, are frequently associated with pelvic fractures, and usually involve the posterior urethra where extraluminal contrast may be seen in the perineum or extraperitoneally in the pelvis.
- **Diaphragmatic rupture** usually occurs on the left side and requires forceful blunt trauma. It is almost always associated with other traumatic lesions.
- **Pancreatic injuries** are relatively uncommon, almost always associated with other abdominal trauma and may have a significant morbidity and mortality.

More information on the imaging findings of abdominal and pelvic trauma is available to registered users online.

27

Recognizing Some Common Causes of Intracranial Pathology

- Advances in neuroimaging have had a remarkable impact on the diagnosis and treatment of neurologic diseases ranging from earlier detection and treatment of stroke to a more timely diagnosis of dementia, from the rapid detection and treatment of cerebral aneurysms to the ability to diagnose multiple sclerosis after a single attack.
- Both CT and MRI are utilized for studying the brain and spinal cord, but MRI is the study of first choice in most clinical scenarios (Table 27.1). Conventional radiography has no significant role in imaging intracranial abnormalities.

NORMAL ANATOMY (FIG. 27.1)

- We will look at the normal anatomy of the brain using CT.
- In the posterior fossa, the **fourth ventricle** appears as an inverted U-shaped structure. Like all cerebrospinal fluid-containing structures on CT, it normally appears black. Posterior to the fourth ventricle are the **cerebellar hemispheres,** anteriorly lie the **pons** and **medulla oblongata.** The **tentorium cerebelli** separates the **infratentorial** components of the posterior fossa (cerebellum and fourth ventricle) from the **supratentorial** compartment.
- The **interpeduncular cistern** lies in the midbrain and separates the paired **cerebral peduncles** (which emerge from the superior surface of the pons). The **suprasellar cistern** is anterior to the interpeduncular cistern and usually has a five- or six-point star-like appearance.
- The **sylvian fissures** are bilaterally symmetric and contain cerebrospinal fluid (CSF). They separate the temporal from the frontal and parietal lobes.
- The **lentiform nucleus** is composed of the **putamen** (laterally) and **globus pallidus** (medially). The **third ventricle** is slit-like and midline. At the posterior aspect of the third ventricle is the **pineal gland.** Farther posterior is the **quadrigeminal plate cistern.**
- The **corpus callosum** connects the right and left cerebral hemispheres and forms the roof of the lateral ventricle. The anterior end is called the **genu** and the posterior end is called the **splenium.**
- The **basal ganglia** are represented by the **subthalamic nucleus** and the **substantia nigra, globus pallidus, putamen, and caudate nucleus.** The putamen and caudate nucleus are called the **striatum.**
- The **frontal** (also known as **anterior**) **horns** of the **lateral ventricles** hug the head of the **caudate nucleus.** The two frontal horns are separated by the midline **septum pellucidum.** The **temporal horns,** which are normally very small, are more

TABLE 27.1	Imaging Studies of the Brain for Selected Abnormalities	
Abnormality	**Study of First Choice**	**Other Studies**
Acute stroke	Diffusion-weighted imaging **(see Table 27.8)** for acute or small strokes, if available	Noncontrast CT can differentiate hemorrhagic from ischemic infarct
Headache, acute and severe	Noncontrast CT to detect subarachnoid hemorrhage	MR-angiography (MRA) or CT-angiography (CTA) if subarachnoid hemorrhage is found in order to detect aneurysm
Headaches, chronic	MRI, without and with contrast	CT, without and with contrast, can be substituted
Seizures	MRI, without and with contrast. Add thin section images through hippocampi in patients with history of childhood seizures	CT, without and with contrast, can be substituted if MRI not available
Blood	Noncontrast CT	Ultrasound for infants
Head trauma	Nonenhanced CT is readily available and the study of first choice in head trauma	MRI is better at detecting diffuse axonal injury, but requires more time and is not always available
Extracranial carotid disease	Doppler ultrasonography	MRA excellent study; CTA best for preoperative stenosis evaluation
Hydrocephalus	MRI as initial study	CT for follow-up
Vertigo and dizziness	Contrast-enhanced MRI	MRA if needed and/or thin section images through internal auditory canals as needed
Masses	MRI, without and with contrast	Contrast-enhanced CT if MRI not available
Change in mental status	MRI, without or with contrast	CT without contrast

Fig. 27.1 Normal Unenhanced CT Scans of the Head. (A) Frontal lobes (F); temporal lobes (T); temporal horns (*white arrows*); fourth ventricle (4); cerebellum (C); pons (P). **(B)** Suprasellar cistern (S); cerebral peduncles (*white arrows*); interpeduncular cistern (*black arrow*). **(C)** Sylvian fissures (S); third ventricle (3); interpeduncular cistern (*solid black arrow*); quadrigeminal plate cistern (*white arrows*). **(D)** Frontal horns of the lateral ventricles (*white arrow*); caudate nuclei (c); third ventricle (3); occipital lobes (O). **(E)** Caudate nuclei (C); lentiform nuclei (L); calcified pineal gland (*white arrow*). **(F)** Genu of corpus callosum (*dotted white arrow*); lateral ventricles (L); septum pellucidum (*dashed white arrow*); parietal lobes (P); occipital horn (*black arrow*); calcified choroid plexus (*solid white arrows*); occipital lobes (O).

inferior and contained in the **temporal lobes**. The posterior horns (**occipital horns**) of the lateral ventricle lie in the occipital lobes. The most superior portion of the ventricular system is the **bodies** of the lateral ventricles.

- The **falx cerebri** lies in the **interhemispheric fissure**, which separates the two **cerebral hemispheres**, and is frequently calcified in adults.
- The surface or **cortex** of the brain is composed of **gray matter** convolutions made up of **sulci** (grooves) and **gyri** (elevations). The medullary **white matter** lies below the cortex.

>> **IMPORTANT POINTS**

- On an unenhanced CT scan of the brain, anything that appears "white" will generally either be **bone (calcium)** density or **blood,** in the absence of a metallic foreign body (Table 27.2).

- **Calcifications that may be seen on CT of the brain that are nonpathologic:**
  - Pineal gland (Fig. 27.2A)
  - Basal ganglia (Fig. 27.2A)

- Choroid plexus (see Fig. 27.1F)
- Falx and tentorium (Fig. 27.2B)
- **Normal structures that can enhance** after administration of iodinated intravenous contrast:
  - **Venous sinuses**
  - **Choroid plexus**
  - **Pituitary gland and stalk**
- **Metallic densities** in the head can cause artifacts on CT scans. Dental fillings, aneurysm clips and bullets can all cause **streak artifacts.**

MRI AND THE BRAIN

>> **IMPORTANT POINTS**

- In general, **MRI is the study of choice** for detecting and staging intracranial and spinal cord abnormalities. It is usually more sensitive than CT because of its **superior contrast** and **soft-tissue resolution.** It is, however, **less sensitive** to CT in detecting **calcification** in lesions or in evaluating **cortical bone,** which appear as signal voids with MR. It cannot be used in most patients with pacemakers.

TABLE 27.2 **CT Densities**		
Hypodense (Dark) **(AKA Hypointense)**	**Isodense**	**Hyperdense (Bright)** **(AKA Hyperintense)**
Fat (not usually present in the head)	Normal brain	Metal (e.g., aneurysm clips or bullets)
Air (e.g., sinuses)	Some forms of protein (e.g., subacute subdural hematomas)	Iodine (after contrast administration)
Water (e.g., CSF)		Calcium
Chronic subdural hematomas/hygromas		Hemorrhage (high protein)

Fig. 27.2 Physiologic Calcifications. (A) There are small punctate calcifications in the basal ganglia (*white circles*) and calcification of the pineal gland (*white arrow*). (B) There is calcification of the falx cerebri (*dotted white arrow*). Physiologic calcifications tend to increase in incidence with advancing age.

- MRI is more difficult to interpret because the same structure or abnormality will appear differently, depending on the pulse sequence, the scan parameters, and the fact that MRI is more variable in its depiction of differences that occur over the **time course of some abnormalities** (e.g., hemorrhage) than is CT.
- **Initial evaluation of an MRI of the brain** might start with a T1-weighted sagittal sequence of the brain. On this sequence,

the brain looks more like the anatomic specimens or diagrams that you are accustomed to looking at (Fig. 27.3). Remember that many structures in the brain are **paired**, so do not forget to compare one side with the other on axial scans of the brain (Fig. 27.4).

- Table 27.3 summarizes the signal characteristics of various tissues seen on MRI.

Fig. 27.3 Normal Midline MRI. Sagittal T1-weighted close-up image demonstrates the midline structures of the brain. For orientation purposes, anterior is to your left (A). The corpus callosum (CC) is located superiorly. The pituitary gland (P) sits in the sella turcica and connects to the hypothalamus via the pituitary stalk or infundibulum (*dotted white arrow*). The mammillary bodies (M) are located anterior to the brainstem. The cerebral aqueduct (*solid white arrow*) is superior to the midbrain. The brainstem is composed of the midbrain (Mi), the pons (Po), and the medulla (Me). The fourth ventricle (4) communicates with the cerebral aqueduct and lies between the cerebellum (Ce) and the brainstem.

Fig. 27.4 Normal MRI of the Brain: T1 and T2. Axial T1-weighted (A) and T2-weighted (B) images of the brain demonstrate that CSF in the lateral ventricles is dark on T1 and bright on T2 (*solid black arrows*). Gray matter, which contains the neuronal cell bodies, is actually gray on T1-weighted images (*open white arrow*) and white matter, which contains myelinated axon tracts, is whiter (*white circle*). The caudate nuclei (*solid white arrows*) and lentiform nucleus (*dotted white arrows*) together form the basal ganglia. The thalamus (*dotted black arrows*) is located posterior to the basal ganglia.

TABLE 27.3 **Signal Characteristics of Various Tissues Seen on T1-Weighted and T2-Weighted MRI Scans**

Bright on T1	Dark on T1	Bright on T2	Dark on T2
Fat	Calcification	Water (edema, CSF)	Fat
Gadolinium	Air		Calcification
High protein	Chronic hemorrhage	Hyperacute hemorrhage	Air
Subacute hemorrhage	Acute hemorrhage is isointense to hypointense on T1	Late subacute hemorrhage	Early subacute hemorrhage
Melanin	Water (edema, CSF)		Chronic hemorrhage
			Acute hemorrhage
			High protein

Fig. 27.5 CT Head: "Brain" and "Bone" Windows. In order to visualize skull fractures, you must view the CT scan using the "bone" windows. (A) Using the "brain window," a lenticular-shaped, hyperintense lesion is seen in the left frontal region displaying the typical appearance of an epidural hematoma (*black arrows*). (B) Viewing the same scan at the "bone window" setting shows a fracture (*white arrow*) of the left frontal bone at the site of the epidural hematoma.

HEAD TRAUMA

- **Traumatic brain injuries** extract a huge cost to the patient and society, not only as a result of the acute injury but for the long-term disability they produce. In the United States, motor vehicle accidents account for nearly half of traumatic brain injuries.
- **Unenhanced CT is the study of choice in acute head trauma.** The primary goal in obtaining the scan is to determine if there is a life-threatening, but treatable, lesion.

> ## ⟩⟩ IMPORTANT POINTS
>
> - **Initial CT evaluation of the brain** in the emergency setting focuses on whether there is (1) **mass effect** and (2) **blood**.

> - To determine if there is **mass effect,** look for a **displacement or compression** of key structures from their normal positions by analyzing the location and appearance of the **ventricles, basal cisterns,** and the **sulci.**
> - **Blood** will usually be hyperattenuating (bright) and might collect in the **basal cisterns, sylvian and interhemispheric fissures, ventricles, the subdural or epidural spaces,** or in the **brain parenchyma (intracerebral).**

Skull Fractures

- Skull fractures are usually produced by **direct impact** to the skull and they most often occur at the point of impact. They are important primarily because their presence implies a **force substantial enough to cause intracranial injury.**
- In order to visualize skull fractures, you must view the CT scan using the "bone window" settings that optimize visualization of the osseous structures (Fig. 27.5).
- Skull fractures can be described as **linear, depressed, or basilar.**

Fig. 27.6 Skull Fractures. (A) There is a depressed fracture of the right parietal bone with the fragment lying deeper than the inner table of the adjacent bone (*white arrow*). Depressed skull fractures occur more often in the frontoparietal region. (B) There is a comminuted fracture of the right temporal bone (*solid white arrows*), fluid in the mastoid air cells (*circle*), and air in the brain (**pneumocephalus**) (*dotted white arrow*). Basilar skull fractures can be associated with tears in the dura mater with subsequent CSF leak. *A*, Anterior.

Linear Skull Fractures

- **Linear skull fractures** are the most common and have little importance other than for the intracranial abnormalities that may have occurred at the time of the fracture, such as an epidural hematoma. Fractures of the cranial vault most likely occur in the **temporal** and **parietal bones** (see Fig. 27.5B).

Depressed Skull Fractures

- **Depressed skull fractures** are more likely to be associated with **underlying brain injury.** They result from a high-energy blow to a small area of the skull (e.g., from a hammer), most often in the **frontoparietal region** and are **usually comminuted.** They may require **surgical elevation** of the depressed fragment when the fragment lies deeper than the inner table adjacent to the fracture (Fig. 27.6A).

Basilar Skull Fractures

> ## ⏩ IMPORTANT POINTS
>
> - **Basilar fractures** are the **most serious** and consist of a linear fracture at the base of the skull. They can be associated with **tears in the dura mater** with subsequent **CSF leak,** which can lead to CSF rhinorrhea and otorrhea. They can be suspected if there is air seen in the brain (**traumatic**

> **pneumocephalus), fluid in the mastoid air cells,** or an **air-fluid level** in the **sphenoid sinus** (Fig. 27.6B).

Facial Fractures

- **CT is the imaging study of choice** for evaluating **facial fractures.** Multislice scanners allow for reconstruction of the images in the sagittal and coronal planes so the patient does not have to be repositioned in the scanner.

> ## ⚠ DIAGNOSTIC PITFALLS
>
> - Care must be taken in diagnosing facial fractures based upon viewing what appears to be a fracture on only one image because CT scans by their nature produce sections so thin, they may not demonstrate the entire contour of the bone in question. Look for a fracture to appear on several contiguous images.

- The most common **orbital fracture** is the **blow-out fracture,** which is produced by a **direct impact on the orbit** (e.g., a ball strikes the eye). It causes a sudden increase in intraorbital pressure leading to a fracture of the **inferior orbital floor** (into the maxillary sinus) or the **medial wall of the orbit** (into the ethmoid sinus). Sometimes the **inferior rectus muscle** can be trapped in the fracture, leading to **restriction of upward gaze** and **diplopia.**

Fig. 27.7 Facial Bone Fractures. (A) **Blow-out fracture**. There is air in the left orbit representing orbital emphysema (*black circle*). There is a fracture of the floor of the orbit and soft tissue (in this case, fat) extends inferiorly into the top of the maxillary sinus (*white arrow*). (B) **Tripod fracture.** There is diastasis of the frontozygomatic suture on the left (*dotted white arrow*), a fracture of the floor of the orbit with orbital emphysema (*dashed white arrow*), and a fracture (*solid white arrow*) through the lateral wall of the maxillary sinus (M), which is filled with blood.

- **Recognizing a blow-out fracture of the orbit** (Fig. 27.7A).
  - **Orbital emphysema.** Air in the orbit from communication with one of the adjacent, air-containing sinuses, either the ethmoid or maxillary sinus.
  - **Fracture** through either the medial wall or floor of the orbit.
  - **Entrapment of fat and/or extraocular muscle** that projects downward as a soft-tissue mass into the top of the maxillary sinus.
  - **Fluid (blood)** in the maxillary sinus.
- A **tripod fracture,** usually a result of blunt force to the cheek, is another relatively common facial fracture. This fracture involves **separation of the zygoma** from the remainder of the facial bones by **separation of the frontozygomatic suture, fracture of the floor of the orbit,** and fracture of the **lateral wall of the ipsilateral maxillary sinus** (Fig. 27.7B).

INTRACRANIAL HEMORRHAGE

- Skull fractures may be associated with **intracranial hemorrhage** and/or **diffuse axonal injury.**
- There are **four types of intracranial hemorrhages** that may be **associated with head trauma:**
  - **Epidural hematoma**
  - **Subdural hematoma**
  - **Intracerebral hemorrhage**
  - **Subarachnoid hemorrhage** (discussed with aneurysms)

Epidural Hematoma (Extradural Hematoma)

- Epidural hematomas represent **hemorrhage** into the potential space **between the dura mater** and the **inner table of the skull** (Table 27.4).
- Most cases are due to injury to the **middle meningeal artery or vein** from blunt head trauma, typically from a motor vehicle accident.

TABLE 27.4	**The Meninges**
Layer	**Comments**
Dura mater	Composed of two layers, an **outer periosteal layer** that cannot be separated from the skull and an **inner meningeal layer;** the inner meningeal layer enfolds to form the tentorium and falx.
Arachnoid	The avascular, middle layer is separated from the dura by a potential space known as the **subdural space.**
Pia mater	Closely applied to the brain and spinal cord, the pia mater carries blood vessels that supply both; separating the arachnoid from the pia is the **subarachnoid space;** together the **pia and arachnoid** are called the **leptomeninges.**

- **Almost all epidural hematomas (95%) have an associated skull fracture, frequently in the temporal bone.** Epidural hematomas may also be caused by disruption of the dural venous sinuses adjacent to a skull fracture.

⯮ **IMPORTANT POINTS**

- **Recognizing an epidural hematoma:**
  - They appear as a **high density, extra-axial, biconvex, lens-shaped "mass"** most often found in the **temporoparietal region** of the brain (Fig. 27.8).
  - Because the dura is normally fused to the calvarium at the margins of the sutures, it is **impossible for an epidural hematoma to cross suture lines (subdural hematomas can cross sutures)**.
  - Epidural hematomas can cross the tentorium, but subdural hematomas do not.

Fig. 27.8 Epidural Hematoma. Findings of an epidural hematoma include a high-density, extraaxial, biconvex, lens-shaped mass-like lesion often found in the temporal-parietal region of the brain (*black arrow*). There is a scalp hematoma (*white arrow*) also present. The patient had a temporal bone skull fracture seen on bone windows.

Subdural Hematoma (SDH)

- **Subdural hematomas are more common** than epidural hematomas and are usually **not associated with a skull fracture.** They are most commonly a result of **deceleration injuries** in motor vehicle or motorcycle accidents (younger patients) **or secondary to falls** (older patients).
- Subdural hematomas are usually produced by **damage to the bridging veins** that cross from the cerebral cortex to the venous sinuses of the brain. SDH represents hemorrhage into the potential space **between the dura mater and the arachnoid.**

> ### 》 IMPORTANT POINTS
>
> - **Acute subdural hematomas** frequently herald the presence of more severe parenchymal brain injury and increased intracranial pressure and are associated with a **higher mortality rate.**

- **Recognizing an acute subdural hematoma:**
  - On CT acute subdural hematomas are **crescent-shaped, extra-cerebral bands of high attenuation** that may **cross suture lines** and **enter the interhemispheric fissure.** They **do not cross the midline.**
  - Typically, a SDH is **concave inward** toward the brain (epidural hematomas are convex inward) (Fig. 27.9A).
  - As time passes and they become subacute, or if the subdural blood is mixed with lower attenuating CSF, they may appear **isoattenuating (isodense)** to the remainder of brain, in

Fig. 27.9 Acute, Isodense, and Chronic Subdural Hematoma. (A) There is a crescent-shaped band of high-density blood concave inward toward the brain (*solid white arrow*). There is mass effect with herniation of the brain as indicated by the dilated contralateral temporal horn (*dotted white arrow*). (B) As they become subacute, subdural hematomas become less dense and may be the same density (isodense) as the normal brain tissue (*white arrow*). You can recognize an isodense subdural hematoma by the unilateral absence or displacement of the sulci away from the inner table of the skull compared with the normal opposite side (*black arrow*). (C) Chronic subdural hematomas (>3 weeks old) are usually of low density (*solid white arrow*) compared with the remainder of the brain. There is still mass effect demonstrated by displacement of the interhemispheric fissure (*dotted white arrow*) and compression of the lateral ventricle.

which case you should look for **compressed** or **absent sulci** or sulci **displaced away from the inner table** as signs of SDH (Fig. 27.9B).

- Subdural collections may demonstrate a **fluid-fluid level** after one week, as the cells settle under serum.
- **Chronic subdural hematoma**
  - Chronic subdural hematomas are those present **more than 3 weeks after injury.**
  - Chronic subdural hematomas are usually **low-density** compared with the remainder of the brain (Fig. 27.9C).

Intracerebral Hematoma (Intracerebral Hemorrhage)

- Trauma is only one of the mechanisms that can lead to intracerebral hemorrhage. Intracerebral hematomas can also occur from ruptures of **aneurysms, atheromatous disease in small vessels, vasculitis, vascular malformations (e.g., cavernoma, arteriovenous malformations, arteriovenous fistulae),** and **amyloid.** Venous thrombosis can also cause parenchymal hemorrhage.
- Injuries occurring at the **point of impact** (called **coup injuries**) and injuries occurring **opposite the point of impact** (called **contrecoup injuries**) are most common following trauma. **Coup** injuries are most often due to **shearing** of small intracerebral vessels. **Contrecoup** injuries are **acceleration/deceleration injuries** that occur when the brain is propelled in the opposite direction, striking the inner surface of the skull.

- Either of these mechanisms can produce a **cerebral contusion. Hemorrhagic contusions** are **hemorrhages** with associated **edema** usually found in the **inferior frontal lobes and anterior temporal lobes on or near the surface of the brain.** Trauma can also produce nonhemorrhagic contusions as well.
- **CT findings of intracerebral hemorrhage change over time** and **may not be immediately evident on the initial scan.** MRI typically demonstrates the lesions from the time of injury, but may not be available on an emergency basis.

> ### ▶▶ IMPORTANT POINTS
>
> - **Recognizing traumatic intracerebral hemorrhage on CT:**
>   - Cerebral hemorrhagic contusions may appear as multiple small, well-demarcated areas of **high attenuation** within the brain parenchyma (Fig. 27.10A).
>   - They may be surrounded by a **hypodense rim** from **edema** (Fig. 27.10B).
>   - **Intraventricular blood** may be present (Fig. 27.11).
>   - **Mass effect is common.** The mass effect may produce **compression** of the **ventricles** and **displacements of the third ventricle** and **septum pellucidum** to the **opposite** side. Such shifts can produce severe brain or vascular damage.
>   - These displacements are called **herniations.** Patients with sufficient mass effect are at risk for **transtentorial** and **subfalcine brain herniation** and death (see Fig. 27.10B).
>   - **The types of brain herniation are described in Table 27.5.**

Fig. 27.10 Cerebral Contusions. (A) Cerebral contusions are usually the result of trauma and can manifest by multiple areas of high attenuation hemorrhage (*white arrows*) within the brain parenchyma on CT. (B) Contusions (*solid black arrow*) are frequently surrounded by a rim of hypoattenuation from edema (*dotted black arrow*) and mass effect is common, as is demonstrated here by amputation of the ipsilateral basilar cisterns (*dotted white arrow*), midline displacement (*solid white arrow*) representing **subfalcine herniation,** and dilatation of the contralateral temporal horn (*circle*). A portion of the left side of the skull has been surgically removed and a large scalp hematoma is present (*dashed white arrow*).

Fig. 27.11 Intraventricular Hemorrhage. Intraventricular hemorrhage (*white arrows*) is common in premature infants, but less common in adults. It usually results from break-through bleeding from a hypertensive basal ganglia hemorrhage, brain contusion, or subarachnoid hemorrhage and requires a considerable amount of force to produce. Therefore it is typically associated with severe brain damage, results in communicating hydrocephalus and has a poor prognosis.

TABLE 27.5	Types of Brain Herniation
Type	**Remarks**
Subfalcine herniation	The supratentorial brain, along with the lateral ventricle and septum pellucidum, herniates beneath the falx and shifts across the midline toward the opposite side (Fig. 27.12A).
Transtentorial herniation	Usually the cerebral hemispheres are displaced downward through the incisura beneath the tentorium compressing the ipsilateral temporal horn and causing dilatation of the contralateral temporal horn (Fig. 27.12B).
Foramen magnum/ tonsillar herniation	Infratentorial brain is displaced downward through the foramen magnum.
Sphenoid herniation	Supratentorial brain slides over the sphenoid bone either anteriorly (in the case of the temporal lobe) or posteriorly (for the frontal lobe).
Extracranial herniation	Displacement of brain through a defect in the cranium.

Fig. 27.12 Brain Herniations. (A) **Subfalcine herniation** occurs when the supratentorial brain, along with the lateral ventricle and septum pellucidum herniate beneath the falx (*solid white arrow*) and shift across the midline toward the opposite side (*dotted white arrow*). (B) **Transtentorial herniation** usually occurs when the cerebral hemispheres are displaced downward through the incisura beneath the tentorium compressing the ipsilateral temporal horn and causing dilatation of the contralateral temporal horn (*white arrow*). Both patients had large cerebral infarcts (I) with cytotoxic edema.

DIFFUSE AXONAL INJURY

- Diffuse axonal injury is **responsible for the prolonged coma following head trauma** and is the head injury with the poorest prognosis.
- Acceleration/deceleration forces **diffusely injure axons deep to the cortex,** producing unconsciousness from the moment of injury. This occurs most often as a result of a motor vehicle accident.
- The **corpus callosum is most commonly affected** and the initial CT scan may be normal or underestimate the degree of injury. CT findings may be similar to those described for intracerebral hemorrhage following head trauma.

> ### ▶▶ IMPORTANT POINTS
>
> - **MR is the study of choice in identifying diffuse axonal injury.**
>   - The **small petechial hemorrhages** may be **bright** on **T1-weighted images.**
>   - Multiple **bright areas on T2-weighted images** at the **temporal or parietal cervicomedullary junction** or in the corpus callosum are common.
>   - **Gradient susceptibility MRI sequences** have the highest sensitivity to detect petechial hemorrhages, which will appear as **punctate dark areas** (Fig. 27.13).

INCREASED INTRACRANIAL PRESSURE

- Some of the clinical signs of **increased intracranial pressure** are **papilledema, headache,** and **diplopia.**

> ### ▶▶ IMPORTANT POINTS
>
> - In general, increased intracranial pressure is caused by either **cerebral edema,** which leads to increased **volume of the brain,** or **hydrocephalus,** which is **increased size of the ventricles.**

Cerebral Edema

- In adults, **trauma, hypertension** (associated as it is with **intracerebral bleeds** and **stroke**), and **masses** are the most common causes of brain edema.
  - Cerebral edema is divided into **two major types: vasogenic** and **cytotoxic.**
    - **Vasogenic edema** represents extracellular accumulation of fluid and is the type that is associated with **malignancy** and **infection.** It is due to **abnormal permeability of the blood–brain barrier.** It predominantly affects the **white matter** (Fig. 27.14A).
    - **Cytotoxic edema** represents cellular edema and is associated with **cerebral ischemia.** It is due to **cell death.** It **affects both the gray and white matter** (Fig. 27.14B).

> ### ▶▶ IMPORTANT POINTS
>
> - **Recognizing cerebral edema:**
>   - There is a **loss** of the **normal differentiation between gray and white matter** in cytotoxic edema, whereas it is retained in vasogenic edema.
>   - There may be **effacement** (compression or obliteration) of the normal **sulci.**
>   - The **ventricles** may be **compressed** (Fig. 27.15).
>   - **Herniation** of the brain may manifest, in part, by **effacement of the basal cisterns** (see Fig. 27.10B).

- Increased intracranial pressure secondary to an increase in the size of the ventricles is discussed under Hydrocephalus.

Fig. 27.13 Diffuse Axonal Injury: MRI. These images were obtained using a pulse sequence extremely sensitive to bleeding at the gray/white matter junction, facilitating visualization of very small lesions. It is particularly helpful for evaluation of the small hemorrhages present in diffuse axonal injury not routinely visible on CT or conventional MR imaging sequences. (A) and (B) are axial images demonstrating innumerable foci of abnormally decreased signal (*black arrows*) in a patient with diffuse axonal injury.

Fig. 27.14 Vasogenic and Cytotoxic Edema. (A) **Vasogenic edema** (*solid white arrow*) is the type that occurs with infection and malignancy, as in this nonenhanced scan of a patient with a glioma. It predominantly affects the white matter. (B) **Cytotoxic edema** (*solid white arrow*) affects both the gray and white matter. Cytotoxic edema is associated with cerebral ischemia, as in this patient with a very large ischemic infarct on the right. In both of these patients, there is increased intracranial pressure as manifest by the herniation of brain to the contralateral side (*dotted white arrows*).

Fig. 27.15 Diffuse Cerebral Edema: CT. Cerebral edema produces loss of normal differentiation between gray and white matter, effacement (narrowing or obliteration) of the normal sulci, and ventricular compression, all of which are visible in this patient with anoxic encephalopathy.

STROKE

General Considerations

- Stroke is a nonspecific term that usually denotes an **acute loss of neurologic function** that occurs when the blood supply to an area of the brain is lost or compromised.

- The diagnosis of stroke is usually made clinically. Patients with suspected stroke are imaged to (**1**) determine if there is **another cause of the neurologic impairment** besides a stroke (e.g., a brain tumor); (**2**) **to identify the presence of blood** so as to distinguish **ischemic** from **hemorrhagic** stroke, which may determine whether or not thrombolytic therapy will be instituted; and (**3**) to **identify** the **infarct** and **characterize it.**

- **Most strokes are embolic in origin**, the emboli arising from the internal **carotid artery** or the common carotid bifurcation. Emboli can also arise in the **heart and aortic arch.**

- The other common cause of stroke is **thrombosis,** representing in situ **occlusion** of the carotid, vertebrobasilar, or intracerebral circulations from **atheromatous lesions.** Thrombosis of the **middle cerebral artery** is particularly common.

✵ IMAGE-GUIDED INTERVENTION

The image is from a cerebral angiogram on a 61-year-old female who developed sudden loss of movement in her left arm 2 hours earlier. The arrow points to something that is missing! How might an image-guided procedure benefit in this case? See the answer in Chapter 29.

- Most **acute strokes** are **initially imaged** by obtaining a **noncontrast-enhanced CT scan of the brain** (within 24 hours of the onset of symptoms), mostly because of its availability. CT findings may be present immediately after a hemorrhagic stroke and within hours after the onset of symptoms for ischemic stroke.
- On MRI, the temporal staging of hemorrhage can be identified based on chemical changes that occur in the hemoglobin molecule as the hemorrhage evolves.
- MRI has become more widely used for early diagnosis. **Diffusion-weighted MRI** is more sensitive and relatively specific for detecting early infarction with the capacity to detect changes within 20 to 30 minutes of the onset of the event (Fig. 27.16).

Ischemic Stroke

- **Thromboembolic disease** as a consequence of **atherosclerosis** is the **most common cause of an ischemic stroke.** The source of the emboli can be from atheromatous debris, arterial stenosis and occlusion, or from emboli arising from the left side of the heart (e.g., atrial fibrillation).

▶ IMPORTANT POINTS

- Strokes are divided into two large groups: **ischemic or hemorrhagic. Ischemic** strokes are much **more common.** The classification is important because rapid treatment of ischemic stroke with **tissue plasminogen activator (tPA)** or another form of intraarterial recanalization technique can substantially improve the prognosis.

▶ IMPORTANT POINTS

- **Vascular watershed** areas are the distal arterial territories that represent the **junctions between areas served by the major intracerebral vessels,** such as the region between the anterior cerebral artery distribution and the middle cerebral artery distribution. **Reduction in blood flow,** for whatever reason, **affects these sensitive and susceptible watershed areas the most.**

Fig. 27.16 CT and Diffusion-Weighted MRI in Acute Stroke. (A) The CT scan in this patient with symptoms for 2 hours prior to the study is normal. (B) A diffusion-weighted MRI scan on the same patient a few minutes later shows an area of abnormally bright signal intensity in the right frontoparietal region (*white arrow*). Diffusion-weighted imaging is an MRI sequence that can be rapidly acquired and which is extremely sensitive to detecting abnormalities in normal water movement in the brain so that it can identify a stroke within 20 to 30 minutes after the event.

- **The most common finding of an acute, nonhemorrhagic stroke is a normal CT scan (<24 hours old).** If multiple vascular distributions are involved, emboli or **vasculitis** should be thought of as the cause. If the stroke **crosses or falls between vascular territories,** then hypoperfusion owing to hypotension (**watershed infarcts**) should be considered.
- **Table 27.6** briefly summarizes the four major vascular distribution patterns of strokes and some of the symptoms associated with each.

>> **IMPORTANT POINTS**

- **Recognizing ischemic stroke:**
  - On CT the findings will depend on the amount of time that has elapsed since the original event.
- **12 to 24 hours:** Indistinct area of low attenuation in a vascular distribution.
- **>24 hours:** Better circumscribed lesion with mass effect that peaks at 3 to 5 days and usually disappears by 2 to 4 weeks (Fig. 27.17A).
- **72 hours:** Although contrast is rarely used in the setting of acute stroke, contrast enhancement typically occurs when the mass effect is waning or has disappeared.
- **>4 weeks:** Mass effect disappears; there is now a well-circumscribed low attenuation lesion with no contrast enhancement (Fig. 27.17B).

TABLE 27.6   Vascular Distribution Territories of Stroke

Circulation	Anatomy Affected	Signs and Symptoms
Anterior cerebral artery (uncommon)	Supplies all of the frontal and parietal lobes (medial surfaces), the anterior four-fifths of the corpus callosum, the frontobasal cerebral cortex, and the anterior diencephalon.	Can result in disinhibition with perseveration of speech; produces primitive reflexes (e.g., grasping or sucking), altered mental status, impaired judgment, contralateral weakness (greater in legs than arms).
Middle cerebral artery (common)	Supplies almost the entire convex surface of the brain, including the frontal, parietal, and temporal lobes (laterally), insula, claustrum, and extreme capsule. Lenticulostriate branches supply the basal ganglia, including the head of the caudate nucleus, the putamen including the lateral parts of the internal and external capsules.	Produces contralateral hemiparesis or hypesthesia, ipsilateral hemianopsia, and gaze preference toward the side of the lesion; agnosia is common; receptive or expressive aphasia may result if the lesion occurs in the dominant hemisphere; weakness of the arm and face is usually worse than that of a lower limb.
Posterior cerebral artery	Supplies portions of the midbrain, subthalamic nucleus, basal nucleus, thalamus, mesial inferior temporal lobe, and occipital and occipitoparietal cortices.	Occlusions affect vision, producing contralateral homonymous hemianopsia, cortical blindness, visual agnosia, altered mental status, and impaired memory.
Vertebrobasilar system	Perfuses the medulla, cerebellum, pons, midbrain, thalamus, and occipital cortex.	Occlusion of large vessels in this system usually leads to major disability or death; small lesions usually have a benign prognosis; may cause a wide variety of cranial nerve, cerebellar, and brainstem deficits; a hallmark of posterior circulation stroke is crossed findings: ipsilateral cranial nerve deficits and contralateral motor deficits (in contrast to an anterior circulation stroke).

Fig. 27.17 CT, Ischemic Stroke, Newer and Older. (A) At about 24 hours, the lesion becomes relatively well-circumscribed (*solid white arrow*) with mass effect evidenced by a shift of the ventricles (*dotted white arrow*) that will peak at 3 to 5 days and disappears by about 2 to 4 weeks. (B) As the stroke matures, it loses its mass effect, tends to become an even more sharply marginated low-attenuation lesion (*solid white arrow*), and may be associated with enlargement of the adjacent ventricle (V) due to loss of brain substance in the infarcted area.

Hemorrhagic Stroke

- Hemorrhage **occurs in about 15%** of strokes. Hemorrhage is **associated with a higher morbidity and mortality** than ischemic stroke. Hemorrhage from stroke can occur into the brain parenchyma or the subarachnoid space.
- In the majority of cases, there is **associated hypertension. About 60% of hypertensive hemorrhages occur in the basal ganglia.** Other areas commonly involved are the thalamus, pons, and cerebellum (Fig. 27.18).
- The decision to utilize **thrombolytic** or another **intraarterial recanalization therapy** is based on algorithms formulated by the initial nonenhanced CT scan findings. The **more rapidly treatment is initiated** (usually <4 to 5 hours after the onset of symptoms), the **greater its potential benefit.**

> ### » IMPORTANT POINTS
>
> - **Recognizing intracerebral hemorrhage (in general):**
>   - Freshly extravasated whole blood with a normal hematocrit will be visible as **increased density** on nonenhanced CT scans of the brain immediately after the event (Fig. 27.18). This is due to the protein in the blood (mostly hemoglobin).
>   - **Dissection** of blood into the **ventricular system** can occur in hypertensive intracerebral bleeds (see Fig. 27.11).
>   - As the clot begins to form, the **blood becomes denser for about 3 days** because of dehydration of the clot.
>   - **After the third day**, the **clot decreases in density** and becomes invisible over the next several weeks. The clot loses density from the **outside in** so that it **appears to shrink.**
>   - **After about 2 months**, only a small hypodensity may remain (Fig. 27.19; Box 27.1).

Fig. 27.18 Intracerebral Hemorrhage: Acute. Freshly extravasated whole blood, such as this bleed into the thalamus (*white arrow*), will be visible as increased density on nonenhanced CT scans of the brain due primarily to the protein in the blood (mostly hemoglobin). The clot will usually become invisible over the next several weeks.

- On MRI the changes in the appearance of hemorrhage over time are more dramatic. MRI is sensitive to changing effects in both the **iron and protein** portions of the hemoglobin molecule in the days and weeks following an acute bleed. Table 27.7 summarizes those changes.

RUPTURED ANEURYSMS

- The most frequent central nervous system aneurysm is the **berry aneurysm,** which develops from a **congenital weakening in the arterial wall,** usually at the sites of vessel branching in the **Circle of Willis** at the base of the brain. They can be familial (about 10% of cases) or associated with connective tissue diseases.
- **Hypertension** and **aging** play a role in the growth of aneurysms. **Larger aneurysms bleed more frequently** than do smaller ones.

> ### BOX 27.1   Lacunar Infarcts
>
> - Small cerebral infarcts produced by occlusion of small end arteries account for up to 20% of all cerebral infarctions.
> - They have a predilection for the basal ganglia, internal capsule, and pons and occur in association with hypertension, atherosclerosis, and diabetes.
> - The term "chronic lacunar infarct" is reserved for low-density, cystic lesions, about 5 to 15 mm in size.

TABLE 27.7   Changes in the Appearance of Blood Over Time on MRI

Phase	Time	T1	T2
Hyperacute	<24 hours	Isointense	Bright
Acute	1–3 days	Isointense	Dark
Early subacute	3–7 days	Bright	Dark
Late subacute	7–14 days	Bright	Bright
Chronic	>14 days	Dark	Dark

Fig. 27.19 Lacunar Infarct. A lacunar infarct, or **lacune**, is a small cerebral infarct produced by occlusion of an end artery. The term **chronic lacunar infarct** is reserved for low-density cystic lesions, 5 to 15 mm in size (*white arrow*).

- The aim is to discover and treat the aneurysm **before** it has undergone a major bleed. In some studies, **10 mm was found to be the critical size for rupture.**
- The classic history a patient who has had a ruptured aneurysm describes is "the worst headache of my life."
- When aneurysms rupture, the **blood usually enters the subarachnoid space.** Rupture of an aneurysm is the **most common nontraumatic cause of a subarachnoid hemorrhage** (80%) but not the only cause. Amyloid, arteriovenous malformations, or breakthrough of an intraparenchymal bleed can also produce subarachnoid hemorrhage.
- Today most aneurysms are detected by **either CT angiography (CTA) or MR angiography (MRA). CT angiography** is performed using a power injector to deliver a rapid bolus intravenous injection of iodinated contrast, a CT scanner capable of rapid acquisition of data, and special computer algorithms and postprocessing techniques that can highlight the vessels and, if desired, display them in three dimensions (Fig. 27.20).

- **MRA** is routinely done without contrast, using a time-of-flight technique. This technique shows flowing blood within the arteries as white. Computerized postprocessing of the imaging generates 3D reconstructions.

> ## IMPORTANT POINTS

- **Recognizing a subarachnoid hemorrhage (from a ruptured aneurysm):**
  - On **CT acute blood** is **hyperdense** and may be visualized **within the sulci and basal cisterns** (Fig. 27.21, A and B).
  - The region of the **falx may become hyperdense,** widened, and irregularly marginated (Fig. 27.21C).
  - Generally the **greatest concentration of blood indicates the most likely location of the ruptured aneurysm.**

Fig. 27.20 Berry Aneurysm: Axial CT and 3D Reconstruction. (A) There is a 2 cm focal out-pouching of contrast in the region of the right internal carotid artery (ICA) on this contrast-enhanced CT of the brain (*white arrow*). This is consistent with an aneurysm. (B) A 3D reconstruction of the circle of Willis from a CT angiogram demonstrates the aneurysm (*solid white arrow*) arising from the supraclinoid segment of the right ICA and another smaller aneurysm (*dotted white arrow*) arising from the supraclinoid segment of the left ICA. Black arrows point to posterior cerebral arteries. *ACA,* Anterior cerebral arteries; *B,* basilar artery; *MCA,* middle cerebral arteries; *V,* vertebral artery.

Fig. 27.21 Subarachnoid Hemorrhage: Unenhanced CT Scans. (A) Blood is most easily visualized within the basal cisterns (*solid white arrows*), (B) in the fissures (*dotted white arrows*), and (C) interdigitated in the subarachnoid spaces of the sulci (*dashed white arrow*). The region of the falx may become hyperdense, widened, and irregularly marginated (*solid black arrow*).

• Other causes of intracerebral hemorrhage besides aneurysms include arteriovenous malformations, tumors, mycotic aneurysms, and amyloid angiopathy (Box 27.2).

HYDROCEPHALUS

• **Hydrocephalus is defined as an expansion of the ventricular system** on the basis of an increase in the volume of CSF contained within it (Box 27.3).

> **IMPORTANT POINTS**

• Hydrocephalus may be caused by several factors:
  • **Underabsorption of CSF (communicating hydrocephalus)**
  • **Restriction of the outflow of CSF from the ventricles (noncommunicating hydrocephalus)**
  • **Overproduction of cerebrospinal fluid** (rare)

• In hydrocephalus the **ventricles** are usually **disproportionately dilated** compared with the **sulci**, whereas **both the ventricles and sulci** are **proportionately enlarged** in **cerebral atrophy**.
• The **temporal horns are particularly sensitive** to increases in CSF pressure. In the absence of hydrocephalus, the **temporal horns are barely visible. With hydrocephalus** the temporal horns may be greater than 2 mm in size (Fig. 27.22).

Obstructive Hydrocephalus

• Obstructive hydrocephalus is divided into two major categories: **communicating (extraventricular obstruction)** and **noncommunicating (intraventricular obstruction)**.
• **Communicating hydrocephalus** is due to abnormalities that **inhibit the resorption of CSF,** most often at the level of the arachnoid villi (Fig. 27.23).

BOX 27.2 Amyloid Angiopathy

• Amyloid is a proteinaceous material that can be deposited with increasing age in the media and adventitia of small and medium-sized intracranial vessels, mostly involving the frontal and parietal lobes.
• This deposit produces a loss of elasticity of the vessels and increases their fragility.
• Amyloid angiopathy plaques may be visible on a special MR gradient sequence. They are too small to see on routine CT or most MR sequences.
• Hemorrhages from amyloid angiopathy are usually large, involving an entire lobe; they may be multiple and occur in several areas simultaneously. They can also present as subarachnoid hemorrhage.
• There is no association with hypertension, and it is not associated with amyloid elsewhere in the body.

BOX 27.3 Normal Flow of Cerebrospinal Fluid

• Most cerebrospinal fluid is produced by the choroid plexuses in the ventricles, primarily the lateral and fourth ventricles.
• The direction of flow is from the lateral ventricles through the Foramina of Monro to the third ventricle, then through the Aqueduct of Sylvius to the fourth ventricle, and then into the basilar subarachnoid cisterns through the two lateral Foramina of Luschka and the medial Foramen of Magendie.
• CSF can then take one of two paths. It can pass upward over the convexities of the brain to be reabsorbed into the bloodstream at the arachnoid villi.
• Or, CSF can also pass inferiorly down the spinal subarachnoid space where it is either reabsorbed directly or ascends back to the brain to the arachnoid villi.

• **CSF flow** through the **ventricles** and **over the convexities** normally occurs **unimpeded.** Reabsorption of CSF through the arachnoid villi can become restricted by such things as **subarachnoid hemorrhage** or **meningitis.**

Fig. 27.22 Noncommunicating Hydrocephalus. (A) There is dilatation of the temporal horns (*solid white arrows*) and the fourth ventricle is compressed and nearly invisible (*dotted white arrow*). A hemorrhagic metastatic lesion (*black arrow*) is obstructing the fourth ventricle. (B) The frontal horns of the lateral ventricles (L) and third ventricle (3) are dilated, but note that the sulci are not dilated. This form of hydrocephalus is the result of obstruction to the outflow of cerebrospinal fluid from the ventricles.

⟫ **IMPORTANT POINTS**

- Classically the fourth ventricle is **dilated** in **communicating hydrocephalus** and **normal** in size in **noncommunicating** hydrocephalus.

- Communicating hydrocephalus is **usually treated with a ventricular shunt.**

- **Noncommunicating hydrocephalus** occurs as a result of **tumors, cysts,** or other physically obstructing lesions that **do not allow CSF to exit from the ventricles.**
  - Congenital hydrocephalus is often produced by a blockage between the third and fourth ventricles at the level of the **Aqueduct of Sylvius (aqueductal obstruction).**
  - When the obstruction is caused by a tumor or a cyst, noncommunicating hydrocephalus is **usually treated by surgically** removing the obstructing lesion (Fig. 27.24).

Fig. 27.23 Communicating Hydrocephalus. Communicating hydrocephalus is caused by abnormalities that inhibit the resorption of cerebrospinal fluid, most often at the level of the arachnoid villi. (A) Classically the fourth ventricle (4) is dilated in communicating hydrocephalus, but normal in size in noncommunicating hydrocephalus. The temporal horns (T) are particularly sensitive to increases in intraventricular volume or pressure and are dilated here. (B) The frontal horns (F), occipital horns (O), and third ventricle (3) are markedly dilated. There is a disproportionate dilatation of the ventricles compared with the sulci (which are normal to small here). Communicating hydrocephalus is usually treated with a ventricular shunt.

Fig. 27.24 Colloid Cyst of the Third Ventricle: CT and MRI. A colloid cyst is an uncommon, benign lesion of the third ventricle that can cause obstructive hydrocephalus. (A) There is a hyperdense mass in the anterior aspect of the third ventricle (*solid white arrow*) causing asymmetric obstruction of the left foramen of Monro compared with the right (*dotted white arrow*). (B) On this T2 FLAIR sequence, the lesion has increased signal (*solid white arrow*) and is causing dilatation of the frontal (*dotted white arrow*) and occipital (O) horns of the lateral ventricle.

- **Nonobstructive hydrocephalus** from overproduction of CSF is rare and can occur with a **choroid plexus papilloma.**

Normal Pressure Hydrocephalus (NPH)

- Normal pressure hydrocephalus is a form of **communicating hydrocephalus** characterized by a classical **triad of clinical symptoms,** including **abnormalities of gait, dementia,** and **urinary incontinence.** The age of onset is typically between 60 and 70 years old.

> **IMPORTANT POINTS**
>
> - Its recognition is important because it is usually amenable to treatment using a one-way **ventriculoperitoneal shunt** that allows the CSF to exit the ventricles and drain into the peritoneal cavity where the CSF is reabsorbed.

- Imaging findings are similar to other forms of communicating hydrocephalus and include **enlarged ventricles,** particularly the temporal horns, with **normal or flattened sulci** (Fig. 27.25).

CEREBRAL ATROPHY

- Disorders associated with **gross cerebral atrophy** are also associated with **dementia, Alzheimer's disease** being one of the most common. Atrophy implies a loss of both gray and white matter.
  - A major finding in patients with Alzheimer's disease (though not specific) is **diffuse cortical atrophy,** especially in the **temporal lobes.**

> **IMPORTANT POINTS**
>
> - As in hydrocephalus, the **ventricles dilate** in cerebral atrophy, but do so because a loss of normal cerebral tissue produces a vacant space that is filled passively with CSF. **Unlike hydrocephalus,** the **dynamics of CSF** production and absorption are **normal in atrophy.**

- In general, cerebral atrophy leads to produce **proportionate enlargement** of both the **ventricles** and the **sulci** (Fig. 27.26).

BRAIN TUMORS

Gliomas of the Brain

- **Gliomas** are a **common, primary supratentorial intraaxial mass in an adult.** They account for **30% of all brain tumors** and 80% of all malignant **primary** brain tumors (**metastases** to the brain from other organs are the most common **malignant** tumors in the brain **overall**).
- **Glioblastoma multiforme** accounts for more than half of all gliomas, astrocytomas for about 20%, with the remainder split between **ependymoma, oligodendroglioma, and mixed glioma** (e.g., oligoastrocytoma).
- **Glioblastoma multiforme** occurs **more commonly in males** between 65 and 75 years of age, especially in the **frontal and temporal lobes.** It has the **worst prognosis** of all gliomas.
- It **infiltrates** adjacent areas of the brain along **white matter tracts** making it difficult to resect but, like most brain tumors, it **does not produce extracerebral metastases.**

Fig. 27.25 Normal Pressure Hydrocephalus. (A) The ventricles are enlarged, particularly the temporal horns (T) as well as the fourth ventricle (4). (B) The bodies of the lateral ventricles (L) are also markedly enlarged, but the sulci are normal or flattened (*white arrow*). The patient had gait disturbances.

Fig. 27.26 Diffuse Cortical Atrophy. Disorders that cause gross cerebral atrophy are also associated with dementia, Alzheimer's disease being one of the most common. (A) The lateral ventricles (*dotted white arrow*) are enlarged. (B) Unlike hydrocephalus, the sulci are also enlarged (*solid white arrows*).

Fig. 27.27 Glioblastoma Multiforme: CT and MRI, Two Different Patients. (A) In this contrast-enhanced CT, the tumor enhances (*solid white arrow*), produces considerable vasogenic edema (*dotted white arrow*), and infiltrates the surrounding brain tissue. Either edema or tumor has crossed over to the left frontal lobe (*solid black arrow*). (B) Axial, T1-weighted, postgadolinium image in another patient demonstrates an enhancing mass in the left temporal lobe (*white arrows*). The internal enhancement of the mass is somewhat heterogeneous (*open black arrow*), which implies intratumoral necrosis or cystic change.

⟫ IMPORTANT POINTS

- **Recognizing glioblastoma multiforme:**
  - Because of its aggressive growth, glioblastoma multiforme frequently demonstrates **necrosis** within the tumor.
  - The tumor **infiltrates** the surrounding brain tissue, frequently **crossing** the white matter tracts of the **corpus callosum** to the **opposite** cerebral hemisphere, producing a pattern called a **butterfly glioma.**

- It tends to produce considerable **vasogenic edema** and **mass effect** and **enhances with contrast**, at least in part (Fig. 27.27).

Metastases

- About **40% of all intracranial neoplasms** are metastases. **Lung, breast, and melanoma** are the most common primary malignancies to produce brain metastases.

Fig. 27.28 Metastases: Contrast-Enhanced CT and MRI. (A) With intravenous contrast, metastases can enhance and show ring enhancement (*white arrows*). Lung, breast, and melanoma are the most common primary malignancies to produce brain metastases. (B) In another patient, MRI shows the characteristic pattern of vasogenic edema (*white arrows*) surrounding a large metastatic lesion (M). Both patients had a lung cancer.

▶▶ IMPORTANT POINTS

- **Recognizing metastases to the brain:**
  - Metastases to the brain are frequently **well-defined round masses near the gray-white junction.**
  - They are **usually multiple, but can be solitary.**
  - They are **typically hypodense or isodense on nonenhanced CT.**
  - With intravenous contrast, they can **enhance,** sometimes with a pattern of **ring-enhancement** (Fig. 27.28A).
  - Most evoke some **vasogenic edema,** frequently disproportionately large to the size of the mass (Fig. 27.28B).

Meningioma

- Meningiomas are the **most common primary brain tumor (benign and malignant) and the most common extraaxial mass,** usually occurring in middle-aged women. Their most frequent locations are **parasagittal,** over the **convexities,** the **sphenoid wing,** and the **cerebellopontine angle** cistern, in decreasing frequency.
- They tend to be **slow-growing** with an **excellent prognosis** if surgically excised.
- When **multiple,** they may have an association with **neurofibromatosis type 2.**

▶▶ IMPORTANT POINTS

- **Recognizing a meningioma on CT scan of the brain:**
  - On unenhanced **CT** over **half are hyperdense** to normal brain and about **20% contain calcification** (Fig. 27.29).
  - On contrast-enhanced studies, **meningiomas enhance markedly.**
  - They **may induce vasogenic edema in the adjacent brain parenchyma.**

Fig. 27.29 Meningioma: Nonenhanced CT. This meningioma is arising from the right sphenoid wing, a relatively common site of origin. On nonenhanced CT, over half are hyperdense to normal brain and about 20% contain calcification, as does this lesion that appears as a dense mass (*white arrow*). On contrast-enhanced studies meningiomas markedly enhance.

Vestibular Schwannoma (Acoustic Neuroma)

- **Vestibular schwannomas** are the most common schwannomas of all of the cranial nerves. Their most frequent symptom is **hearing loss,** but they also produce **tinnitus** and disturbances in **equilibrium.**

- They usually occur along the **course of the eighth cranial nerve** within the **internal auditory canal** at the **cerebellopontine angle** (Fig. 27.30).
- Like meningiomas, when they are multiple (i.e., **bilateral**) they are usually associated with **neurofibromatosis type 2.**

Fig. 27.30 Vestibular Schwannoma: T1-Weighted MRI With Contrast. A homogeneously enhancing soft-tissue mass is seen at the right cerebellopontine angle (*white arrow*), classical for a vestibular schwannoma. These tumors occur most commonly along the course of the eighth nerve. Hearing loss is the most common presenting symptom.

> **IMPORTANT POINTS**

- **Contrast-enhanced MRI** is the **most sensitive** imaging study for detecting vestibular schwannomas which virtually **always enhance**, usually **homogeneously.** They may also be seen on certain MRI sequences through the internal auditory canal.

OTHER DISEASES

Multiple Sclerosis (MS)

- Multiple sclerosis is considered to be **autoimmune** in origin and is the **most common demyelinating disease.** Any neurologic function can be affected by the disease, with some patients having mostly cognitive changes, whereas others present with ataxia, paresis, or visual symptoms.
- Characterized by a **relapsing and remitting course,** there are specific clinical criteria that must be met to establish this diagnosis, but imaging by MRI along with ancillary tests now permit the diagnosis to be made after a single clinical episode.
- MS characteristically affects **myelinated (white matter) tracts** with lesions known as **plaques.** Lesions of MS have a predilection for the **periventricular area, corpus callosum and optic nerves.**

> **IMPORTANT POINTS**

- **MRI is the study of choice** in imaging MS because of its greater sensitivity than CT in demonstrating plaques, both in the brain and in the spinal cord.
  - The lesions produce **discrete globular foci of high-signal intensity (white) on T2-weighted images.**
  - On T1-weighted nonenhanced images, they are isointense to hypointense, but in **acute MS, the lesions enhance with gadolinium on T1-weighted images.**
  - The lesions tend to be oriented with their long axes perpendicular to the ventricular walls (Fig. 27.31).

Fig. 27.31 Multiple Sclerosis: Axial and Sagittal MRI. Lesions of multiple sclerosis have a predilection for the periventricular area, corpus callosum, and optic nerves (*white arrows*). (A) The lesions produce discrete globular foci of high signal intensity (white) on T2-weighted images. (B) Ovoid lesions with their long axis perpendicular to the ventricular surface seen in multiple sclerosis are called **Dawson's finger's** (*white arrows*). MRI is the study of choice in imaging multiple sclerosis because of its greater sensitivity than CT in demonstrating plaques, in both the brain and the spinal cord.

TERMINOLOGY

- Table 27.8 defines some of the terms used in this chapter.

TABLE 27.8 Terminology

Intraaxial/extraaxial	Intraaxial lesions originate in the brain parenchyma and extraaxial lesions originate outside of the brain substance (i.e., meninges, intraventricular).
Infratentorial	Beneath the tentorium cerebelli, which includes the cerebellum, brainstem, fourth ventricle, and cerebellopontine angles.
Supratentorial	Above the tentorium cerebelli, which includes the cerebral hemispheres (frontal, parietal, occipital, and temporal lobes) and the sella.
Transient ischemic attack (TIA)	Sudden neurologic loss that persists for a short time and resolves within 24 hours.
Completed stroke	Neurologic deficit lasts for >21 days.
Open versus closed head injuries	*Open* = communication of intracranial material outside of the skull. *Closed* = no external communication.
Increased attenuation/ hyperattenuation/hyperdense/ hyperintense	On CT, tissue that is of increased attenuation, hyperattenuates, or hyperdense is **whiter** than surrounding tissues. Hyperintense refers to **increased signal** on MRI imaging.
Decreased attenuation/ hypoattenuation/hypodense/ hypointense	On CT, tissue that is of decreased attenuation, hypoattenuates, or hypodense is **darker** than surrounding tissues. Hypointense refers to **decreased** signal on MRI imaging.
Diffusion-weighted imaging (DWI)	An MRI sequence that can be rapidly acquired and which is extremely sensitive to detecting abnormalities in normal water movement in the brain so that it can identify a stroke within 20 to 30 minutes after the event. DWI also helps differentiate acute infarction from more chronic infarction

TAKE HOME POINTS

- The anatomy of the brain can be demonstrated on either CT or MRI scans, although MRI is generally the study of choice for detecting and staging intracranial and spinal cord abnormalities because of its superior contrast and soft-tissue resolution.
- Unenhanced-CT is usually the study of first choice in acute head trauma. The search for findings should initially focus on finding mass effect or blood.
- **Linear skull fractures** are important mainly for the intracranial abnormalities that may have occurred at the time of the fracture; **depressed skull fractures** can be associated with underlying brain injury and may require elevation of the fragment; **basilar skull fractures** are more serious and can be associated with CSF leaks.
- **Blow-out fractures** of the orbit result from a direct blow and may present with orbital emphysema, fracture through either the floor or medial wall of the orbit, and entrapment of fat and/or extraocular muscles in the fracture.
- There are four types of intracranial hemorrhages that may be associated with trauma: epidural hematoma, subdural hematoma, intracerebral hemorrhage, and subarachnoid hemorrhage.
- **Epidural hematomas** represent hemorrhage into the potential space between the dura mater and the inner table of the skull and are usually due to injuries to the middle meningeal artery or vein from blunt head trauma; almost all (95%) have an associated skull fracture. When acute, epidural hematomas appear as hyperintense collections of blood that typically have a lenticular shape.
- **Subdural hematomas** most commonly result from deceleration injuries or falls; acute subdural hematomas portend the presence of more severe brain injury. They are crescent-shaped bands of blood that may cross suture lines and enter the interhemispheric fissure, although they do not cross the midline.
- Traumatic **intracerebral hematomas** are frequently from shearing injuries and present as petechial or larger hemorrhages in the frontal or temporal

lobes; they may be associated with increased intracranial pressure and brain herniation.
- **Brain herniations** include subfalcine, transtentorial, foramen magnum/tonsillar, sphenoid, and extracranial herniations.
- **Diffuse axonal injury** is a serious consequence of trauma in which the corpus callosum is most commonly affected; CT findings are similar to those for intracerebral hemorrhage following head trauma; MRI is the study of choice in identifying diffuse axonal injury.
- In general, **increased intracranial pressure** is due to either increased volume of the brain (cerebral edema) or increased size of the ventricles (hydrocephalus).
- There are two major categories of **cerebral edema:** vasogenic and cytotoxic.
- **Vasogenic edema** represents extracellular accumulation of fluid and is the type that occurs with malignancy and infection and affects the white matter more.
- **Cytotoxic edema** represents cellular edema, is due to cell death, and affects both the gray and white matter; cytotoxic edema is associated with cerebral ischemia.
- **Stroke** denotes an acute loss of neurologic function that occurs when the blood supply to an area of the brain is lost or compromised. MRI is more sensitive to the early diagnosis of stroke than CT.
- Strokes are usually due to **embolic** (more common) or **thrombotic** events and are typically divided into **ischemic** (more common) and **hemorrhagic** varieties (poorer prognosis); hypertension is frequently associated.
- **Intracerebral hemorrhage** will display increased density on nonenhanced CT scans of the brain; after about 2 months, only a small hypodensity may remain.
- **Berry aneurysms** are usually formed from congenital weakening in the arterial wall; when they rupture, the blood typically enters the subarachnoid space

TAKE HOME POINTS—cont'd

presenting in the basilar cisterns and in the sulci. The aneurysm itself can be detected on either CTA or MRA.

- **Hydrocephalus** represents an increased volume of CSF in the ventricular system and may be due to overproduction of CSF (rare), underabsorption of CSF at the level of the arachnoid villi (**communicating**), or obstruction of the outflow of CSF from the ventricles (**noncommunicating**).
- **Normal-pressure hydrocephalus** is a form of communicating hydrocephalus characterized by a classical triad of symptoms that include abnormalities of gait, dementia, and urinary incontinence, which may be reduced by insertion of a ventricular shunt.
- **Cerebral atrophy** is a loss of both gray and white matter that may resemble hydrocephalus, except that the CSF fluid dynamics are normal in atrophy and, in general, cerebral atrophy produces proportionate enlargement of both the ventricles and the sulci.
- **Glioblastoma multiforme** is a highly malignant glioma that occurs most commonly in the frontal and temporal lobes producing a very aggressive infiltrating, partially enhancing, sometimes necrotic mass, which may cross the corpus callosum to the opposite cerebral hemisphere.

- **Metastases to the brain** are frequently well-defined round masses near the gray-white junction and are usually multiple, typically hypodense or isodense on non-enhanced CT that enhance with contrast; they can provoke vasogenic edema out of proportion to the size of the mass. Lung, breast, and melanoma are the most frequent sources of brain metastases.
- **Meningiomas** usually occur in middle-aged women in a parasagittal location; they tend to be slow-growing with an excellent prognosis if surgically excised; on CT they characteristically can be dense without contrast because of calcification within the tumor and may enhance dramatically.
- **Vestibular schwannomas** occur most commonly along the course of the eighth cranial nerve within the internal auditory canal at the cerebellopontine angle and are best identified on MRI, where they homogeneously enhance.
- **Multiple sclerosis** is the most common demyelinating disease, characterized by a relapsing and remitting course and a predilection for the periventricular area, corpus callosum, and optic nerves; it is best visualized on MRI and produces discrete globular foci of high signal intensity (white) on T2-weighted images.

 More information on recognizing some common causes of intracranial pathology is available to registered users online.

28

Recognizing Pediatric Diseases

- Children differ physiologically from adults and are susceptible to abnormalities in development and maturation not seen in adults. They differ in anatomy (e.g., the thymus) and are more susceptible to the harmful effects of ionizing radiation. This chapter highlights some of the more common pediatric diseases associated with imaging findings.

DISEASES DISCUSSED IN THIS CHAPTER

- **Newborn respiratory distress**
  - Transient tachypnea of the newborn
  - Neonatal respiratory distress syndrome (hyaline membrane disease)
  - Meconium aspiration syndrome
  - Bronchopulmonary dysplasia
- **Childhood lung disease**
  - Reactive airways disease/bronchiolitis
  - Asthma
  - Pneumonia
- **Soft tissues of the neck**
  - Enlarged tonsils and adenoids
  - Epiglottitis
  - Croup (laryngotracheobronchitis)
  - Ingested foreign bodies
- **Other diseases**
  - Cardiomegaly in infants
  - Salter-Harris epiphyseal plate fractures
  - Child abuse
  - Necrotizing enterocolitis
  - Esophageal atresia with/without tracheoesophageal fistula

NEWBORN RESPIRATORY DISTRESS

- Respiratory distress is one of the **most common** presenting problems of **newborns.** Clues to its etiology include the infant's **gestational age**, the severity and the progression of symptoms, and the appearance on the chest radiograph. There are many etiologies of respiratory distress including those produced by cardiac, metabolic, hematologic, and anatomic causes. Four pulmonary causes will be discussed.

Transient Tachypnea of the Newborn (TTN)

- Occurring in **full-term** or **larger, slightly preterm** infants, **transient tachypnea of the newborn** is the **most common cause of respiratory distress in the newborn**. It is thought to be due to delay in the resorption of fetal lung fluid. TTN is more common in shortened labor, when delivery is by cesarean section and in mothers with diabetes or asthma.

- Clinically TTN is marked by the **immediate onset** of tachypnea and mild respiratory distress. Infants typically **improve over several hours** with oxygen and supportive therapy and completely recover by 48 hours.

> ### ▸▸ IMPORTANT POINTS
>
> - **Imaging findings of TTN:**
>   - The lungs are usually **hyperinflated**. There may be **streaky perihilar linear densities**. There may be **fluid in the fissures** and/or **laminar pleural effusions** (Fig. 28.1).

Respiratory Distress Syndrome (RDS) of the Newborn (Hyaline Membrane Disease)

- **Respiratory distress syndrome (RDS)** is a disease of **premature infants**, usually in those fewer than 34 weeks of gestation. The incidence and severity of the disease worsen with increasing prematurity. There are numerous risk factors, including perinatal asphyxia and hypoxia and maternal diabetes.
- The major cause of this disorder is **surfactant deficiency.** Without surfactant, the alveolar sacs have an increased tendency to collapse, leading to widespread atelectasis.
- Typically, these premature infants have **severe respiratory distress after birth,** which **progressively worsens.** Clinical findings include cyanosis, grunting, nasal flaring, intercostal and subcostal retractions, and tachypnea.

Fig. 28.1 Transient Tachypnea of the Newborn (TTN). In this disease, there may be streaky perihilar linear densities (*circle*). There may be fluid in the fissures (*black arrow*) and/or laminar pleural effusions (*white arrow*). The lungs are usually hyperinflated.

> **IMPORTANT POINTS**

- **Imaging findings of RDS** (Fig. 28.2):
  - There is typically a diffuse **ground-glass** or **finely granular** appearance to the lungs in a **bilateral** and **symmetric** distribution. The granularity seen in the lungs is the interplay of air-distended bronchioles and ducts against a background of atelectasis of alveoli.
  - **Air bronchograms are common,** especially extending peripherally.
  - **Hypoaeration** is seen in nonventilated lungs. **Hyperinflation** (in nonventilated lungs) **excludes RDS.**

- **Oxygen requirements progressively increase** over the first few hours after birth. The treatment of RDS generally includes **positive pressure ventilation** and may include **intratracheal surfactant replacement.**
- Infants who are very premature (23 to 28 weeks gestation) may require positive pressure respiratory support for several weeks. They are at increased risk for the development of **bronchopulmonary dysplasia** (also known as **chronic respiratory insufficiency of the premature; see later**). The ductus may fail to close, leading to **patent ductus arteriosus,** and **pulmonary hemorrhage** can occur.
- Sudden worsening in symptoms suggests the possibility of an **air leak**—a complication of positive pressure ventilation in relatively noncompliant lungs. There are four manifestations of an air leak (Table 28.1).
- The **mortality rate** from RDS in the newborn varies by country and is dependent, in part, on the rate of premature births and the availability of appropriate treatment interventions in those who develop the disease. In the United States, the mortality rate has declined dramatically in the last several decades.

Meconium Aspiration Syndrome

- Meconium aspiration syndrome is the **most common cause of neonatal respiratory distress in postmature infants.**
- Meconium is found in the amniotic fluid in approximately 15% to 20% of pregnancies. As a consequence, **meconium aspiration** as such is considered to be a **relatively common**

event. Meconium products produce bronchial obstruction, air trapping, and a chemical pneumonitis.
- There is **severe respiratory distress almost immediately,** differentiating it from RDS, whose onset is slightly later. However, whereas many infants have the onset of symptoms at birth, some infants have an asymptomatic period of several hours and then worsen over time.
- Clinically, there may be tachypnea, hypoxia, and hypercapnia. Small airways obstruction may produce a ball-valve effect, leading to **air trapping, overdistension,** and **air leaks.**

> **IMPORTANT POINTS**

- **Imaging findings of meconium aspiration** (Fig. 28.3):
  - The lungs are hyperinflated with **diffuse "ropey" densities** (similar in appearance, but not in timing, to bronchopulmonary dysplasia). There may be patchy areas of **atelectasis** and **emphysema** from air trapping. Spontaneous **pneumothorax** and **pneumomediastinum** occur in 25% (Fig. 28.4). There may be an associated **pneumonia**, usually without air bronchograms. Small **pleural effusions** may be present in 20%.

Fig. 28.3 Meconium Aspiration Syndrome. The lungs are hyperinflated with diffuse "ropey" densities (*white circles*). The patchy pattern is a mosaic of areas of atelectasis along with emphysema from air trapping. This is a baby of 40+ weeks gestation with meconium staining.

Fig. 28.4 Meconium Aspiration Syndrome With Pneumothorax. Spontaneous pneumothorax and pneumomediastinum occur in 25% of babies with meconium aspiration syndrome. The lungs show a coarse interstitial pattern (*white circle*). There is a large right pneumothorax (solid *white arrows*). A "deep sulcus sign" (see Chapter 25) is also present (*dotted white arrow*). The pneumothorax is a tension pneumothorax because the heart and trachea (*black arrow*) are pushed to the left.

Fig. 28.2 Respiratory Distress Syndrome (RDS) of the Newborn (Hyaline Membrane Disease-HMD). There is a diffuse **ground-glass** or finely granular appearance (*white circle*) in a bilateral and symmetric distribution. Hypoaeration is seen in nonventilated lungs (*double black arrow*).

• Treatment is **supportive,** consisting of **antibiotics** and **oxygen,** inhaled nitric oxide, or extracorporeal membrane oxygenation (ECMO), if needed.

Bronchopulmonary Dysplasia (BPD) (Chronic Respiratory Insufficiency of the Premature)

• BPD is a **consequence of early acute lung disease,** frequently **respiratory distress syndrome.** It is a clinical diagnosis and has been defined as **oxygen dependence at 28 days of life to maintain arterial oxygen tensions >50 mm Hg** accompanied by **abnormal chest radiographs.** Associated with most cases of BPD is the prior use of oxygen that was administered under positive pressure.

• BPD may also complicate meconium aspiration syndrome and neonatal pneumonia.

• Clinically, infants with BPD have **oxygen dependence,** hypercapnia, and a compensatory metabolic alkalosis. They may develop pulmonary arterial hypertension and right-sided heart failure. BPD more often manifests in a milder form now than the severe manifestations of the disease when it was first described.

⤻ IMPORTANT POINTS

• **Imaging findings of BPD** (Fig. 28.5):
  • It may be impossible to distinguish early stages of bronchopulmonary dysplasia from later stages of RDS. The lungs are usually **hyperaerated** overall. They may contain **coarse, irregular, rope-like linear densities** representing **atelectasis** or, later, **fibrosis**. These areas of atelectasis may be intermixed with **lucent cyst-like** foci representing hyperexpanded areas of **air trapping**. Together, these processes give the lung a **sponge-like** appearance.

TABLE 28.1 Complications of Treatment: Barotrauma (Air Leaks)

Assisted ventilation with high peak inspiratory pressures and positive end-expiratory pressures may cause overdistension and rupture of alveoli

Complication	Remarks
Pulmonary interstitial emphysema	Rupture of an alveolus with dissection of the air back along the bronchovascular and perilymphatic interstitium may produce multiple small pockets of air in the lung called pulmonary interstitial emphysema (Fig. 28.6).
Pneumothorax	Rupture of an alveolus adjacent to the visceral pleural surface of the lung may dissect outward into the pleural space producing a pneumothorax (Fig. 28.7).
Pneumomediastinum	Air leaks along the bronchovascular bundles of the lung will eventually reach the mediastinum and may produce a pneumomediastinum (Fig. 28.8).
Pneumopericardium	In infants, there may be connections between the mediastinum and the pericardial sac. Air that surrounds the heart, but does not extend above the level of the great vessels, may be a sign of pneumopericardium (Fig. 28.9).

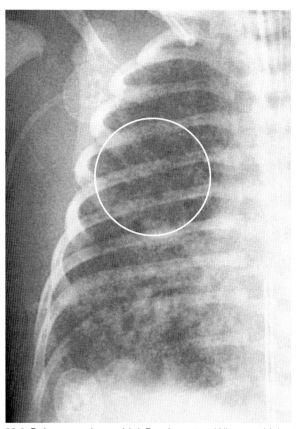

Fig. 28.6 Pulmonary Interstitial Emphysema. When multiple small collections of air (*white circle*) are seen in the interstitial tissues of the lung, it is called pulmonary interstitial emphysema. This is most likely the result of an alveolus rupturing and the air tracking back along the bronchovascular bundles of the lung. This baby has underlying respiratory distress syndrome.

Fig. 28.5 Bronchopulmonary Dysplasia (BPD). The lungs in this radiograph have a typical "sponge-like" appearance. They contain coarse linear densities representing atelectasis (*black arrows*) intermixed with lucent cyst-like foci from areas of air trapping (*white arrows*). BPD is also called **chronic respiratory insufficiency of the premature.**

Fig. 28.7 Respiratory Distress Syndrome of the Newborn With Pneumothorax. Rupture of an alveolus adjacent to the visceral pleural surface of the lung may dissect outward into the pleural space, producing a pneumothorax. There is a ground-glass appearance to the lungs (*circle*). A left-sided pneumothorax is present (*solid white arrows*). There is a **deep-sulcus sign** of a pneumothorax on the left (*dotted white arrow*).

Fig. 28.9 Pneumopericardium. This is a premature infant with underlying Respiratory Distress Syndrome who is on a ventilator. There is a lucency surrounding the heart (*black arrows*) representing air in the pericardial space. Notice how the air does not extend above the reflection of the aorta and main pulmonary artery. The tip of the endotracheal tube extends too far and is in the right main bronchus (*white arrow*).

Fig. 28.8 Spinnaker Sail Sign From Pneumomediastinum. Air leaks may produce a pneumomediastinum. The right and left lobes of the thymus normally rest on the base of the heart. When pneumomediastinum forces the thymic lobes upward and outward, they can form a characteristic appearance, shown here, that has been likened to the **spinnaker sail** on a boat (*white arrows*).

- Infants with BPD may require mechanical ventilation for months. Changes of BPD will revert to normal on the chest radiograph in most patients after 2 years of age, although abnormalities may remain visible on CT of the chest.

CHILDHOOD LUNG DISEASE

Reactive Airways Disease/Bronchiolitis

- Reactive airways disease is a general term for a group of diseases in the pediatric population featuring **wheezing, shortness of breath,** and **coughing**. Initial episodes are frequently referred to as **bronchiolitis.** Unlike asthma, which is chronic, reactive airways disease is usually **transient,** although it can progress over time to asthma.
    - The **clinical findings** of reactive airways disease/bronchiolitis are tachypnea, retractions, cough, fever, and rhinorrhea.

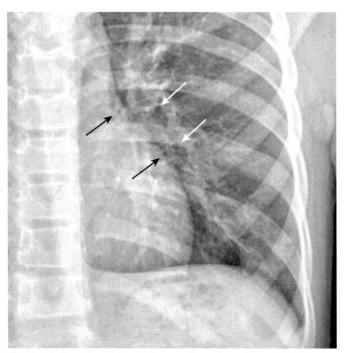

Fig. 28.10 Reactive Airways Disease. There is peribronchial thickening that involves primarily the lobar and segmental bronchi and is manifest by visualization of the walls of the bronchi on conventional radiographs. Here they are seen as small circles or doughnuts near the hilum of a child (*white and black arrows*). Adults may normally demonstrate bronchi on-end in the hilar regions, but children usually do not.

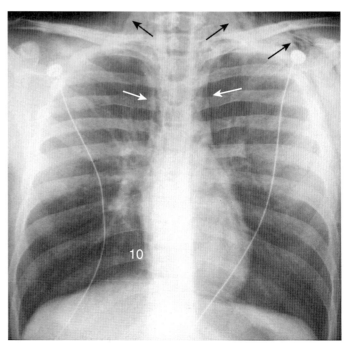

Fig. 28.11 Asthmatic With Pneumomediastinum. The edges of the mediastinum are visible as white lines (*white arrows*) because there is now air in the mediastinum. There is also subcutaneous emphysema (*black arrows*) in this patient who was having an asthmatic attack. This patient has more than 10 posterior ribs visible, in this case a pathologic inspiratory effort.

▶ IMPORTANT POINTS

- **Imaging findings of reactive airways disease** (Fig. 28.10):
  - **Peribronchial thickening,** which involves primarily the lobar or segmental bronchi, is manifest by **visualization of the walls of the bronchi on conventional radiographs.**
  - Bronchi viewed on end appear as **small doughnut-like** densities.
  - Peribronchial thickening may also produce **tram-track linear densities** in the lungs from the thickened bronchial walls visualized in profile.
  - There may be **hyperinflation** of the lungs. **Atelectasis** from mucus plugging may be present.

- **Treatment** includes bronchodilators, steroids and oxygen.

Asthma

- Asthma is a clinical, not a radiologic, diagnosis. Chest radiographs can help in determining either the **cause** or the **complications** of an asthmatic episode.
- Inciting events include **pneumonia,** usually accompanied by a fever that provides a clue to its presence. Complications include **atelectasis** secondary to plugging by mucus (see Fig. 7.2), **pneumothorax,** and **pneumomediastinum** (Fig. 28.11).
- During or after an acute attack, the lungs may be **overaerated** with **flattening of the diaphragm.** There may be **peribronchial thickening** as is seen with reactive airways disease.

Pneumonia

- Age is a determining factor in both the etiology and clinical presentation of childhood pneumonia.
- In **neonates,** group B beta hemolytic streptococcus is the most common cause of pneumonia. Its imaging appearance can mimic respiratory distress syndrome of the newborn.
- In **older infants,** the most common causes are **respiratory syncytial virus (RSV), respiratory viruses** (parainfluenza, influenza, and adenoviruses), **and *Mycoplasma pneumoniae*** in children **older than 5 years.**
- Clinically, neonates may have only a fever. In older infants and children, **bacterial** pneumonia tends to produce **fever, chills, tachypnea, cough, pleuritic chest pain, and shortness of breath.** Viral pneumonia is more often associated with cough, wheezing, and stridor than with fever.

▶ IMPORTANT POINTS

- **Imaging findings of pneumonia:**
  - **Bacterial pneumonia**
    - It characteristically produces **lobar consolidation** or a **round pneumonia,** with **pleural effusion** in 10% to 30% of cases (see Fig. 9.6).
  - **Viral pneumonia**
    - It characteristically shows **interstitial infiltrates** or **patchy areas** of consolidation suggestive of bronchopneumonia.

Fig. 28.12 Normal Soft Tissue Lateral Neck Radiograph, 4-Year-Old. The adenoids (A) are seen at the base of the skull and are adjacent to the nasopharyngeal airway (N). More distally is the pharynx (P). The epiglottis (*solid white arrow*) is bounded superiorly by air in the vallecula. The aryepiglottic folds are thin, paired structures (*dotted white arrow*). The normal-sized laryngeal ventricle (*black arrow*) separates the false vocal cords above from the true cords below. The trachea (T) starts below the true cords.

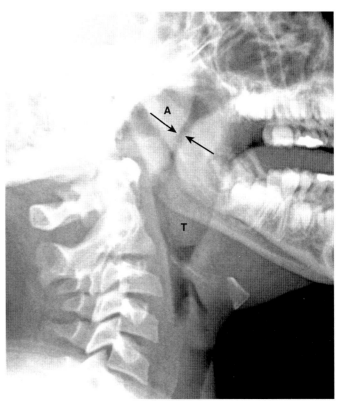

Fig. 28.13 Enlarged Adenoids. There is marked narrowing of the nasopharynx (*black arrows*) by the enlarged adenoids (A). The palatine tonsils (T) are also enlarged. The tonsils and adenoids frequently enlarge at the same time.

- **Treatment** is supportive with antibiotics, as needed.

SOFT TISSUES OF THE NECK

Enlarged Tonsils and Adenoids

- **Newborns do not have visible adenoids,** even though the adenoids are present at birth. They are usually not visible radiographically **until 3 to 6 months.** The adenoids can grow until about age 6 years. They then involute through adulthood. **Adults normally do not have visible adenoids** (Fig. 28.12).
- The **palatine tonsils and adenoids** frequently enlarge at the same time. As with enlarged adenoids, the significance of enlarged tonsils is best made in light of clinical symptoms and compression of the airway.
- **Clinical findings** of enlarged tonsils and adenoids include nasal congestion, mouth-breathing, chronic or recurrent otitis media due to their proximity to the eustachian tubes, painful swallowing, and sleep apnea.

IMPORTANT POINTS

- **Imaging findings of enlarged adenoids** (Fig. 28.13):
  - The lateral neck radiograph is the main imaging study; the neck should always be extended at the time of exposure.
  - **Measurements of the adenoids are not reliable.** The size of the adenoids is less of a consideration than the degree to which they do or do not impinge on the nasopharyngeal airway. **Look for marked narrowing or obliteration of the nasopharyngeal airway.**

Epiglottitis

- Acute bacterial epiglottitis can be a **life-threatening medical emergency** leading to airway obstruction due to infection with edema of the epiglottis and aryepiglottic folds.
- The most frequent causative organism had been *Haemophilus influenzae* type B, but introduction of the vaccine in 1985 has led to a marked decrease in the number of cases of epiglottitis. *H. influenzae* **still remains the most common cause,** although it may also be caused by pneumococcus, streptococcus group A, viral infection such as herpes simplex 1, parainfluenza, thermal injury, or angioneurotic edema. Chemical irritation has also been reported from the ingestion of laundry detergent pods.

- Epiglottitis typically has a **peak incidence from about 3 to 6 years of age**.
- **Clinically,** epiglottitis resembles **croup**, but the clinician should think of epiglottitis if the child cannot breathe unless **sitting up**, what appears to be "croup" seems to be **worsening** or if the child cannot swallow saliva and **drools**. Cough is rare.
- The classical triad of epiglottitis is **drooling, severe dysphagia, and respiratory distress with inspiratory stridor.**
- The patient should be accompanied everywhere by someone experienced in endotracheal intubation. Imaging studies are not always necessary for the diagnosis and may be falsely negative in early stages.
- The imaging study of choice is the **lateral neck radiograph**, which should be exposed in the **upright position only**, as the supine position may close off the airway.

> ## ►► IMPORTANT POINTS
>
> - **Imaging findings of epiglottitis:**
>   - **Enlargement of the epiglottis.** The epiglottis should not be "larger than your thumb," no matter what the size of your thumb. There is **thickening of the aryepiglottic folds** (which is an important component of airway obstruction and the true cause of stridor) and, sometimes, circumferential **narrowing of the subglottic portion of trachea** during inspiration (Fig. 28.14).

- **Treatment** includes securing the airway, which may require intubation or emergency tracheostomy; some treatment

protocols call for administering intravenous steroids and starting empiric antibiotic therapy.

Croup (Laryngotracheobronchitis)

- Croup is usually **viral in etiology**, the most common causes being parainfluenza viruses (types 1, 2, and 3). Respiratory syncytial virus, influenza, and mycoplasma are other common causes. It typically occurs from age **6 months to 3 years,** which is a younger age range than epiglottitis. It **frequently follows a common cold.**
- The diagnosis of croup usually is made on the basis of **clinical findings**. It may be difficult to distinguish from early retropharyngeal abscess; the differential diagnosis can be aided by imaging. There is characteristically a **harsh cough** described as **"barking" or "brassy,"** associated with hoarseness, inspiratory stridor, low-grade fever, and respiratory distress.

> ## ►► IMPORTANT POINTS
>
> - **Imaging findings of croup** (Fig. 28.15):
>   - The **three key findings,** seen on the lateral soft-tissue neck radiograph, are **distension of the hypopharynx, distension of the laryngeal ventricle,** and haziness and/or **narrowing of the subglottic trachea.** The **steeple sign,** which may be seen on the frontal radiograph of the neck, is, by itself, an **unreliable** sign of croup.

- **Treatment** can consist of steroids, aerosolized epinephrine, and humidification.

Fig. 28.14 Epiglottitis. The epiglottis (E) should not be thumb-like in appearance. It is very enlarged in this case. There is thickening of the aryepiglottic folds (*white arrow*). Care must be taken to protect the airway from complete closure in any patient with epiglottitis.

Fig. 28.15 Laryngotracheobronchitis (Croup). There is distension of the hypopharynx (H), distension of the laryngeal ventricle (*white arrow*), and haziness with narrowing of the subglottic space (i.e., proximal trachea) (*black arrows*). This was an 11-month-old with a characteristic barking cough.

INGESTED FOREIGN BODIES

- The majority of foreign body ingestions occurs between **6 months and 6 years of age.** Over **80% pass spontaneously.** Food or true foreign body ingestions include coins, toys, chicken bones (opaque), and fish bones (nonopaque).
- Most often the foreign body impacts at a point at which the esophagus naturally narrows—**just below** the **cricopharyngeus** at the level of C5-C6 (70%), at the level of the **thoracic inlet,** at the **aortic arch** (20%), or at the level of the **esophagogastric junction** (10%). Once past the esophagus, most foreign bodies will pass through the gastrointestinal (GI) tract.
- The **major complications** of ingested foreign bodies are perforation, obstruction, or stricture formation.
- **Disk (button) batteries** and **magnets** pose **particular hazards.** Button batteries should be removed from the esophagus emergently because of their ability to produce perforation (Fig. 28.16). Multiple small magnets also pose the risk of perforation by drawing apposing loops of bowel together and should be removed, if possible.
- **Clinical findings** of an impacted esophageal foreign body include **dysphagia** and **odynophagia**, most commonly. Even after the foreign body passes, many complain of pain occurring in the cervical esophagus regardless of the actual site of impaction.

> ### 》 IMPORTANT POINTS
>
> - **Imaging findings of an impacted foreign body:**
>   - The imaging findings will depend on whether the foreign body is opaque or not. **Conventional radiographs** of the **neck** and **chest** are usually obtained **first**. If no foreign body is visualized, the abdomen may also be radiographed.

- A coin may appear differently on conventional radiographs, depending on whether it is impacted in the **esophagus** or in the **trachea** (Fig. 28.17).
- If conventional radiographs are negative and a very high suspicion remains for a nonopaque ingested foreign body, then either contrast esophagram or CT may be considered.

Fig. 28.16 Ingested Disk Battery in Colon. This is an extreme close-up of the right lower quadrant where the outline of a round metallic foreign body can be seen. It was in the approximate position of the right colon. The dark band (*white arrow*) inside the whiter rim and the object's size and shape identify it as a disk or button battery.

Fig. 28.17 Ingested Coin in the Esophagus. A coin impacted in the esophagus will usually appear round on the frontal view (A, *white arrow*) and flat on the lateral view (B, *black arrow*) because of its orientation in the esophagus. A coin in the trachea more likely will appear on-end in the frontal view and round in the lateral view because of the shape of the trachea. This coin was a US nickel and it passed uneventfully a day later.

- Because children who ingest foreign bodies may also be predisposed to eating **other foreign material (pica),** such as paint, **always look for** dense lines in the metaphyses of visible bones on any foreign body study, a sign of **lead poisoning.**
- **Treatment**
  - Under most circumstances, **watchful waiting** will result in elimination of the foreign body. Endoscopy is performed if removal is considered clinically necessary (e.g., sharp objects, disk batteries, magnets).

OTHER DISEASES

Recognizing Cardiomegaly in Infants

- In **newborns and infants** it is important to remember that the **heart will normally appear larger** relative to the size of the thorax than it does in adults. Whereas a cardiothoracic ratio greater than 50% is considered abnormal in adults, the **cardiothoracic ratio may reach up to 65% in infants and still be normal** because newborns cannot take as deep an inspiration as adults and the relative proportions in the size of their abdomen to chest are not the same as for adults (Fig. 28.18).
- Any assessment of cardiac enlargement in an infant should take into account other factors, such as the appearance of the **pulmonary vasculature,** and any **associated clinical signs or symptoms** (e.g., a murmur, tachycardia, or cyanosis).

> **! DIAGNOSTIC PITFALLS**
>
> - In a child the **thymus gland** may overlap portions of the heart and sometimes mimic cardiomegaly. The normal thymus may be seen on conventional chest radiographs in a child up to 3 years of age and sometimes later. The **normal thymus** gland has a somewhat **lobulated** appearance, especially where it is indented by the ribs (Fig. 28.19).

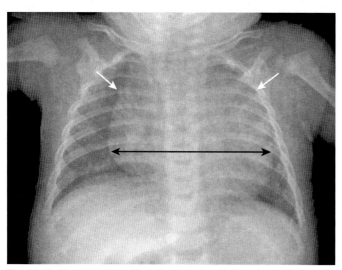

Fig. 28.18 Normal Infant Chest. In the normal infant, the cardiothoracic ratio may be as large as 65% (compared with 50% in adults). Here the heart appears enlarged (*black arrows*), but is normal for a newborn. The thymus gland (*white arrows*) accounts for some of the apparent cardiomegaly.

Fig. 28.19 Normal Thymus Gland. One aid in identifying the thymus gland is that it is frequently lobulated in appearance (*white arrows*). Although the thymus gland will usually involute with age, it may still be normally visible in children as old as 3 years of age on conventional radiographs.

SALTER-HARRIS FRACTURES: EPIPHYSEAL PLATE FRACTURES IN CHILDREN

- In growing bone, the **hypertrophic zone** in the **growth plate (epiphyseal plate** or **physis)** is most vulnerable to shearing injuries. Epiphyseal plate fractures are **common** and account for as many as 30% of childhood fractures. By definition, because these are all fractures through an **open** epiphyseal plate, they **can occur only in skeletally immature** individuals.
- The **Salter-Harris classification of epiphyseal plate injuries** is a commonly used method of describing such injuries that helps identify the type of treatment required and predicts the likelihood of complications based on the type of fracture (Fig. 28.20) (Table 28.2).

Fig. 28.20 Salter-Harris Classification of Epiphyseal Plate Fractures. All of these fractures involve the epiphyseal plate (growth plate). **Type I** are fractures of the epiphyseal plate alone. **Type II** fractures, the most common, involve the epiphyseal plate and metaphysis. These first two types have a favorable prognosis. **Type III** are fractures of the epiphyseal plate and the epiphysis and have a less favorable prognosis. **Type IV** is a fracture of the epiphyseal plate, epiphysis, and metaphysis. It has an even less favorable prognosis. **Type V** is a crush injury of the epiphyseal plate. It has the worst prognosis.

» IMPORTANT POINTS

- Type I and II **heal well**.
- Type III can develop **arthritic changes** or **asymmetric growth plate fusion**.
- Type IV and V are more likely to develop **early fusion** of the growth plate with **angular deformities** and/or **shortening** of that bone.

- **Type I: fractures of the epiphyseal plate alone**
  - Salter-Harris type I fractures are often **difficult to detect without the opposite side for comparison.** Fortunately these fractures have a **favorable prognosis.**
  - **Slipped capital femoral epiphysis (SCFE)** is a manifestation of a Salter-Harris type I injury.
    - Slipped capital femoral epiphysis occurs most often in **taller and/or heavier teenage boys.** It can occur during periods of rapid growth, from trauma, renal osteodystrophy, and endocrine disorders, such as hypothyroidism.
    - The proximal (capital) femoral epiphysis slips **inferior, medial, and posterior** relative to the neck of the femur (Fig. 28.21).
    - It is **bilateral in about 25% of cases** and can result in **avascular necrosis** of the slipped femoral head because of interruption of the blood supply in up to 15% of cases.
- **Type II: fracture of the epiphyseal plate and fracture of the metaphysis**
  - This is the **most common type of Salter-Harris fracture (75%),** seen especially in the distal radius. Healing is typically rapid and growth is rarely disturbed, except in the distal femur and proximal tibia where a residual deformity may occur.
  - The **small metaphyseal fracture fragment** of a Salter-Harris type II fracture produces the so-called **corner-sign** (Fig. 28.22).

Fig. 28.21 Slipped Capital Femoral Epiphysis (SCFE). SCFE produces inferior, medial, and posterior slippage of the proximal femoral epiphysis relative to the neck of the femur (*black arrow*). A line drawn parallel to the neck of the femur, called **Klein's line** (*white lines*), should intersect the lateral portion of the femoral head. It does so on the normal left side, but does not on the right side because the epiphysis has slipped.

Fig. 28.22 Salter-Harris II Fracture. In Salter type II fractures, there is a fracture of the epiphyseal plate and a fracture of the metaphysis. The small metaphyseal fracture fragment (*white arrow*) produces the so-called **corner-sign.**

Type	What's Fractured	Remarks
I	Epiphyseal plate	Seen in phalanges, distal radius, SCFE; good prognosis
II	Epiphyseal plate and metaphysis	Most common of all Salter-Harris fractures; frequently distal radius; displays **corner-sign;** good prognosis
III	Epiphyseal plate and epiphysis	Intraarticular fracture; especially distal tibia; prognosis: less favorable
IV	Epiphyseal plate, epiphysis, and metaphysis	Seen in distal humerus and distal tibia; poor prognosis
V	Crush injury of epiphyseal plate	Worst prognosis; difficult to diagnose until healing begins

TABLE 28.2 Salter-Harris Classification of Epiphyseal Plate Fractures

SCFE, Slipped capital femoral epiphysis.

- **Type III: fracture of the epiphyseal plate and the epiphysis**
  - There is a **longitudinal fracture through the epiphysis itself,** which means the fracture invariably enters the joint space and fractures the articular cartilage.
  - This type of injury can have long-term implications for the development of **secondary osteoarthritis** and can

Fig. 28.24 Salter-Harris Type IV Fracture. In type IV fractures, there is a fracture of the epiphyseal plate, metaphysis (*white arrow*), and the epiphysis (*black arrow*). These have an increased likelihood of premature and possibly asymmetric closure of the epiphyseal plate.

Fig. 28.23 Salter-Harris III Fracture. With Salter type III fractures, there is a fracture of the epiphyseal plate as well as a longitudinal fracture through the epiphysis itself (*white arrow*). This fracture has a poorer prognosis than types I and II.

Fig. 28.25 Salter-Harris Type V Fracture. Type V fractures are crush fractures of the epiphyseal plate. In this child, the medial portion of the distal radial epiphyseal plate has fused (*solid black arrow*), whereas the lateral portion remains open (*dotted black arrow*). This premature fusion of the medial growth plate has resulted in an angular deformity of the distal radius (*black line*).

result in **asymmetric** and **premature fusion of the growth plate** with subsequent deformity of the bone (Fig. 28.23). Its treatment requires early recognition for appropriate reduction.

- **Type IV: fracture of the epiphyseal plate, metaphysis, and epiphysis**
  - Type IV fractures have a **poorer prognosis** than other Salter-Harris fractures (i.e., premature and possibly asymmetric **closure of the epiphyseal plate**), especially in bones of the lower extremity, that may lead to differences in leg length, angular deformities, and secondary osteoarthritis (Fig. 28.24).
  - If the fracture is displaced, open reduction and internal fixation is usually performed, although growth deformities can occur even with perfect reduction.
- **Type V: crush fracture of epiphyseal plate**
  - Type V Salter-Harris fractures are **rare**, crush-type injuries of the epiphyseal plate that are **associated with vascular injury** and almost always **result in growth impairment** through early focal fusion of the growth plate.

- They are **most common** in the **distal femur, proximal tibia,** and **distal tibia.** They are **difficult to diagnose** on conventional radiographs until later in their course when complications ensue (Fig. 28.25).

CHILD ABUSE

- Salter-Harris fractures are examples of **accidental** injuries in children. Certain fractures at other sites or fractures of other types can be highly suggestive for **nonaccidental** injuries produced by abuse. **Radiologic evaluations are key in diagnosing child abuse.**

although ischemia and/or reperfusion injury have been implicated along with poorly developed intestinal motility with resultant stasis.

- It is **more common in premature** infants, but can also be seen in term babies. Usually its **onset** occurs within the **first week** of life. Term infants have an increased risk for the disease if they have congenital heart disease or there is a history of maternal cocaine use.

> ### » IMPORTANT POINTS
>
> - There are several fracture sites and characteristics should raise the suspicion for child abuse (Table 28.3).
>   - **Metaphyseal corner fractures.** Small avulsion-type fractures of the metaphyses due to rapid rotation of ligamentous insertions, corner fractures are considered **diagnostic of physical abuse.** They parallel the metaphysis and can have a **bucket-handle appearance** (Fig. 28.26A).
>   - **Rib fractures,** especially multiple fractures and/or fractures of the posterior ribs (which rarely fracture because of accidental trauma) (Fig. 28.26B).
>   - **Head injuries** are the most common cause of death in child abuse in those under 2 years of age. Findings include **subdural and subarachnoid hemorrhage** and **cerebral contusions. Skull fractures** tend to be comminuted, bilateral, and may cross suture lines.

TABLE 28.3 Skeletal Trauma Suggestive of Child Abuse

Site(s)	Remarks
Distal femur, distal humerus, wrist, ankle	Metaphyseal corner fractures
Multiple sites	Fractures in different stages of healing
Femur, humerus, tibia	Spiral fractures in children <1 year of age
Posterior ribs, avulsed spinous processes	These are unusual "naturally occurring" fractures in children <5 years of age
Multiple skull fractures	Multiple fractures of occipital bone should suggest child abuse
Fractures with abundant callous formation	Implies repeated trauma and no immobilization
Metacarpal and metatarsal fractures	These are unusual "naturally occurring" fractures in children <5 years of age
Sternal and scapular fractures	
Vertebral body fractures and subluxations	

NECROTIZING ENTEROCOLITIS (NEC)

- NEC is the **most common GI** medical and/or surgical **emergency** occurring in **neonates.** Its etiology remains unknown,

Fig. 28.26 Child Abuse. (A) There are metaphyseal **corner fractures** (*solid white arrows*), small avulsion-type fractures of the distal radius, a finding characteristic of child abuse. (B) There are several healing rib fractures (*dotted white arrows*), as evidenced by callus formation, including one involving the left sixth posterior rib. Fractures of the posterior ribs should raise suspicion for child abuse.

- **Clinical findings** may be subtle and can include feeding intolerance, delayed gastric emptying, abdominal distention and/or tenderness, and decreased bowel sounds.
- Box 28.1 describes the imaging findings of a **normal infant abdomen.**

> ## IMPORTANT POINTS
>
> - **Imaging findings of necrotizing enterocolitis**
>   - **Conventional radiographs** of the abdomen remain the modality by which the disease is diagnosed most often. The acute disease **most commonly affects the terminal ileum.**
>   - Early findings may be a few **distended loops of bowel.** A **persistently dilated** loop that remains **unchanged** in appearance is a marker of advanced disease, although it can be seen earlier in its course.
>   - **Thickened bowel walls** are manifest by **separation of the bowel loops.**
>   - **Pneumatosis intestinalis** is **pathognomonic of NEC in the newborn.** A **linear radiolucency** within the bowel wall parallels the bowel lumen and represents **subserosal** air that has entered from the lumen (Fig. 28.28A).Cystic collections of air are submucosal in location, but also a sign of pneumatosis.
>   - Abdominal **free air** is an ominous finding that usually requires emergency surgical intervention.
>   - **Portal venous gas,** originally thought to be ominous, is now considered less so. It appears as linear branching tubular-structures of air density over the periphery of the liver and represents air in the portal venous system **(**Fig. 28.28B).

Fig. 28.27 Normal Infant Abdomen. Because most infants swallow a great deal of air, there are many air-filled polygonal-shaped loops of bowel (*circle*) with walls that closely appose each other (*white arrows*).

> ## BOX 28.1 Normal Infant Abdomen: Conventional Radiographs
>
> - Almost all infants will demonstrate gas in the stomach by 15 minutes after birth and air in the rectum by 24 hours of age.
> - It is virtually impossible on radiographs to differentiate small from large bowel in infants as the haustra do not develop in the colon until about 6 months of age.
> - Most infants swallow a great deal of air so expect to see many air-filled polygonal-shaped loops of bowel with walls that closely appose each other (Fig. 28.27).

- **Complications**
  - Of those who survive, 50% develop a long-term complication. The two most common complications are **intestinal stricture** and **short-gut syndrome.** Mortality rates range from 10% to 44% in infants weighing less than 1500 grams.

ESOPHAGEAL ATRESIA WITH/WITHOUT TRACHEOESOPHAGEAL FISTULA (TEF)

- The etiology of esophageal atresia is not completely understood. By far the most common form is a **blind-ending esophagus (esophageal atresia)** with a **fistulous connection between the trachea** and the **distal esophageal remnant.**
- Esophageal atresia is commonly associated with **other abnormalities of the GI tract,** including imperforate anus; duodenal atresia or stenosis; in 25% of cases, there are 13 or more pairs of ribs or 6 or more lumbar vertebral bodies. Infants with isolated esophageal atresia have an increased incidence of trisomy 21 and duodenal atresia.
- In up to 50% of cases of esophageal atresia with/without TEF there may be **associated congenital abnormalities. VACTERL** is an acronym to help remember a constellation of congenital abnormalities that may occur together and stands for **V**ertebral anomalies, **A**nal atresia, **C**ardiac abnormalities, **TE** fistula and/or esophageal atresia, **R**enal agenesis or dysplasia, and **L**imb defects.
- **Clinical findings usually occur early in life** and include choking, drooling, difficulty handling secretions, regurgitation, aspiration, and respiratory distress.

> ## IMPORTANT POINTS
>
> - **Imaging findings** will depend on the geometry of the atresia and fistula:
>   - With **esophageal atresia** and **no fistula**, **no air** enters the GI tract so the **abdomen is airless.** Normally there should be air in the stomach within 15 minutes after birth.
>   - With a **distal fistula** between the esophagus and trachea (the most common type), there is **gas in the bowel,** which entered via the trachea, and a radiolucent **blind-ending, dilated pouch of upper esophagus** may be seen on chest x-ray, representing the atretic esophagus. Further imaging studies are usually not necessary, but introduction of a soft catheter into the blind-ending pouch will confirm the diagnosis (Fig. 28.29).
>   - There may be **aspiration pneumonia.** Aspiration pneumonia often involves the right upper lobe when there is esophageal atresia.
>   - Prenatal ultrasound can suggest the diagnosis as early as 24 weeks because of polyhydramnios.

Fig. 28.28 Necrotizing Enterocolitis: Portal Venous Gas. This is a 1-week-old infant. (A) The bowel is dilated (*double white arrows*). There is a linear radiolucency paralleling the bowel wall representing air in the bowel wall (*dotted white arrow*) and abnormal separation of the loops of bowel from wall thickening (*double black arrows*). Numerous, small, peripherally located air-containing vessels are seen in the liver (see [B] for inset), representing portal venous gas. (B) Close-up of the liver shows multiple tubular lucencies representing air in the portal venous system (*white oval*). There is air in the bowel wall (*black arrow*).

Fig. 28.29 Esophageal Atresia With a Tracheoesophageal Fistula. The tip of an orogastric tube is kinked in a blind-ending pouch in the upper esophagus and can pass no farther in the atretic esophagus (*circle*). The air throughout the bowel (*black arrow*) arrived via a fistula that connects the trachea with the distal end of the esophagus (not visible on plain films).

- **Treatment**
  - Primary anastomosis of the proximal and distal esophagus is usually done when the infant is a few months old. Colonic interposition may be used if primary anastomosis is impossible.

🏠 TAKE HOME POINTS

- **Transient tachypnea of the newborn** is the most common cause of respiratory distress in the newborn, occurring in **full-term** or larger, slightly preterm infants. The lungs are usually hyperinflated with streaky perihilar linear densities, fluid in the fissures, and/or laminar pleural effusions.
- **Respiratory distress syndrome** is a disease of premature infants. There is typically a diffuse "ground-glass" or finely granular appearance in a bilateral and symmetric distribution with air bronchograms. The lungs are frequently hypoaerated.
- **Meconium aspiration syndrome** is the most common cause of neonatal respiratory distress in full-term/postmature infants. The lungs are hyperinflated with diffuse "ropey" densities. There may be patchy areas of atelectasis along with emphysema from air trapping.
- **Bronchopulmonary dysplasia (BPD)** is a consequence of early acute lung disease, frequently respiratory distress syndrome. Infants with BPD have a supplemental oxygen dependence. The lungs are usually hyperaerated and "sponge-like" in appearance, containing both coarse linear densities from atelectasis intermixed with lucent foci from hyperexpanded areas of air trapping.
- Complications of treatment of respiratory distress in the newborn are usually from **barotrauma (air leaks)** and include pulmonary interstitial emphysema, pneumomediastinum, pneumothorax, and pneumopericardium.
- **Reactive airways disease/bronchiolitis** is a general term for a group of diseases in the pediatric population featuring wheezing, shortness of breath, and coughing. There may be peribronchial thickening and hyperaeration.
- **Asthma** is a clinical diagnosis. Chest radiographs can help in determining either the cause or the complications of an asthmatic episode. Pneumonia is one cause and pneumothorax and atelectasis are among the complications of an asthmatic attack.
- Clinically, neonates with **pneumonia** may have only a fever. Bacterial pneumonia characteristically produces lobar consolidation or a round pneumonia, with pleural effusion in some cases. Viral pneumonia characteristically shows interstitial infiltrates or patchy areas of consolidation suggestive of bronchopneumonia.
- The **adenoids** can grow until about age 6 years and then involute through adulthood. The key imaging finding for enlarged adenoids is marked narrowing or obliteration of the nasopharyngeal airway on a soft-tissue lateral neck radiograph. The tonsils and adenoids frequently enlarge together.
- Acute bacterial **epiglottitis** can be a life-threatening medical emergency. The epiglottis should not normally be thumb-like in size or appearance. It occurs at an older age (3 to 6 years) than croup (6 months to 3 years).
- **Croup** is usually viral in etiology and the diagnosis is most often made on the basis of clinical findings. The three key imaging findings, seen on the lateral soft-tissue neck radiograph, are distension of the hypopharynx, distension of the laryngeal ventricle, and haziness and/or narrowing of subglottic trachea.
- Most **foreign body ingestions** occur between 6 months and 6 years of age with the vast majority passing spontaneously. They impact at several different landmarks where the esophagus naturally narrows. Disk (button) batteries and magnets pose particular hazards and should generally be removed.
- The **cardiothoracic ratio** may reach up to 65% in infants and still be normal. In a child, the thymus gland may overlap portions of the heart and sometimes mimic cardiomegaly.
- **Epiphyseal plate fractures** are common in childhood. The Salter-Harris classification of epiphyseal plate injuries is a commonly used method of describing these injuries.
- Certain kinds of fractures can be highly suggestive for nonaccidental injuries produced by **child abuse**. Included among injuries pointing to child abuse are metaphyseal corner fractures, rib fractures, and head injuries. Radiologic evaluations are key in diagnosing child abuse.
- **Necrotizing enterocolitis** is the most common GI medical and/or surgical emergency occurring in neonates, especially premature infants. There may be dilated loops of bowel, thickened bowel walls, pneumatosis intestinalis, and portal venous gas.
- **Esophageal atresia** may occur with or without a tracheoesophageal fistula (TEF). The most common form is a blind-ending esophagus with a fistulous connection between the trachea and the distal esophageal remnant.
- TEF may be associated with other congenital anomalies signified by the acronym VACTERL, which stands for **V**ertebral anomalies, **A**nal atresia, **C**ardiac abnormalities, **TE**F and/or esophageal atresia, **R**enal agenesis or dysplasia, and **L**imb defects.

📶 More information on recognizing diseases in pediatric patients is available to registered users online.

29

Using Image-Guided Interventions in Diagnosis and Treatment: Interventional Radiology

Jeffrey L. Weinstein, MD, and Trevor Lewis, MD

- **Interventional radiology (IR),** also known as **vascular and interventional radiology (VIR),** is a medical specialty that utilizes **image-guidance** (i.e., fluoroscopy, ultrasound, computed tomography [CT], or magnetic resonance imaging [MRI]) to perform **minimally invasive diagnostic or therapeutic procedures.**
- Interventional radiologists perform a wide variety of procedures that can be characterized as **vascular** or **nonvascular** and subdivided into the vascular distribution or organ system for the procedure being performed.
- With specific examples from the case scenarios in prior chapters, this chapter will discuss the **indications, techniques, and benefits** of image-guided interventions that cover a wide gamut of interventional procedures.

ARTERIAL ACCESS AND ARTERIOGRAPHY

- **Arterial access and arteriography** are fundamentals of interventional radiology, allowing for diagnostic evaluation of a myriad of arterial pathologies (e.g., arteriovenous fistula, aneurysm, vascular occlusion, or vascular stenosis).

> ### ▶▶ IMPORTANT POINTS
>
> - The **Seldinger technique** is the basis for modern vascular access, both arterial and venous. This method, first described by Dr. Sven Seldinger (a Swedish radiologist), uses a hollow needle to gain entry into a blood vessel. A wire is then passed through this needle, which is then removed and exchanged for a catheter placed over the wire. This exchange is the basis for the initial steps in a **majority** of **endovascular interventional radiology procedures** (Fig. 29.1).

Indications for Arterial Access

- Arterial access is utilized to facilitate **image-guided arterial interventions** (e.g., **embolization** for active bleeding, **angioplasty** for arterial stenosis and arteriovenous malformation **sclerotherapy**).

Procedure for Arterial Access

- Arterial access is most commonly performed from a **femoral or radial artery approach,** though other arteries can be utilized, the selection of which depends on a variety of parameters,

including the type of intervention, the anatomic orientation of the vasculature, and the presence of a coagulopathy, among others.
- Arterial access is traditionally performed over a **bony landmark,** which aids in **compression** of the artery to obtain hemostasis **after** the procedure is complete. In the case of femoral artery access, the segment of artery **over the femoral**

Fig. 29.1 Seldinger Technique. (A) Percutaneous puncture of a blood vessel with a hollow needle. (B) Introduction of an atraumatic guidewire through the needle into the blood vessel lumen. (C) Needle is removed while guidewire remains in place. Compression over the puncture secures the guidewire and prevents bleeding. (D) Angiographic catheter is advanced into vessel over the guidewire. (From: Kadir S. *Diagnostic Angiography.* Philadelphia: WB Saunders, 1986:186. Also appeared with permission in Kaufman JA, Lee, Michael J. *The Requisites: Vascular and Interventional Radiology,* 2nd ed. Philadelphia: Saunder, 2014:26.)

TABLE 29.1 Short Glossary of Interventional Tools

Device	Description
Access needle	The entry needle used at the puncture site for percutaneous procedures; all contain a central channel for introduction of a guidewire.
Guidewires	Thin wires of varying lengths, composition, and flexibility, that are fed through the channel of the access needle, over which other devices, which themselves contain a hollow channel, can be fed.
Catheters	Tubular structures usually made of some kind of plastic with varying lengths, diameters, shapes, and coatings through which substances can be either withdrawn from or introduced into the body.
Sheath	A vascular access hollow tube, usually made of plastic, which allows for the exchange of catheters during a given procedure while maintaining vascular access through the same puncture site.
Dilator	Short, tapered catheters used to increase the diameter of the hole from percutaneous access to an organ, space, or vessel to allow easier passage of a catheter, sheath, or other device; sometimes used in a serial fashion from smaller to larger.

head is targeted with palpatory, fluoroscopic, and/or ultrasound guidance.

- Utilizing the Seldinger technique, an access needle is ultimately exchanged over a wire for a vascular sheath (Table 29.1).
- **Ultrasound guidance** during the arterial puncture can sometimes facilitate vascular access, especially in cases of weakly palpable pulses or challenging anatomy.
- Radial artery or brachial artery access is similar to the femoral artery approach. In the case of brachial artery access, care must be taken to choose an access site that would allow for **compression** to obtain **hemostasis after the procedure.**

- Once arterial access is obtained and a catheter or sheath is in place, the injection of iodinated contrast can be performed for **arteriography** in the desired location.

Benefits and Potential Risks of Arterial Access

- Arterial access and arteriography allow for **diagnostic evaluation** and **localization** of abnormalities and provide a route for endovascular **treatment** by minimally invasive means.
- **Risks** of arterial access include bleeding and injury to tissues and organs adjacent to the vessels as attempts are made to gain access, such as a **pseudoaneurysm** at the groin access site from puncture and arterial extravasation (see Fig. 20.6).
- Arterial access carries the further risk of **dissection**, **bleeding**, or **thrombosis** of the accessed vessel. There is a risk of **infection** and **injury** to the surrounding structures at the access site. Meticulous technique and experience can help mitigate many of these complications.

CENTRAL VENOUS ACCESS: IMAGE-GUIDED VENOUS ACCESS

▶▶ IMPORTANT POINTS

- **Central venous access,** a fundamental technique used throughout medicine, which allows for entry into the venous system either for **intervention** (e.g., thrombolysis or stenting) or for **placement** of a catheter for pharmaceutical treatment or hemodialysis/**pheresis** (i.e., procedures in which blood is filtered, separated, and returned to the patient, as in **plasmapheresis**).

Indications for Central Venous Access

- Central venous access is attempted when a **venous intervention** is indicated for a specific pathology (e.g., thrombolysis for an occlusive venous thrombus or inferior vena caval filter placement for prevention of pulmonary embolus).
- Additionally, central venous catheter placement is indicated when medical treatment necessitates the need for **pharmacotherapy** (i.e., port placement for oncologic therapy) or hemodialysis (Fig. 29.2).

Fig. 29.2 Central Venous Access. A 55-year-old with a known history of kidney failure presented with shortness of breath from pulmonary edema. (A) The chest radiograph demonstrates cardiomegaly and pulmonary edema (*white arrows*). (B) A tunneled hemodialysis line (highlighted in *circle*) was placed utilizing image-guided intervention in the radiology department, allowing the clinicians to perform dialysis and facilitating a net removal of fluid from the patient. The tip of the hemodialysis catheter (*black arrow*) is in the right atrium.

Procedure for Central Venous Access

- For venous access, **ultrasound guidance** is utilized to **locate** and **gain entry into the central veins** without injury to adjacent tissues/organs. Nearby anatomic landmarks or the relationship to a known artery may be used instead of ultrasound.
- The venous access site of choice depends on the type of procedure performed.
    - For **central venous** catheter placement, the internal jugular, femoral, and subclavian veins are commonly used as access points.
    - **Peripherally inserted central venous catheters (PICCs)** are placed in the upper extremity veins, above the elbow, with the tip of the catheter usually located in the superior vena cava (see Fig. 10.8).
    - Most commonly, a needle is inserted into the selected vein with subsequent exchange for a catheter via a wire, using the Seldinger technique.

> ### » IMPORTANT POINTS
>
> - Central venous catheters can be **tunneled**, which requires an additional procedure in which a segment of the catheter is placed (tunneled) **under** the adjacent **soft tissues.** These catheters may have a segment in the subcutaneous tract wrapped in material to encourage cellular ingrowth to secure the catheter, which is referred to as a **cuff.**
>   - **Tunneled** central venous catheters are considered to be more **resistant** to **central line infections** compared with nontunneled central venous catheters. They are used for **long-term** hemodialysis or pharmacotherapy (e.g., chemotherapy or parenteral nutrition) (see Fig. 29.2B).

Benefits and Potential Risks of Central Venous Access

- Central venous catheter placement allows for venous access, intervention, and pharmacotherapy. Tunneled or subcutaneous central venous access may obviate the need for repeated central access procedures if multiple treatments are needed.
- Risks of venous access include **bleeding** and **injury** to tissues and organs adjacent to the vessels as attempts are made to gain access. Access from the neck can be complicated by pneumothorax, hemothorax, and inadvertent subclavian and carotid puncture. Arteriovenous fistula formation is a rare, but reported, complication.

PULMONARY EMBOLISM: THROMBOLYSIS

- **Massive pulmonary embolism (PE)** is defined as **PE with sustained hypotension.** This is irrespective of the radiologic **burden of clot** in the pulmonary arterial tree. The "burden of clot" generally refers to the qualitative assessment of thrombus in the pulmonary arteries. Quantitative scoring methods exist, but are used infrequently.

> ### » IMPORTANT POINTS
>
> - **First-line treatment** for massive PE, in the absence of a known contraindication, is **intravenous thrombolysis** where a medication, such as **tissue plasminogen activator (tPA),** is administered in large doses to dissolve the clot (Fig. 29.3 shows similar results using thrombectomy).

Indications for Catheter-Directed Pulmonary Embolism Thrombolysis

- Patients who have massive PE and are at high risk for developing a bleeding complication if they were to receive **systemic intravenous thrombolytic medication.**
- Those who have active bleeding, are perioperative from major surgery, or who have known metastatic cancer in the brain, for example, are at high risk to receive systemic thrombolytic therapy. They may be candidates for a more focal **catheter-based intervention,** such as catheter clot fragmentation, aspiration of clot, or lysis catheter placement.

Fig. 29.3 Pulmonary Embolism With Thrombectomy. This is a 56-year-old woman with chest pain and hemoptysis. (A) CT angiography of the chest demonstrates a thrombus in the right main pulmonary artery (*solid white arrow*) and a smaller embolus on the left (*dotted white arrow*). (B) The same patient is now status, post-percutaneous mechanical thrombectomy of the right pulmonary artery which opacifies with contrast because it is now free of thrombus (*dotted white arrow*). There has been an interval increase in bilateral pleural effusions (*solid white arrows*).

- **Submassive pulmonary embolism** is defined as **PE without hemodynamic instability.** There is a wide spectrum of disease in this category, from a clinically asymptomatic subsegmental PE that was incidentally noted on chest CT to a large burden of clot in a patient who is tachycardic and may be short of breath.
  - Although the traditional treatment for submassive PE is intravenous anticoagulation, there has been research and a clinical movement toward **catheter-based therapies** for the subgroup with high-risk features for **progressing to massive PE.**
    - Among others, these features include **elevated biomarkers** (troponin and brain natriuretic peptide) and evidence of **right heart strain** on imaging.

Procedure for Catheter-Directed Thrombolysis

- Under fluoroscopic guidance, a flexible catheter is inserted in the **common femoral vein** or **internal jugular vein** and threaded through the **heart** to access the **pulmonary arteries.**
- Various types of catheters with multiple holes can be placed into the **clot itself** to administer medications (**thrombolytic medication**) that can be infused over time to dissolve the clot. Other catheters that use technologies to accelerate clot lysis, such as ultrasound, are also in use clinically. Still other devices can also be introduced that fragment or aspirate the thrombus.

Benefits and Potential Risks of Catheter-Directed Thrombolysis

- **Catheter-based thrombolysis** or **thrombus removal** can **decrease the right heart pressure** rapidly and may prevent the patient from developing further hemodynamic compromise compared with anticoagulation alone.
- In the case of massive pulmonary embolism, catheter-based therapies may be **life-saving** when systemic thrombolysis is contraindicated or is utilized but is unsuccessful in improving the patient's clinical status.
- Risks of catheter-based lysis include **bleeding** at **other sites** remote to the lytic infusion due to the systemic circulation of the medication after it passes through the lungs back to the left heart.
- Additional risks include **arrhythmias** when passing catheters and wires through the heart, and, rarely, **injury to the pulmonary artery, cardiac valves,** or **heart** itself.

PULMONARY EMBOLISM: INFERIOR VENA CAVAL (IVC) FILTER PLACEMENT

Indications for IVC Filter Placement

- IVC filter placement is a controversial topic, but is generally accepted for the following US Food and Drug Administration–approved indications:
  - **Pulmonary thromboembolism** when **anticoagulation is contraindicated**
  - **Progression of venous thromboembolic disease** despite use of anticoagulation
  - **Following massive PE** when anticipated benefits of conventional therapy are reduced

- **Chronic, recurrent PE** when anticoagulant therapy has **failed**
- Many vena caval filters may be placed "off-label" on a case-by-case basis for other indications, such as prolonged immobility after trauma; prior to some types of surgery where the postoperative risk of PE is felt to be high; and as protection for proximal iliac or IVC deep venous thrombosis.
- Contraindications to filter placement include an **inability to access the IVC** (e.g., due to thrombosis or anatomic anomalies) or a vena caval size **too large** or **too small** for a filter to deploy properly.
- IVC filters are most commonly placed in the **infrarenal IVC** in proximity to the renal vein inflow. This is felt to promote **lysis of clot** captured in the **filter** and **prevent filter thrombosis.** A **suprarenal filter** is sometimes placed above the renal veins when required during **pregnancy,** when there is **insufficient room** below the renal veins to accommodate a filter and in instances where there is variant renal vein anatomy (Fig. 29.4).

Procedure for IVC Filter Placement

- Central venous access is obtained via a jugular or femoral vein. The right jugular or right femoral is preferred given the typical rigidity of the IVC delivery system, but the left common femoral vein is commonly used and placement via the upper extremity veins has been described.
- **IVC venography** is **first performed** with a diagnostic catheter to allow for:
  - Visualization of the **venous anatomy**, including location of the renal veins, and to see if any venous variants are present

Fig. 29.4 Inferior Vena Caval Filter. A filter (*solid white arrow*) is deployed in the inferior vena cava (IVC) as seen on this close-up of a conventional radiograph of the lower abdomen. Hooks on the filter are designed to anchor it in the vena cava to prevent filter migration. The dotted white arrow indicates the direction of blood flow in the IVC.

- Determination of the **size of the IVC**, which can affect filter type
- Determination of **IVC patency**
- After the IVC anatomy and desired filter location have been determined, the catheter is exchanged for an **IVC filter-delivery sheath**. The filter is deployed from inside the sheath and the sheath is withdrawn.
- Postplacement venograms are sometimes performed to confirm appropriate positioning. The catheter and wire are removed. Pressure is then applied to the access site until hemostasis is achieved.

Benefits and Potential Risks of IVC Filter Placement

- The intended benefit is to potentially decrease the incidence of new clinically significant emboli to the lungs. IVC filters **do not prevent** new deep-venous thrombus formation nor do they decrease the amount of thrombus burden already present. The actual clinical benefit, which is still under investigation, is a source of debate.
- Potential **risks** include **filter migration, filter fracture, or filter element penetration through** the IVC wall. Caval and renal vein thrombosis are other rare, but significant, complications. Some of the risks can be mitigated by retrievable filters, if they are removed promptly after caval filtration is no longer medically necessary.
- Although counterintuitive, IVC filters have been associated with an increased risk of deep vein thrombosis in the lower extremities.

PULMONARY NODULE: IMAGE-GUIDED BIOPSY

- **Image-guided biopsy** is a means of accurately obtaining a tissue sample of a lesion for diagnostic analysis.

- Sampling of a lesion can determine its characteristics (benign or malignant) or provide additional information about a known lesion (cytogenetics).

Indications for Image-Guided Biopsy

> ### ▶ IMPORTANT POINTS
>
> - Image-guided biopsy is indicated for the **minimally invasive sampling** of a lesion previously identified on an imaging study or when **pathology is in question** to aid in yielding a definitive diagnosis.

- The lesion to be sampled should be reliably visualized on at least one imaging modality.

Procedure for Image-Guided Biopsy

- The modality that most reliably demonstrates the lesion should be used for the biopsy, if feasible; if the lesion was best seen on CT, then CT localization will probably be used for the biopsy.
- A trajectory from a cutaneous entry point, along a percutaneous tract to the lesion should be determined. Sometimes a course through a natural orifice may be used.
- Careful understanding of the anatomy is necessary to avoid injuring structures (e.g., blood vessels or nerves) that can lead to increased morbidity.
- In the case of a **pulmonary nodule biopsy**, a path that limits the number of pleural surfaces crossed by the biopsy needle and avoids large blood vessels is usually chosen.
- Under image guidance (CT, ultrasound, fluoroscopy, or MRI), a needle is advanced into the lesion with visual confirmation that the tip of the needle is in the lesion.
- Samples for pathology may be obtained for cytology through **aspiration** or by using a **biopsy device** to take needle-sized pieces of tissue (Fig. 29.5).

Fig. 29.5 Pulmonary Nodule Biopsy. A 68-year-old man with extensive pulmonary disease and a long smoking history presented with worsening cough with hemoptysis. (A) Chest CT demonstrates a solitary pulmonary nodule in the posterior aspect of the left upper lobe (*white arrow*), which is consistent with a malignancy. (B) A percutaneous biopsy of the lesion for a tissue diagnosis was requested. The biopsy needle (*dotted arrow*) traverses the nodule (*solid white arrow*) from a posterior approach. The patient is lying in the right lateral decubitus position to enable the biopsy needle to pass through the shortest path to reach the lesion and potentially reduce the risk of pneumothorax. *A,* Anterior; *P,* posterior.

- Samples for analysis may be taken at the same time, if clinically indicated.
- If the need exists for **multiple samples** in a challenging location, a coaxial system is often used, which involves placing a **larger needle** into the lesion (called the **access needle**) and performing the biopsy using **smaller needles/devices** through the larger access needle.

Benefits and Potential Risks of Image-Guided Biopsy

- Image-guided biopsy provides a minimally invasive means of tissue sampling that can **obviate the need for surgical biopsy** in many cases.
- **Risks** include bleeding, infection, injury to surrounding organs and structures, and a false–negative biopsy result.
- In the case of pulmonary nodule biopsies, risks also include pneumothorax, hemothorax, pulmonary hemorrhage, chest wall hematoma, intercostal nerve injury, and even, very rarely, stroke from air embolism.

> ## ▶▶ IMPORTANT POINTS
>
> - For **small** and **stable** pneumothoraces on serial images, the treatment is **conservative management** with observation.
> - **Chest-tube insertion** is indicated for a **large or symptomatic** pneumothorax or one that is **enlarging** on serial imaging studies.

HEPATIC/RENAL/PULMONARY TUMOR: THERMAL ABLATION

- **Thermal ablation** is an umbrella term for tissue destruction using extreme heat or cold. Common forms of thermal ablation include **radiofrequency** and **microwave ablation** through tissue heating and **cryoablation**, which has a cytotoxic effect through tissue cooling. Other forms of thermal ablation using laser and high-intensity focused-ultrasound are in practice at some centers.
- **Nonthermal ablation** techniques include **chemical ablation** (e.g., using acetic acid or ethanol) and newer technologies, such as irreversible **electroporation**, a process that increases the permeability of the cell membranes causing cell death.

Indications for Thermal Ablation

- **Pulmonary tumor ablation** is indicated for **early-stage lung cancer** (usually non–small-cell lung cancer) in patients who are **not candidates for resection** or who **refuse** surgical resection. Thermal ablation using either radiofrequency or microwave is most commonly used.
  - Pulmonary tumor ablation for **metastatic disease** may be considered for small, limited disease to the lungs in an otherwise controlled cancer.
- **Hepatic tumor ablation** was first performed using chemical ablation but thermal means, predominately using heat in the form of radiofrequency ablation and microwave ablation, is most commonly used now. Microwave usage is newer, and its use has increased because of its ability to produce an ablation zone of similar size to radiofrequency, but in less time (Fig. 29.6).
  - Hepatic tumor ablation is most efficacious in **early-stage small, hepatocellular carcinomas** (≤3 cm), oligometastatic disease in patients who are not surgical candidates, or as a bridge to transplantation for patients with hepatocellular carcinoma. **Oligometastatic** is defined as a state of highly localized and limited metastatic tumors for which local ablative therapy might be curative.

Fig. 29.6 Preablation and Postablation of a Hepatocellular Carcinoma (HCC). (A) This 62-year-old male with history of hepatitis C presented with abdominal pain and was found to have a mass in the liver consistent with a hepatocellular carcinoma as shown on this postcontrast T1-weighted MRI image. The lesion in the right lobe of the liver enhances on the arterial phase (*white arrow*). (B) CT imaging immediately following microwave ablation of the tumor demonstrates a geographic area of hypoattenuation with a peripheral enhancing rim (*black arrows*) representing expected postablation changes.

- **Renal tumor ablation** is generally performed with radiofrequency or **cryoablation**, with the latter more frequently used because of the ability to monitor the active ablation zone that is appropriate to treat the tumor while sparing as much normal kidney parenchyma as possible.
  - Renal tumor ablation is indicated for **small renal masses** in patients who have: **comorbid conditions** that prevent surgery, have a condition that requires sparing of renal parenchyma (e.g., a **solitary kidney**), or who **refuse surgical** removal and desire a minimally invasive treatment.

Procedure for Thermal Ablation

- Ablation probes can be placed using ultrasound, CT, or MRI.
- Depending on the modality of ablation utilized, the type of tumor to be ablated (i.e., pulmonary, hepatic, or renal), and the morphology of the tumor, **multiple probes or multiple overlapping ablations may be used** to ablate the entire tumor effectively.
- Imaging is obtained before and during the procedure to ensure the probes are placed for effective treatment and to monitor the ablation margin, depending on the modality used (Fig. 29.7).
- Adjustments in the ablation settings and time are based on the intraprocedural imaging.
- Postablation imaging is often performed to evaluate for procedural complications (e.g., bleeding or pneumothorax) and the adequacy of ablation.

▶▶ IMPORTANT POINTS

- An adequate margin beyond the visibly involved tissue is recommended to reduce the chance of incomplete ablation or residual tumor. In the case of hepatocellular carcinomas, a 1-cm margin or more is usually desired.

Benefits and Potential Risks of Thermal Ablation

- Thermal ablation provides a minimally invasive approach for treatment of primary or metastatic tumors. In the appropriate setting, ablation may **obviate the need for surgery** and reduce morbidity in patients who are not candidates for surgical treatment.
- **Risks** of thermal ablation include infection, bleeding, and injury to adjacent tissues or solid organs through unintended thermal injury, or injuries caused by the probe itself (including pneumothorax). Although controversial, a potential risk exists of spreading the tumor (known as **seeding**), but certain ablation techniques may mitigate such an occurrence.

PORTAL HYPERTENSION: TRANSJUGULAR INTRAHEPATIC PORTOSYSTEMIC SHUNT (TIPS)

▶▶ IMPORTANT POINTS

- **TIPS** placement (usually shortened to just "TIPS") is a minimally invasive procedure for **lowering the portal pressure** by decompression through the creation of a **portal-hepatic venous shunt**. This shunt allows blood to **bypass** the **parenchyma of the liver** in order to return to the **heart**. By doing so, the shunt **decreases** the pressure in the portal venous system and can help control the sequelae of sinusoidal or postsinusoidal portal hypertension, most especially **varices**. TIPS can also act as a conduit for portal, splenic, or superior mesenteric vein thrombectomy/thrombolysis.

Indications for TIPS

- The major indications for TIPS are the control of **recurrent variceal bleeding** refractory to endoscopic and medical management and **control of abdominal ascites** and/or **hepatic hydrothorax** that does not respond to medical management (Fig. 29.8). Additional indications include treatment of hepatic congestion from Budd-Chiari syndrome and as a means of access for portomesenteric thrombectomy/thrombolysis.

Fig. 29.7 Hepatocellular Cancer Ablation. This CT image was obtained for localization confirmation during the microwave ablation of the right hepatic lobe HCC in the patient shown in Fig. 29.6. The ablation probe (*white arrow*) is implanted within the tumor (*circle*).

Fig. 29.8 Cirrhosis with Varices: Pre-TIPS. A 48-year-old woman with cirrhosis presented with refractory ascites and a history of recurrent variceal bleeding. There is a large volume of ascites (A), nodular contour of the liver (L), as well as varices (*circle*), all sequelae of portal hypertension. Oral contrast opacifies the stomach.

Procedure for TIPS

- Traditionally, right-sided internal jugular venous access is obtained with subsequent catheterization of a hepatic vein, classically the right hepatic vein.
- A long needle is placed through a curved cannula in the hepatic vein to direct the needle **through the hepatic parenchyma toward the portal vein.** From the right hepatic vein, the right portal vein is anatomically anterior and inferior.
- Gentle aspiration is performed with slow withdrawal of the needle or catheter and blood return indicates that the needle or catheter is in a blood vessel. Contrast is then injected to **confirm portal venous access.**
- A wire is passed from the hepatic vein catheter/needle into the portal vein over which a **stent** is ultimately passed and **deployed across the tract from the portal vein back to the hepatic vein-IVC junction.** A specialized TIPS stent is available that is partially covered in a material to act as a barrier to tissue ingrowth and to line the parenchymal tract.
- Pressure measurements of the portal vein and right atrium are obtained both before and after placing the TIPS to assess for decrease in the gradient between the portal system and the systemic venous system.
  - A **decrease** in the pressure gradient below 12 mm Hg is recommended to reduce the chance of bleeding from varices.
- **Embolization** of esophageal and gastric **varices** may be performed before or after placing a TIPS stent, based on operator preference.
- Repeat venography is done to assess flow through the TIPS, which should demonstrate preferential flow **through the TIPS** as opposed to through the varices. Pressures are rechecked with the expectation of a reduction in the gradient between the portal pressure and right atrial pressure (Fig. 29.9).

Benefits and Potential Risks of TIPS placement

- **TIPS** can provide relief of portal hypertension and often reduce or eliminate symptoms of variceal bleeding or recurrent ascites.
- Risks of TIPS are generally divided into **procedural complications/risks** and **postprocedural complications/risks.**
  - Procedural risks include hepatic injury/infarction, hemoperitoneum, pneumothorax, skin radiation injury (from prolonged radiation exposure), hemobilia, and injury to the biliary system or adjacent organs.

> ### ▶▶ IMPORTANT POINTS
>
> - **Hepatic encephalopathy** is a **common postprocedural complication** as blood flow after TIPS is shunted through the liver without being detoxified. Although the exact cause is not well-known, the increased blood ammonia levels and other byproducts are thought to play a role. Hepatic encephalopathy can often be **managed medically.**
> - Additional postprocedural complications include **recurrent variceal bleeding** or **ascites,** as well as shunt dysfunction, including TIPS thrombosis.
> - Heart failure from increased volume of blood return to the right heart and progressive liver failure from decreased perfusion are also known complications.

ABSCESS: PERCUTANEOUS ABSCESS ASPIRATION AND DRAIN PLACEMENT

- **Abscess aspiration and drain placement** can provide definitive diagnosis and help bring curative relief for infected collections that are accessible with image guidance.
- The abscess or fluid collection can be targeted for **sampling** with aspiration if diagnosis is unclear, or a drain may be

Fig. 29.9 Transjugular Intrahepatic Portosystemic Shunt (TIPS) Procedure. (A) A catheter (*white arrow*) has been placed through the TIPS tract connecting the hepatic vein, via the liver parenchyma, to the portal vein. Opacification of the left gastric vein (*dotted black arrow*) and gastric varices (*solid black arrow*) are secondary to elevated portal venous pressures promoting flow through the varices. (B) A stent (*dotted black arrow*) has now been placed through the parenchymal tract connecting the hepatic and portal venous systems. The varices are no longer filling with contrast (*white oval*), illustrating the desired physiologic change in the pressure gradient through the portal venous system.

Fig. 29.10 Periappendiceal Abscess With Drain. (A) Abdominal/pelvic CT demonstrates a large abscess (*white arrow*) in a 34-year-old female patient with severe right lower quadrant pain. This abscess was secondary to perforated appendicitis. (B) The patient subsequently underwent percutaneous drain placement (*dotted white arrow*) that was left in place to allow for resolution of the abscess while she simultaneously received antibiotic therapy.

placed through the percutaneous tract used to access the abscess to allow for **drainage.**

- Common regions for abscess drainage include the mediastinum, abdomen (intraperitoneal and retroperitoneal), pelvis, gluteal region, and solid organs, such as the liver, kidney and spleen.

Indications for Abscess Aspiration and Drain Placement

- Imaging modalities used for aspiration and drain placement include ultrasound, fluoroscopy and/or CT.

> ## ⟫ IMPORTANT POINTS
>
> - In general, any complex fluid collection diagnosed as an abscess or suggestive of an abscess on imaging that includes some component that can be drained (i.e., is **liquid in character**) is a candidate for image-guided aspiration and possible drain placement.

Procedure for Abscess Aspiration and Drain Placement

- Preprocedural imaging is reviewed to determine if there is **enough fluid** present to place a needle and catheter into the collection for safe aspiration and drainage.
- The skin and subcutaneous tract are anesthetized and, under image guidance, a needle is passed through the tract into the collection.
- The target location is confirmed by imaging and aspiration is performed, at which time aspirate may be sent to the laboratory for analysis, if desired.
- Once the determination has been made that a drain will be left in place, a wire is placed into the abscess cavity through the needle that was used to access it.
- The **drainage catheter** is placed into the abscess cavity over the wire and the wire is removed, with the subsequent creation of a **retaining loop** to keep the drainage catheter seated within the cavity (Fig. 29.10). Another technique utilizes a **trocar,**

Fig. 29.11 Postabscess Drainage Resolution. The previously demonstrated abscess (see Fig. 29.10A) from a perforated appendix is almost completely resolved (*solid white arrow*). Note the subcutaneous tract that remains from the abscess drain (which has been removed) made visible by scarring and inflammatory changes along the drain's path (*dotted white arrow*).

which functions as the access needle from which the drain is fed directly into the collection.

- The drainage catheter is then **anchored** in place with subcutaneous sutures and is connected to a drainage bag.
- The drain is left in place **until the infection has cleared**, as demonstrated by clinical factors (e.g., symptoms abate or patient is afebrile), laboratory values normalize, and no significant drainage (e.g., <10 mL/day) (Fig. 29.11).
- The precise drainage removal parameters are dictated by a clinical assessment of the patient on a case-by-case basis. In some centers the tube is injected under fluoroscopy to confirm patency of the drain and exclude the presence of any residual collection or fistula to adjacent structures prior to removal.

Benefits and Potential Risks of Abscess Aspiration and Drain Placement

- **Abscess aspiration and drainage** provide diagnostic information and curative treatment to those affected. Percutaneous drainage can obviate the need for surgery in many cases
- **Risks, depending on location, include:**
  - **Spread of infection**, including septic shock, peritonitis, or mediastinitis
  - **Bleeding**, hematoma, hemoperitoneum, or hemothorax
  - **Fistula formation** by forming a tract into adjacent structures or forming a tract into the subcutaneous soft tissues, creating a cutaneous fistula

GASTROINTESTINAL (GI) BLEEDING: ARTERIOGRAPHY AND EMBOLIZATION

- **GI bleeding** from either an upper or lower GI source can cause symptomatic anemia or hemodynamic instability and could result in death if not treated.
- Presenting symptoms can vary from hematemesis, melena, or frank bright-red blood per rectum (hematochezia).
- The initial **imaging study of choice** for a **lower GI bleed (LGIB)** is **CT angiography** (see Fig. 18.17) or, possibly, a radionuclide tagged-red blood cell scan to assess for the location and presence of active bleeding.
- Frequently **endoscopic evaluation** is the first diagnostic/therapeutic maneuver in patients with **upper GI bleeding (UGIB)** (proximal to the ligament of Treitz) to identify the source of bleeding that, if located, may be treated by the endoscopist.

Indications for GI Arteriography and Embolization

Fig. 29.12 CT Angiogram Showing Lower GI Bleed. A 36-year-old male presented to the emergency department with bright red blood per rectum. CT angiography of the abdomen and pelvis demonstrates focal, active extravasation of contrast in the terminal ileum (*solid white arrow*). The cecum is distended with dense contents representing stool and blood products (*dotted white arrow*). A partially visualized percutaneous jejunostomy tube (*black arrow*) is seen within the left upper abdomen and used for nutritional support.

> ## ▶▶ IMPORTANT POINTS
>
> - **Positive bleeding scan** (abdominal CT angiography or tagged-red blood cell study demonstrating active lower GI bleeding [Fig. 29.12]).
> - **Active upper GI bleeding** demonstrated on endoscopy with an inability to satisfactorily treat the bleeding from an endoscopic approach.
> - **Massive lower GI hemorrhage** with **hemodynamic instability** generally warrants immediate interventional radiology and surgery consult and may bypass noninvasive diagnostic imaging.
> - Angiography may be valuable in those who have ongoing symptomatic **anemia** with **melena**, requiring **frequent blood transfusions** despite negative or equivocal body imaging studies.

Procedure for GI Arteriography and Embolization

- After preprocedural CT angiography, tagged RBC scan or endoscopy is reviewed to aid in localization of the bleeding, arterial access is obtained and arteriography is performed in the branch arteries supplying the area of concern.
- If **initial arteriography is negative**, a stepwise approach can be performed to interrogate major branch vessels of the upper and lower arterial anatomy (e.g., the gastroduodenal artery in upper GI bleeding and the right colic artery in a LGIB).

- In the case of **upper GI bleeding, prophylactic embolization** of the blood vessel supplying the anatomic area of reported bleeding may be performed because of the **rich collateral supply** to the organs of the upper abdomen and the low incidence of visualizing active bleeding on angiography despite ongoing active bleeding.
- In the case of **lower GI bleeding, embolization** is usually **only performed if the source of active bleeding is identified.** This is due to the increased risk of ischemia compared with the upper GI tract (Fig. 29.13).
- The type of embolic material used (e.g., metallic coil, cyanoacrylate glue, or Gelfoam) depends on the location of the bleed, the patient's hemodynamic status and comorbidities, as well as operator preference.
- Once embolization of the bleeding is complete, a **postembolization arteriogram** is performed to ensure the bleeding has stopped.

Benefits and Potential Risks of GI Arteriography and Embolization

> ## ▶▶ IMPORTANT POINTS
>
> - **GI arteriography and embolization** can provide diagnostic confirmation of the location and then intervention that can lead to symptomatic relief and may be lifesaving in severe cases of GI bleeding.

Fig. 29.13 Digital Subtraction Angiogram (DSA) and Occlusion of Lower GI Bleed (LGIB). These digital subtraction images are produced by imaging an area before contrast is given and then using that image to electronically mask-out all but the contrast in subsequent images. (A) Delayed DSA imaging of the ileocolic artery (*black arrow*) demonstrates a focal blush of contrast (*white circle*) in the region of the cecum and terminal ileum corresponding to the region of active extravasation on the previous CTA (see Fig. 29.12), originating from a branch of the ileocolic artery. (B) Status post-insertion of a coil for embolization of the bleeding vessel (*white circle*) shows no further extravasation.

- **Risks** of GI arteriography and embolization consist of the standard risks of arteriography, including vessel dissection from manipulation with guidewires, bleeding, and/or access site hematoma.
- **Nontarget embolization** can occur and refers to placement of embolic material in an unintended vessel because of catheter malpositioning or a technical issue in deploying the embolic agent.
- **Ischemia** can occur after embolization, which can result in bowel infarction, which can lead to perforation and may require surgical resection. This is more common after embolization of lower GI bleeding, where the collateral blood supply is less robust compared with the upper GI tract.

OBSTRUCTIVE UROPATHY: PERCUTANEOUS NEPHROSTOMY (PCN)/NEPHROURETEROSTOMY (PCNU)

- **Obstructive uropathy,** or obstruction of the renal collecting system, can cause symptoms of renal colic and radiating flank pain and can lead to renal failure or urosepsis, if not recognized and treated promptly.
- **Renal obstruction** can be secondary to **renal calculi** that become lodged within the ureter (Fig. 29.14), **malignancy** within the abdomen or pelvis (including bladder or urothelial tumors of the ureter), or secondary to **ureteral inflammatory changes** (e.g., Crohn disease, diverticulitis, or retroperitoneal fibrosis). Renal obstruction will demonstrate varying degrees of hydronephrosis on imaging.

Fig. 29.14 Hydronephrosis and Calculi. This 75-year-old woman presented with severe abdominal and flank pain in addition to hematuria. Noncontrast CT of the abdomen shows moderate hydronephrosis (*solid white arrow*) and multiple renal calculi (*dotted white arrows*). She also had ureteral calculi with an obstructing stone at the ureteropelvic junction causing the hydronephrosis (not shown).

Indications for Percutaneous Nephrostomy/Nephroureterostomy

- **Hydronephrosis,** either with or without signs of **renal failure**, infection, or secondary to renal/ureteral stones, malignancy, or inflammation
- **Urinary diversion** that is not amenable to urologic intervention in cases of ureteral rupture, leak, or fistula formation between the ureter and adjacent organs

- **Preoperative access** to the urinary collecting system prior to ureteroplasty (dilation of the ureter) or nephrolithotomy (stone removal)

Procedure for Percutaneous Nephrostomy/ Nephroureterostomy

- Preprocedural imaging is reviewed to determine the best approach for percutaneous access to the desired renal calyx.
- **Ultrasound and/or fluoroscopic guidance** is used to help determine the approach to the target so as to deliver superficial and subcutaneous anesthetic along the approach route.
- An **access needle** is then used to course along the anesthetized tract under image guidance until the tip lies within the **renal calyx,** which is confirmed by aspiration of urine and often an injection of contrast.
- A guidewire is then inserted through the needle into the renal pelvis with subsequent **dilation** of the access tract prior to catheter placement.
- If **percutaneous nephrostomy** placement is desired, the nephrostomy catheter is inserted over the wire with a **locking loop** formed within the renal pelvis (Fig. 29.15).
- For **percutaneous nephroureterostomy (PCNU)**, a series of catheters and guidewires is maneuvered to **cross** the stricture/ stenosis/obstruction until access is gained into the urinary bladder, at which time the PCNU is advanced into the bladder and loops are formed in the bladder and renal pelvis.
- In both cases, the catheter is secured to the skin and is **connected to a drainage bag** for urine collection. Alternatively, a **cap** may be placed on the external portion in order to **promote internal drainage**, through the bladder and urethra so long as there is antegrade drainage.

Benefits and Potential Risks for Percutaneous Nephrostomy/ Nephroureterostomy

> ### ⟩⟩ IMPORTANT POINTS
>
> - PCN and PCNU placement can provide symptomatic relief of **obstructive uropathy,** allow for **urinary diversion,** decompress an obstructed, infected collecting system, or for preprocedural access in a minimally invasive manner.

- **Risks** of PCN and PCNU placement are bleeding, bacteremia through spread of infection during placement, peritonitis, and pneumothorax in cases where the approach is high enough to cross the pleura.
- Renal hemorrhage, pseudoaneurysm formation or renal arteriovenous fistula formation can cause severe symptoms and in rare cases may require additional surgical or interventional radiology intervention (e.g., embolization of a bleeding vessel).

AORTIC ANEURYSM: ENDOVASCULAR ANEURYSM REPAIR (EVAR)

- An **aortic aneurysm** is a focal or segmental enlargement of the aorta resulting from weakening of all three layers of the arterial wall.
- **True aortic aneurysms** are defined by an enlargement that is greater >1.5 to 2 times the normal size and can occur anywhere along the course of the aorta, although they are more common in the abdominal aorta.

> ### ⟩⟩ IMPORTANT POINTS
>
> - Small aortic aneurysms are usually periodically imaged because of the increasing risk of rupture if they enlarge. **Intervention** usually occurs if the patient is symptomatic or when the abdominal aortic aneurysm reaches **5.5 cm in diameter** or the aneurysm **grows** over a **short period** of time.
> - **Aneurysm repair** can be achieved either with **open surgical repair** or through an **endovascular approach** with a covered stent placement (**endograft**), which forms an **endoluminal channel** through which the blood flows with the purpose of **excluding flow** through the aneurysm sac itself. **Covered stents** are generally metal stents wrapped with a fabric or graft material that is designed to **inhibit** the eventual growth of tissue that may occlude the stent and prevent flow of blood through the interstices of the stent.

Indications for EVAR

- A thoracic or abdominal aneurysm that is **asymptomatic and ≥5.5 cm** or has a growth rate of >1 cm/year or > 0.5 cm in 6 months
- **Symptomatic** thoracic or abdominal aneurysm, regardless of size
- Thoracic or abdominal aneurysm with **known or impending rupture**

Fig. 29.15 Percutaneous Nephrostomy (PCN). (A) Image from fluoroscopically guided placement demonstrates a looped (*solid white arrow*) right PCN tube (*dotted white arrow*) with contrast injected through the tube showing the proximal ureter (*solid black arrow*) in the same patient as Fig. 29.14. (B) The right-sided PCN (*solid white arrow*) remains in place on this follow-up CT image without contrast. Hydronephrosis (*circle*) is no longer seen. The renal calculi remain (*dashed white arrow*).

Procedure for EVAR

- In general, preprocedural imaging entails CT or MR angiography to fully characterize the aortic aneurysm and best determine the ideal location to place the endovascular stent graft.
- Either unilateral or bilateral common **femoral artery access** is achieved utilizing the Seldinger technique **percutaneously** or by performing surgical **cut-downs** (surgical opening of subcutaneous tissues to expose the arteries).
- A **marking catheter** is advanced into the aorta and an **aortogram** is performed, which also allows for length measurement of the stent graft needed for adequate coverage of the aneurysm.
- The stent graft is deployed over stiff guidewires to allow maximal control during placement (Fig. 29.16).
- The ideal placement ensures **no vital aortic branch vessels are occluded** during placement (e.g., superior mesenteric artery or renal arteries) or that a fenestrated stent graft is deployed to allow for patency of major arteries (e.g., renal arteries). The inferior mesenteric artery is often covered by the graft.
- A **completion aortogram** is performed to ensure **no leak** around or through the new endograft exists.
- Surveillance imaging will look for any residual flow into the excluded part of the aneurysm, referred to as the **aneurysm sac.** Continued **flow** into the **excluded portion** of the aneurysm is referred to as an **endoleak.**
- Occasionally blood vessels that were excluded by the endograft can continue to bring blood **into** the **aneurysm sac.** This is most commonly seen with lumbar and inferior mesenteric arteries in abdominal endografts.

Risks and Benefits of EVAR

- EVAR placement provides a minimally invasive option for repair of thoracic and abdominal aortic aneurysms, allowing patients to experience less intraprocedural blood loss and shorter hospital stays, all with comparable results to open repair in appropriately selected patients.
- Risks of EVAR placement are generally divided into two categories: **procedural-based** and **device-related.**
  - **Procedural-based risks** include aneurysm perforation, organ ischemia, and groin and/or retroperitoneal hematoma.
  - **Device-related risks** include stent-graft migration, stent fracture, stent thrombosis, and/or stenosis, and endoleak.

UTERINE FIBROIDS: UTERINE FIBROID EMBOLIZATION (UFE)

- **Uterine fibroids (leiomyomas)** are benign uterine tumors. They may be highly symptomatic and may be responsible for heavy menstrual bleeding (either menorrhagia or menometrorrhagia), abdominal and/or pelvic bloating, heaviness or discomfort, as well as urinary symptoms, and dyspareunia. They may also cause infertility.
- Uterine fibroids can be treated with **hormonal therapy,** excised individually through surgery (**myomectomy**), removed through a **hysterectomy**, or treated through **uterine fibroid embolization.**

Fig. 29.16 Endovascular Aneurysm Repair (EVAR). An 80-year-old male patient with a history of abdominal aortic aneurysm (AAA) presented with a pulsatile abdominal mass and pain. (A) Sagittal CT angiogram of the abdomen and pelvis demonstrated interval growth of a fusiform infrarenal AAA (*solid white arrow*) that measured about 6 cm in maximum dimension (anterior to posterior). The aneurysm does not fill with contrast because it contains plaque/thrombus. The normal aortic caliber and appearance are seen at the level of the celiac and superior mesenteric arteries (*dotted white arrow*). (B) CT angiogram in the same patient after endovascular aneurysm repair. A stent (*dotted white arrow*) that extends above and below the aneurysm sac (*solid white arrows*) was placed in the aneurysm to exclude it from the flow of blood.

Fig. 29.17 Uterine Fibroids and Uterine Fibroid Embolization (UFE). (A) This 44-year-old woman, who presented with abdominal pain and menometrorrhagia, had multiple, hypoenhancing uterine masses consistent with uterine fibroids (*white arrows*) on a T1-weighted, postcontrast MRI of the pelvis. (B) Left uterine artery angiogram demonstrates significant arterial filling of the largest uterine fibroid (*solid black arrows*) when correlated with the preprocedural MRI. At the superior aspect of the image, the catheter (*dotted black arrow*) traverses the common iliac and internal iliac arteries, terminating in the uterine artery.

Indications for UFE

> ### ▶ IMPORTANT POINTS
>
> • UFE is indicated in women with documented uterine fibroids causing symptoms of heavy menstrual bleeding, abdominal/pelvic pain/pressure/discomfort, urinary frequency or retention, dyspareunia, or any combination of these.

• UFE is **not indicated** in pregnant patients. Although fertility is less impacted than in those patients who undergo hysterectomy, UFE is generally **discouraged** in patients who **plan on pregnancy in the near future.** This is an area of controversy and the impact on fertility is still being studied.
• In addition, UFE should not be performed if a uterine **leiomyosarcoma** is suspected or in patients who may have **another cause** for their uterine bleeding (e.g., endometrial cancer).
• UFE can be performed in patients with adenomyosis; however, current information shows that it is less effective than treating fibroids.

Procedure for UFE

• Preprocedural evaluation includes review of imaging, which in most cases should include a gadolinium-enhanced pelvic MRI to best characterize the uterine fibroids and confirm their viability.
• Arterial access is achieved and uterine arteriography is performed bilaterally to establish the arterial distribution supplying the fibroids. The **uterine arteries** are usually a branch of the anterior division of the **internal iliac arteries** (Fig. 29.17).
• UFE is performed by injecting **embolic material** into the uterine arteries bilaterally to **slow** arterial flow. **Tris-acryl gelatin microspheres (nonabsorbable)** are a common product used for this purpose, but other materials, such as polyvinyl alcohol, have been described. The microspheres are injected until **stasis** within the artery is achieved, using angiography as a guide.

Fig. 29.18 Postuterine Fibroid Embolization: MRI. The same patient seen in Fig. 29.17 after uterine fibroid embolization for treatment of her fibroids. A follow-up pelvic MRI done 4 months after the embolization shows the fibroids are smaller in size (*dotted white arrows*) and do not enhance now, a desired outcome that is consistent with the fibroids having undergone necrosis.

> ### ▶ IMPORTANT POINTS
>
> • **Pain control** is an important part of intra- and postprocedural care. Moderate to severe **cramping** is common in the first 8 to 24 hours and can be treated with antiinflammatory and opioid pain medications. Patient-controlled analgesia may be used and some interventional radiologists perform a **hypogastric nerve block** as part of the UFE procedure.

• Patients may undergo follow-up pelvic MRI as well as clinical evaluation to document fibroid size and character changes and interval change in symptoms (Fig. 29.18).

Risks and Benefits of UFE

• UFE provides a minimally invasive approach toward treatment of uterine fibroids in patients who experience symptoms of heavy menstrual bleeding, abdominal pain, and/or discomfort, as well as urinary symptoms.

- The general **risks** of UFE are much the same as other arterial interventions, including bleeding, infection, and vascular injury, exist in uterine artery embolization.
- Endometritis, uterine ischemia, and necrosis are also **rare** but reported complications that may require surgical intervention or hysterectomy and could be life-threatening, especially in the setting of infection.
- **Amenorrhea/early menopause** have been described as complications and tend to become more common as a woman gets closer to menopause. This may be caused by inadvertent ovarian embolization
- **Fibroid passage** may occur in those individuals that have **intracavitary (endometrial cavity) or submucosal fibroids**, as the ischemic changes cause the sloughing of the fibroid. This may necessitate evaluation by a gynecologist to facilitate removal. Likewise **pedunculated subserosal fibroids** may detach from the uterus and migrate into the pelvis with infarction of their stalk.

ACUTE ISCHEMIC STROKE: MECHANICAL THROMBECTOMY

- **Stroke** is the result of brain tissue death from a hemorrhagic or ischemic insult. It can result in permanent neurologic deficits or death.

▶▶ IMPORTANT POINTS

- **Ischemic stroke,** if recognized early, can be treated with intravenous thrombolytics, most commonly **tissue plasminogen activator (tPA)** or **mechanical thrombectomy** to aid in revascularization of the affected brain before the infarct enlarges or undergoes hemorrhagic transformation, as neurons die quickly from ischemia.

Indications for Thrombectomy in Stroke

- Therapy for acute ischemic stroke is a widely debated subject and is the topic of many research trials.
- Current data suggest that **mechanical thrombectomy,** with either a **stent retriever** (see below) or **thrombus aspiration,** may be performed in patients:
  - Who had a **good prestroke** functional status
  - When there is **large-vessel occlusion** (internal carotid, middle cerebral, or first-branch of the middle cerebral arteries)
  - Whose onset of symptoms occurred <6 hours previously or who did not respond to intravenous thrombolytic infusion (which is administered in ischemic stroke in patients with onset of symptoms within 4.5 hours of presentation). For posterior and possibly anterior circulation strokes, the intervention window may be considerably longer. With new studies, these intervals may change.
  - **Significant neurologic deficit without** an extensive **infarct core** or **hemorrhage** on imaging of head. The **infarct core** is that portion of the infarct that will not likely improve with reperfusion.

Procedure for Mechanical Thrombectomy in Stroke

- Preprocedure imaging is **critical in directing therapy** in acute stroke and may entail noncontrast CT, CT-angiography, or

CT or MRI perfusion imaging to identify the offending thrombus to be targeted for mechanical thrombectomy.
- Arterial access is obtained and a catheter is advanced into the internal carotid artery on the affected side. Angiography is performed. The thrombus is traversed using a microcatheter, microwire, and a stent retriever device (see below) is passed through the microcatheter and unsheathed over the clot. The stent is allowed to dwell for a period of time and then pulled out through a larger guiding catheter. Aspiration systems also exist, which use suction to remove thrombus (Fig. 29.19).

Fig. 29.19 Embolic Stroke Treated With Thrombectomy. A patient who presented with acute stroke symptoms was referred to angiography for evaluation. (A) This is a selective catheterization of the right internal carotid artery (ICA) that demonstrates abrupt cutoff (*solid white arrow*) of the right middle cerebral artery (MCA) with no flow to most of the MCA's distribution. This correlates with an occlusive embolus in this segment, which was a potential target for intervention. Note that the anterior cerebral artery (ACA) and its branches are opacified. Because this is a selective catheterization of the right ICA, the left-sided vessels are not visualized. (B) In the same patient following mechanical thrombectomy, repeat right ICA arteriography shows perfusion of the entire right MCA distribution (*dotted white arrow*) beyond the previously occluded point (*circle*), signifying a technically successful intervention.

- A **stent retriever** is a small stent that is permanently fused to a long wire. The stent can be deployed over a thrombus; it will incorporate the thrombus in its interstices and can then be removed while open to **pull the clot out** with it. Most devices can be used three times (three pulls) to remove clot.
- **Postprocedural arteriography** is performed to demonstrate **revascularization** and follow-up CT imaging is done to assess the effects on the brain parenchyma following clot retrieval (e.g., hemorrhage).

Risks and Benefits of Mechanical Thrombectomy in Stroke

- Mechanical thrombectomy is a critical treatment for eligible patients to prevent further neurologic deficits and salvage that part of the brain at risk of dying but is not already dead. Patient selection is key to having satisfactory clinical outcomes.
- **Risks** for mechanical thrombectomy are **significant** and include intracranial hemorrhage, arterial dissection or perforation during thrombectomy, embolization of clot fragments, reperfusion hemorrhage, and groin hematoma.

TAKE HOME POINTS

- The indications, procedures, and risk/benefits are described for a variety of procedures that form a part of **interventional radiology**, a medical specialty that uses image guidance to perform minimally invasive diagnostic and therapeutic procedures.
- Each procedure chosen highlights a different facet of the specialty: arterial access, central venous access, thrombolysis, image-guided biopsy, tumor ablation, shunt placement, percutaneous drainage, embolization, endovascular repairs, and thrombectomy.
- A **glossary** of terms applied to some of the more widely used tools in interventional radiology is included.
- **Arterial access** facilitates many other image-guided arterial interventions (e.g., embolization for active bleeding and angioplasty for arterial stenosis).
- **Central venous access** is used for venous intervention, pharmacotherapy, or hemodialysis. Tunneled catheters are used for long-term hemodialysis or pharmacotherapy (e.g., chemotherapy or parenteral nutrition).
- Patients who have a life-threatening, massive pulmonary embolism and are at high risk for developing a bleeding complication if they receive systemic intravenous thrombolytic medication may benefit from **catheter-directed thrombectomy/thrombolysis.**
- **Inferior vena caval filters** may be placed in patients with a pulmonary embolus when anticoagulation is contraindicated or when progression of the thromboembolic disease occurs despite use of anticoagulation or in chronic, recurrent PE when anticoagulant therapy has failed.
- **Image-guided biopsy** is indicated for the minimally invasive sampling of a lesion previously identified on an imaging study or when the pathology of a lesion is in question.
- Common forms of **image-guided ablations** include radiofrequency and microwave ablation (through tissue heating), cryoablation (cooling), and chemical ablation. Pulmonary, hepatic, and renal tumors are those most frequently targeted.
- **Transjugular Intrahepatic portosystemic shunt (TIPS)** placement is a minimally invasive procedure for lowering the portal pressure by creation of a portal-hepatic venous shunt. It is used most often to control recurrent variceal bleeding refractory to endoscopic and medical management and to control abdominal ascites secondary to cirrhosis.
- **Abscess aspiration and drain placement** can provide definitive diagnosis and offer curative relief for infected collections in locations accessible with image guidance.
- **GI bleeding,** either from upper or lower GI sources, can cause symptomatic anemia or possible hemodynamic instability and could result in death if not treated. In the case of lower GI bleeding, **embolization** can be performed if the source of active bleeding is identified.
- **Percutaneous nephrostomy (PCN)/nephroureterostomy (PCNU)** can alleviate hydronephrosis secondary to renal/ureteral stones, malignancy, or inflammation. It can also be used for urinary diversion and preoperative access to the urinary collecting system.
- **Aneurysm repair** can be achieved with either open surgical repair or through an endovascular approach with a covered stent placement (endograft), which forms a new endoluminal channel through which the blood flows, the purpose being to exclude flow through the aneurysm itself.
- **Uterine fibroid embolization** may be useful in women with documented uterine fibroids causing symptoms of heavy menstrual bleeding, abdominal or pelvic pain, pressure, discomfort, urinary frequency or retention, dyspareunia, or any combination of these symptoms.
- Image-guided intervention is used in patients with **strokes.** Mechanical thrombectomy may be performed in patients with a good prestroke functional status, large-vessel occlusion, and in those in whom certain temporal requirements from the onset of stroke symptoms are met.
- Each procedure described comes with its attendant **benefits** and certain **potential risks,** including—but not limited to—bleeding, infection, vessel or other organ injury, pneumothorax, and, rarely, radiation overexposure. In all cases, the potential benefits should outweigh the potential risks for a procedure to be performed.

More information on using image-guided interventions in diagnosis and treatment (interventional radiology) is available to registered users online.

30

Recognizing the Findings in Breast Imaging

Debra Copit, MD

- Breast imaging is the field of radiology dedicated to the detection and management of breast abnormalities, especially breast cancer.
- **Breast cancer** is second only to **skin cancer** as the **most common cancer** diagnosed in **women** and is the **second leading cause of cancer death in women,** behind lung cancer.
- Medicine increasingly relies on assessments of efficacy in the diagnosis and management of disease. Toward that end, one of the key parameters in diagnosis and management of breast disease is assessment of the **lifetime risk of breast cancer,** which is defined as the likelihood that a woman will develop cancer over an 80-year life span. For example, a woman with **no known risk factors** has a lifetime risk of developing breast cancer of **approximately 12%.**
- **Risk factors** for breast cancer include **early menarche, late menopause,** and other factors, some of which are shown in Table 30.1. Certain **histopathologic findings** also increase the risk of breast cancer.

BREAST IMAGING MODALITIES: OVERVIEW

Mammography

- The most widely studied and utilized of all breast imaging studies is **mammography.** A mammogram is a type of **low-dose**

x-ray imaging developed to evaluate breast abnormalities, most importantly to diagnose breast cancer (Fig. 30.1).
- Mammograms are performed on specialized radiographic units that produce **low-energy x-rays.** A device that applies **compression** to the breast is used to improve image quality

BOX 30.1 *BRCA1* and *BRCA2* Genes

- The most common cause of hereditary breast cancer is an inherited mutation in the *BRCA1* or *BRCA2* gene. **BRCA1** and **BRCA2** are human genes that are tumor suppressors. *BRCA* is an abbreviation for **BR**east **CA**ncer.
- Mutations in these genes correlate with an increased risk of breast cancer. If *BRCA1* or *BRCA2* itself is damaged by a mutation, damaged DNA is not properly repaired.
- Females with an abnormal *BRCA1* or *BRCA2* gene have up to an 80% risk of developing breast cancer by age 90. The increased risk of developing ovarian cancer is about 55% for females with *BRCA1* mutations and about 25% for females with *BRCA2* mutations.
- **CHEK2** (Checkpoint kinase 2) is a tumor suppressor gene that encodes the protein CHK2. Inherited mutations in the *CHEK2* gene have been linked to certain cases of breast cancer.

TABLE 30.1 Lifetime Risk Categories for Breast Cancer

Category	Percent Risk	Factors Affecting Risk
Average	<15%	No known risk factors
Intermediate	15% to 25%	Strong family history of breast cancer, but no *BRCA* mutation; those with a mutation in *CHEK2* (Box 30.1); those in the highest category of mammographic density; and those with a past history of lobular carcinoma in situ or atypical hyperplasia
High	>20%	*BRCA* mutation carriers and their untested first-degree relatives, such as a sister, mother, or daughter; women with histories of chest radiation between the ages of 10 and 30; a personal history of invasive breast cancer or ductal carcinoma in situ (DCIS)

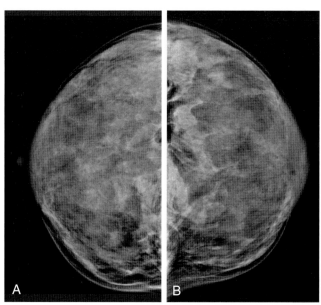

Fig. 30.1 Mammogram. Mammography, like all of radiography, utilizes the differential absorption of x-rays by fat, soft tissues, and calcifications to yield diagnostic images of the breast. It does this by using a very low dose of radiation. In this example of a right (on your left) and left (on your right) craniocaudal view of both breasts, the breast tissue is dense, which has diagnostic implications discussed in this chapter.

by reducing the **thickness** of the tissue x-rays must penetrate, decreasing radiation **scatter**, reducing the required radiation **dose**, and **holding** the breast in place. The images today are typically captured **digitally** rather than on film.

- Mammographic examinations are divided into **screening mammography** and **diagnostic mammography**. They are different, but related.
  - The purpose of **screening mammography** is to try to detect breast cancer in **asymptomatic** patients.
  - **Diagnostic mammography** is used for either a patient with **breast symptoms** (e.g., pain, lumps, nipple discharge) or those who are asked to undergo more extensive examination for **potential abnormalities detected** at the time of their **screening mammogram**. Diagnostic mammograms are also often performed on women with a **history of breast cancer** and on those with **breast implants**.
- **Digital breast tomosynthesis (DBT)** (sometimes called "3D mammography") is a type of mammography in which images are obtained at multiple different angles to create **thin slices** through the breast. It has been shown to reduce false–positive diagnoses while increasing invasive cancer detection.
- We discuss the differences between screening and diagnostic examinations later in this chapter.

Ultrasound (US)

- **Breast ultrasound** is most commonly used in conjunction with **diagnostic mammography,** but may also be performed as an **additional screening method**.
- Ultrasound is the initial study used in **average-risk, symptomatic patients under 30 years of age**.
- The primary use of ultrasound is to distinguish **cystic** from **solid** breast masses. It is also an extremely important **problem-solving tool** for patients **recalled** for additional breast imaging and in **symptomatic patients** (Fig. 30.2).
- Studies have shown that screening **high-risk patients** and patients with **dense breasts** with **ultrasound increases breast cancer detection** over mammography alone.

Magnetic Resonance Imaging (MRI)

- **Breast MRI** is used for screening certain **high-risk patients** as well as evaluating patients who have received **breast implants** (Fig. 30.3). Other indications for MRI include evaluating response to **neoadjuvant chemotherapy** or in patients with positive lymph nodes and an **unknown primary** site.
  - *Neoadjuvant chemotherapy* refers to treatment that is given to reduce the size of a tumor in advance of more definitive therapy, such as surgery.
- Breast MRI is the **most sensitive** of all breast imaging modalities, but also the most expensive. Some patients cannot tolerate an MRI because of feelings of **claustrophobia** from the scanner or because they have certain **medical devices**, such as pacemakers, or ferromagnetic foreign bodies, such as surgical clips.
- **MRI** is the **gold standard** for evaluating the **structural integrity** of **silicone breast implants,** which is discussed later in this chapter.
- The other modalities included under the umbrella of breast imaging include **contrast-enhanced mammography, molecular**

Fig. 30.2 Ultrasound of the Breast. Because, in part, of the relatively superficial nature of breast lesions and sonography's absence of ionizing radiation, ultrasound is an ideal modality to study the breast. This patient displays a mass consistent with a breast cancer (*white arrow*) discussed later in this chapter (see Fig. 30.14B).

Fig. 30.3 Breast MRI. For a breast MRI, the patient lies prone with a gap in the table for the breasts, which are surrounded by a special magnetic coil dedicated to this type of imaging. Both breasts are imaged simultaneously. The MRI images can be reconstructed by computer to be visualized in any plane. Almost all studies use gadolinium-enhancement as part of the protocol.

breast imaging, positron-emission tomography (PET), and even CT.
- We will concentrate on **mammography, ultrasound,** and **MRI**, the studies used most widely today.

MAMMOGRAPHY: SCREENING VERSUS DIAGNOSTIC

Screening Mammography

- The **sensitivity of mammography** in detecting a breast abnormality depends on breast density: as **density increases** (tissue becomes whiter) **sensitivity decreases.** As with all conventional radiography, **fat appears gray** on mammography, whereas the imaging **signs of breast cancer are whiter**. This is why the denser ("whiter") a patient's underlying breast tissue is, the more difficult it is to detect a cancer among normal tissue. Finding cancer in a dense breast has been likened to looking for a polar bear in a snowstorm.

- Breast density is divided into several categories, ranging from almost entirely fatty to very dense (see Fig. 30.1).
- Every screening mammogram consists of two views of each breast, the **craniocaudal (CC) view** and the **mediolateral oblique (MLO) view** (Fig. 30.4). As with every x-ray study, these views are named by the direction the x-ray beam passes through the tissue from the **source** to the **detector**. Thus, for the craniocaudal view the x-ray passes **from** the source above the breast (cranio-) **to** the detector that sits below the breast (caudal). As with almost all images in radiology, images are viewed with the patient's right on your left and the patient's left on your right.

Screening Recommendations

- Multiple **randomized controlled trials (RCTs)** have shown a **22% reduction in breast cancer mortality** in women who undergo screening mammography versus those who do not. **More recent and larger scale observational studies** report a

Fig. 30.4 Routine Mammographic Images. (A) Craniocaudal (CC) views are displayed with the right side on your left (RCC) and the left on your right (LCC), just as most images in radiology. (B) Right and left mediolateral oblique (MLO) views. Normal structures include areas of fat (*solid white arrows*), fibroglandular tissue (*dotted white arrows*), and the suspensory Cooper's ligaments (*white circle*).

TABLE 30.2 **Mammography Screening Recommendations—American College of Radiology**		
Risk Factors	**Start Screening**	**Frequency**
Average	Age 40	Annual screening
Women with certain *BRCA1* or *BRCA2* mutations or who are untested, but have first-degree relatives (mothers, sisters, or daughters) who are proved to have *BRCA* mutations	Age 30	Annual screening
Women with histories of mantle radiation (usually for Hodgkin disease) received between the ages of 10 and 30	Starting 8 years after the radiation therapy, but not before age 25	Annual screening
Women with ≥20% lifetime risk for breast cancer on the basis of family history (both maternal and paternal)	Starting by age 30 (but not before age 25), or 10 years earlier than the age of diagnosis of the youngest affected relative, whichever is later	Annual screening
Women with mothers or sisters with premenopausal breast cancer	Starting by age 30 (but not before age 25), or 10 years earlier than the age of diagnosis of the youngest affected relative, whichever is later	Annual screening
Women with biopsy-proven lobular neoplasia (lobular carcinoma in situ and atypical lobular hyperplasia), atypical ductal hyperplasia (ADH), ductal carcinoma in situ (DCIS), invasive breast cancer, or ovarian cancer	From time of diagnosis, regardless of age	Annual screening

38% mortality reduction from breast cancer among those screened.

- The American College of Radiology (ACR) recommends **annual mammographic screening beginning at age 40** for women at **average risk** and for **intermediate-risk women,** such as women with a personal history of breast cancer (Table 30.2). Other organizations also have guidelines.[a]

- Some organizations point to the "risks" or "harms" of mammography. These include mammograms that are interpreted as abnormal, but turn out to be normal, or biopsy recommendations that reveal benign disease (false–positive) as well as the issue of "overdiagnosis," meaning detecting cancers that may not be lethal. The ACR contends that overdiagnosis should not be a factor in deciding when to start screening or the interval between examinations.
- The ACR recommends that women should be aided in the understanding of the risks of screening, but that women themselves should weigh the benefits and risks of screening in guiding their decision to undergo screening.
- For **intermediate-risk women**, such as women with a history of breast cancer, MRI may be used as an adjunct test. Ultrasound may also be considered.
- At what age should screening mammograms stop? The randomized controlled trials that proved the mortality reduction from screening stopped at age 74, but there have been numerous studies that show continued benefit for women over the age of 74. The ACR recommends that screening be stopped based on a woman's health status and not on her age.

Diagnostic Mammography

- **Diagnostic mammograms** are performed on **symptomatic patients** (those with lumps, pain, nipple discharge), women **recalled** for **additional imaging** because of an abnormal screening mammogram, and often women with a **history of breast cancer** or **implants.**
- Any patient with **breast symptoms** who is **age 30 years or older** is first evaluated with **routine mammographic views** as described under the section above on screening mammography.
- Patients **recalled** because of prior screening mammography findings may be evaluated using a variety of **additional mammographic views.** Some of these additional views are spot compression images, spot compression magnification views, true lateral or 90 degree lateral views, rolled views, exaggerated views, and cleavage views, as well as ultrasound.
- Patients with an appropriate history (e.g., breast symptoms) who present for a diagnostic imaging examination who are **less than 30 years** of age undergo an **ultrasound** before a mammographic evaluation. Occasionally in this age group, a mammogram will be performed after the ultrasound if the sonographic findings are suspicious.
- If a patient has a **focal symptom** (e.g., pain in one spot), the technologist identifies it with a **radiopaque metal marker** placed on the breast surface prior to imaging. This helps the radiologist interpreting the images to identify the patient's area of concern. If the mammogram reveals anything **other** than a finding that is definitively benign, patients with a **focal** symptom will then undergo breast ultrasound. Patients with **generalized symptoms,** such as nonfocal pain, do not need further imaging after the mammogram.
- Although the majority of **symptomatic** breast cancers **will** display an abnormality on mammography, ultrasound, or both, some cancers will have no imaging correlate to a clinically palpable finding or a reported symptom. For example, invasive lobular carcinomas are classically difficult to detect with imaging and can also be subtle clinically (Table 30.3).

TABLE 30.3 Types of Breast Cancer

Preinvasive	Ductal Carcinoma in situ (DCIS)	Lobular Carcinoma in situ (LCIS)[a]
25%	80%	20%
Limited to basement membrane	Spreads through ducts / 1% progress to invasive cancer per year / Usually unilateral / Usually does not produce palpable mass	Does not distort breast architecture; not visible mammographically / 1% progress per year / Can be bilateral / Typically incidental finding on biopsy and almost never palpable

Invasive	Invasive Ductal Carcinoma (IDC)	Invasive Lobular Carcinoma (ILC)
75%	79%	10%
Extends beyond basement membrane	Usually originates from DCIS or LCIS precursor / Causes fibrous reaction leading to palpable mass / Metastasizes through lymphatics and bloodstream	Usually arises from LCIS precursor / Minimal fibrous response; less often produces palpable mass / May metastasize to GI tract, ovaries, uterus

Inflammatory Breast Cancer
Uncommon type of invasive carcinoma (1% to 3%), seen more in younger women and those of African ancestry
Can resemble mastitis in early stages
More aggressive; lymph node metastases common; can be bilateral in 30% to 55%

Medullary Breast Cancer
Uncommon form of invasive carcinoma (3%) associated with *BRCA* gene abnormalities; more common in Japanese women
Tends to affect women <50 years of age
Produces palpable mass; usually unilateral
Despite its pathologic appearance, it has a good prognosis

Tubular Carcinoma
Accounts for about 1% to 4% of all invasive cancers
Usually affects women older than 50 years
Smallest spiculated mass on mammography
Very favorable prognosis

Other Types of Cancer
Mucinous, papillary, and medullary carcinoma with not otherwise specified (NOS)

[a]Also known as **lobular neoplasia. Lobular carcinoma in situ** is not thought to represent a cancer by many but to serve as a precursor for breast cancer. Between 20% and 40% of women with this condition will develop a separate invasive breast cancer within the next 15 years (IDC or ILC). The use of the drugs tamoxifen and raloxifene have been shown to lower the risk of developing invasive breast cancer in these patients.

Therefore, anything that is clinically palpable, but has a negative imaging work-up, should be evaluated **clinically**, often by a breast surgeon. The clinician can then decide whether to do follow-up studies or a biopsy.
- Patients who undergo diagnostic mammography typically receive their results at the conclusion of the examination(s)

so that they understand what to do next and also have the opportunity to ask questions.

FUNDAMENTAL MAMMOGRAPHY FINDINGS

- There is **no "typical" appearance of the breast in any age group**. All breasts are composed of fat, fibroglandular tissue and connective tissue (Cooper's ligaments) (see Fig. 30.4). Depending on the amount of fat and fibroglandular tissue, the breast will appear **less dense (more fat), more dense (less fat), or a combination of both.**
- There is a tendency for breasts to become less dense with age, but there are a large number of younger women with fatty breasts and a large number of elderly women with dense breasts.
- **Four basic signs of breast disease** can be seen on mammography. They are:
  - **Masses**
  - **Asymmetry**
  - **Architectural distortion**
  - **Calcifications**
  - Other important findings are **skin changes** and **abnormal lymph nodes** (Fig. 30.5).
- Great overlap exists between the appearance of benign and malignant conditions. The ACR uses a standardized system called **BI-RADS,** which stands for **Breast Imaging Reporting and Data System,** to help describe findings, standardize reporting, and provide greater clarity to breast imaging interpretations. The final BI-RADS assessment categories help guide recommendations for biopsy or follow-up.

Masses

- A **mass** is defined as a space-occupying lesion seen in at least two different radiographic projections. Masses are described by their **shape** (e.g., oval), **margins** (e.g., spiculated), and **density**

(e.g., fat-containing). These appearances help radiologists decide how suspicious a mass is for malignancy (Table 30.4).
- In general, a mass that is **irregular, spiculated,** and **high-density** is more likely to be **malignant** (Fig. 30.6), whereas a mass that is **oval, circumscribed,** and **low-density** is more

TABLE 30.4	**How Masses Are Described**
Shape	Oval, round, irregular
Margins	Circumscribed, obscured, microlobulated, indistinct, spiculated
Density	High-density, equal density, low-density, fat-containing

Fig. 30.5 Skin Thickening and Abnormal Lymph Nodes. (A) Skin thickening (*white arrows*) in a patient with breast cancer. Compare the skin here with the normal skin thickness in Fig. 30.4. (B) Abnormal axillary lymph node (*solid black arrow*) adjacent to a normal lymph node (*dotted white arrows*). The fatty interior (hilum) of the normal lymph node is visible.

Fig. 30.6 Spiculated Mass: Invasive Ductal Carcinoma. There is a dense mass with spiculated margins (*white arrow*). A spiculated mass is a principal finding in invasive ductal carcinoma, the most frequently encountered breast malignancy. They are most common in women ages 50 to 60 years.

likely to be **benign** (Fig. 30.7). **Any fat-containing mass is typically benign** (Fig. 30.8).

Asymmetry

- **Asymmetry** is a **unilateral** deposit of **fibroglandular tissue** that does not meet the definition of a mass. Asymmetries

on mammography appear as an area of tissue that **does not** have a corresponding similar-appearing pattern in the **opposite breast**. Asymmetries can be described as **global, focal, developing,** or simply **asymmetric**. Most asymmetry is **benign,** but it **may be a sign of breast cancer** (Fig. 30.9).

Fig. 30.7 Cyst: Mammogram. Craniocaudal (CC) and mediolateral oblique (MLO) views of the left breast show a small oval low-density mass (*white arrow* in [A] and *white circle* in [B]). Cysts are benign, may be single or multiple, and may change in size over time. They are most common in premenopausal women in their 30s or 40s.

Fig. 30.8 Hamartoma. This mass (*solid white arrow*) contains fat (*dotted white arrow*), a finding that typically indicates benignity. Hamartomas are composed of benign dysplastic breast tissue that usually contains fat and may contain calcifications.

Fig. 30.9 Asymmetry as a Sign of Cancer. (A) A bilateral mammogram reveals a focal asymmetry in the right breast (*solid white arrow*). (B) A special view called a **spot compression view** over the area of asymmetry (*dotted white arrow*) again demonstrates and confirms the finding. (C) An ultrasound image shows a corresponding suspicious mass (*solid white arrow*).

Architectural Distortion

• **Architectural distortion** describes an alteration in the expected architecture of a breast with **no discrete mass** visible. It is one of the most subtle signs of breast cancer. It can be thought of as spiculation without a mass or a "tethering in" of the tissue (Fig. 30.10). **Digital breast tomosynthesis** has been shown to be particularly helpful in identifying architectural distortion (Fig. 30.11).

Fig. 30.10 Architectural Distortion as a Sign of Cancer. Architectural distortion can be a sign of breast cancer. It is caused by a desmoplastic reaction—a growth of fibrous or connective tissue presumably in response to the neoplasm. (A) This craniocaudal view shows such distortion (*solid white arrow*) described as "tethering-in" and associated retraction of the areola (*dotted white arrow*). (B) Ultrasound shows corresponding distortion (*solid white arrow*).

Fig. 30.11 Digital Breast Tomosynthesis (DBT) Revealing Distortion. In DBT multiple views are acquired while the x-ray source traverses an arc, in most cases spanning about ≤60°. The views acquired are reconstructed to provide multiple "sections/slices" of the breast, which can be as thin as 1 mm. (A) The two-dimensional mediolateral oblique mammogram view shows dense fibroglandular tissue, but no abnormality. (B) A single tomosynthesis slice reveals an area of distortion (*solid white arrow*) that proved to be an invasive carcinoma.

Calcifications

- **Calcifications** in the breast fall into two major categories: those that appear **typically benign** (e.g., rod-like) and those that are **suspicious for malignancy** (e.g., pleomorphic). They are also described by their arrangement or **distribution** in the breast: **diffuse calcifications** throughout the breast are less likely associated with malignancy than **grouped** or **clustered** calcifications (Table 30.5; Fig. 30.12).

ULTRASOUND

- Ultrasound is very important in the evaluation of breast lumps. It plays a key role in the differentiation between **cystic** and **solid** breast masses. A special high-frequency transducer is necessary for breast ultrasound because of the superficial nature of breast findings.
- For a **cyst** to meet the definition of **benign** by ultrasound, it must have the following criteria: **anechoic** (echo-free), **enhanced through transmission**, and a **thin back wall** (Fig. 30.13). If the ultrasound does **not** demonstrate these criteria or shows a **solid mass**, then the lesion may still be benign or malignant (Fig. 30.14).
- Ultrasound may also reveal a prominent "ridge" of fibroglandular tissue that explains a lump (Fig. 30.15). However; these patients should also be evaluated by a clinician, such as a breast surgeon, to ensure that the clinical findings correlate with the imaging results.

Fig. 30.12 Breast Calcifications. This image shows two examples of calcifications in degenerating fibroadenomas in the same breast. One has coarser calcifications (*solid white arrow*) than the other (*dotted white arrow*). Fibroadenomas are common benign tumors that form during adolescence, may enlarge during pregnancy and lactation, and regress—frequently with calcification—after menopause.

Fig. 30.13 Benign Cyst: Ultrasound. The cyst (C) itself is anechoic (contains no echoes), has a sharp back wall (*solid white arrow*), and has enhanced through transmission, as demonstrated by the strong echoes posterior to the cyst (*solid black arrow*). Cysts are the most common cause of a breast lump in women between ages 35 and 55 years.

TABLE 30.5	Types of Breast Calcifications	
Classification	**Morphology**	**Distribution**
Typically benign	Skin, vascular, coarse or "popcorn-like," large rod-like, round, rim, dystrophic, milk of calcium, suture	Diffuse Regional
Suspicious	Amorphous, coarse heterogeneous, fine pleomorphic, fine linear, or fine-linear branching	Grouped, linear, segmental

Fig. 30.14 Sonograms of Solid Masses. (A) The margins of the mass are well circumscribed (*solid white arrow*). This represents a **fibroadenoma**. (B) In another patient, there are two adjacent **malignant** masses with both circumscribed (*solid white arrows*) and spiculated margins (*dotted white arrow*). Malignant lesions on ultrasound are commonly hypoechoic lesions with poorly defined borders. Typically a malignant lesion has spiculated margins and may have microcalcification. Compare these lesions to the appearance of the cyst in Fig. 30.13.

Fig. 30.15 Fibroglandular Ridge. Fibroglandular changes in the breast can produce lumps and ridges that may be worrisome to the patient. Here an ultrasound demonstrates a ridge of normal fibroglandular tissue (*solid white arrows*) that accounts for a patient's lump.

- A lesion that can be seen using ultrasound that requires a biopsy is best biopsied under image guidance utilizing ultrasound (Fig. 30.16). A clip is placed to document the site of the biopsy. A variety of biopsy devices and needle sizes are available to do these procedures.

MAGNETIC RESONANCE IMAGING

- When breast MRI is used to diagnose breast cancer, gadolinium-based intravenous contrast is administered and images are acquired over a period of several minutes (see Fig. 30.3).
- Breast cancer **typically enhances within the first two minutes** after injection (Fig. 30.17). Similar to mammography, an evaluation of the mass's morphology is important in diagnosis. Also, how quickly the mass picks up the contrast agent and how long the contrast remains in the mass are important

Fig. 30.16 Ultrasound-Guided Biopsy. (A) Ultrasound shows a suspicious mass with an irregular contour and internal echoes (*solid white arrow*). (B) The area is first anesthetized prior to biopsy (*dotted white arrow*). (C) The biopsy needle (*solid white arrow*) passes through the mass. (D) A postbiopsy mammogram shows a clip in place (*white circle*) within the mass (*dotted white arrow*).

Fig. 30.17 Breast Cancer: MRI. (A) This axial image shows a gadolinium-enhancing mass (*white circle*). This patient had a history of *BRCA1* mutation. This was a breast cancer. (B) A different patient with a larger mass (*solid white arrow*) that extends forward, involving the nipple (*dotted white arrow*). Most breast cancers show a 90% increase in their signal intensity 90 seconds after gadolinium injection. A technique called fat suppression is used to reduce the signal from any fatty tissues in the breast and improve the ability to visualize masses **(see Chapter 21).**

factors to evaluate. Cancers typically will have **early enhancement** and the contrast will **"wash-out" rapidly.**

MANAGEMENT OF BREAST ABNORMALITIES

- In general, breast abnormalities are managed with **percutaneous procedures,** such as cyst aspiration, ultrasound-guided biopsy, and stereotactic biopsy, prior to any surgical procedure.

Cyst Aspiration

- **Any cyst that does not fulfill strict criteria for a cyst** (see **Ultrasound section** earlier) **should undergo aspiration.** Cysts may also be aspirated to relieve symptoms such as pain.
- Aspiration is performed under ultrasound guidance after cleansing of the skin and use of a skin anesthetic (Fig. 30.18). The color of cyst fluid varies; it may be blue, green, or yellow. Pure blood is sent for cytology, assuming the procedure was not traumatic (i.e., ruptured a blood vessel), but otherwise the fluid does not need to be sent for cytologic evaluation.
- After an **ultrasound-guided procedure, a postprocedure mammogram** is typically obtained to first ensure that the

aspirated cyst corresponded to the original mammographic finding and, second, that the marker clip placed under ultrasound guidance did deploy and corresponds to the site of the mammographic lesion.

Stereotactic Biopsies

- **Stereotactic biopsies** are performed **predominantly on calcifications** because most soft-tissue abnormalities can be seen and biopsied with ultrasound. A stereotactic biopsy uses x-ray to obtain images of the lesion at angles that are 30 degrees apart. A computer determines how much the lesion "shifts" on those images, allowing the **location** and **depth** of the lesion to be determined (Fig. 30.19).
- After a percutaneous image-guided biopsy, the radiologist determines if the pathology is concordant or discordant. If it is **concordant** (i.e., the radiologist thought the lesion looked like a fibroadenoma and the results revealed a fibroadenoma), then the patient may return to a routine screening protocol. If the result is **discordant** (i.e., the radiologist was expecting carcinoma and the results showed fibrocystic changes) rebiopsy or excisional biopsy is performed.

Fig. 30.18 Cyst Aspiration. This patient presented with a tender lump in the left breast. (A) Craniocaudal view of the left breast demonstrates a round mass (*solid white arrow*). (B) Ultrasound revealed a cyst (*dotted white arrow*). (C) Another image during an ultrasound-guided aspiration of the cyst shows the needle (*solid white arrow*) entering the cyst (*dotted white arrow*). (D) A postaspiration mammogram shows resolution of the mass.

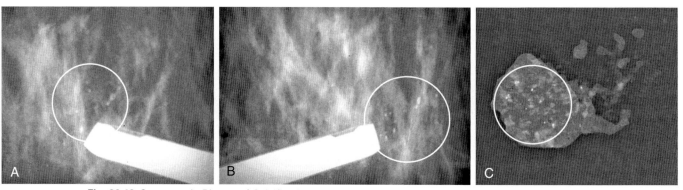

Fig. 30.19 Stereotactic Biopsy of Calcifications. (A) and (B) A close-up pair of prebiopsy images taken at an angle of 30 degrees from each other demonstrates the needle tip adjacent to multiple calcifications (*white circles*). (C) A radiograph of the excised specimen confirms that the tissue with numerous calcifications (*white circle*) has been obtained. Biopsy results showed ductal carcinoma in situ. Stereotactic breast biopsy is used especially for microcalcifications or nonpalpable lesions visible only on mammograms.

Fig. 30.20 Needle Localization for Surgical Excision. The patient had a prior stereotactic biopsy for calcifications that revealed ductal carcinoma in situ. (A) An image with a special alpha-numeric paddle shows the marker clip from the previous biopsy (*white circle*). (B) After needle placement, the hub of the needle is seen (*white circle*). (C) The orthogonal (90 degree) view shows the needle (*dotted white arrow*) passing adjacent to the clip and the tip of the hookwire engaged (*solid white arrow*). The hook on the wire keeps the wire in place without moving and guides the surgeon in removing the correct tissue. (D) A specimen radiograph demonstrates the hookwire in the removed tissue with the surgical marker clip (*solid white arrow*) and several calcifications (*white circle*).

Surgical Excision

- Certain lesions (Box 30.2) require needle localization followed by surgical excision (Fig. 30.20). Other lesions such as **papillary lesions** and **radial scars** may also need excision.
- The goal of needle localization is to guide the surgeon to the nonpalpable abnormality so that it may be successfully excised. General rules of needle localization include choosing the **shortest distance** from the skin to the lesion and obtaining a **specimen radiograph** after surgery to ensure that the lesion was removed.

SPECIAL CONSIDERATIONS

Masses During Pregnancy

- Any **breast lump during pregnancy** needs to be evaluated, starting with a **mammogram** if the patient is **30 years of age or older** or with an **ultrasound** if **younger than 30**. The differential diagnosis includes benign etiologies such as normal breast tissue, cysts, fibroadenomas (which are hormone sensitive and therefore, may grow with pregnancy), **galactoceles** (Fig. 30.21), and carcinoma.

Nipple Discharge

- Most nipple discharges result from **benign** etiologies. Important clinical considerations are if the discharge is spontaneous, unilateral, or bilateral, emanates from a single or from multiple ducts; and what color it is.
- In general, pathologic discharge is **spontaneous, unilateral,** and either **clear/serous or bloody.** The most common cause of bloody nipple discharge is a **solitary papilloma.** As with other breast symptoms, imaging starts with mammography if the patient is 30 years of age or older and often includes an ultrasound directed at the subareolar breast.

Fig. 30.21 Galactocele. This patient was breastfeeding and felt a lump in the left breast. Galactoceles typically occur during breastfeeding, but may also be seen during pregnancy; they will contain fat on mammography. They represent the retention of fat in areas of cystic ductal dilatation. (A) Craniocaudal and (B) mediolateral oblique views show a mass (*solid white arrows*) that contains fat (*dotted white arrows*).

BOX 30.2 Breast Lesions Requiring Surgical Excision

- Invasive carcinoma
- Ductal carcinoma in situ (DCIS)
- Atypical ductal hyperplasia
- Flat epithelial atypia
- Cellular fibroadenomas
- Fibroepithelial lesions

- A **ductogram** is a study that involves injecting a small amount of iodinated contrast into the duct from which discharge can be expressed and subsequently taking mammographic images looking for a filling defect(s) or areas of narrowing or irregularity of the duct.

Mastitis and Breast Abscess

- **Mastitis** is inflammation of the breast and can be either infectious or noninfectious. The **most common cause of infectious mastitis** is *Staphylococcus aureus*. Mastitis and breast abscesses are defined as **puerperal (related to childbirth)** or **nonpuerperal**. Risk factors for nonpuerperal infections include smoking, diabetes, and obesity.
- Mastitis is often **treated initially before any imaging.** It can look identical to **inflammatory carcinoma** of the breast, both clinically and mammographically, so if the patient does not completely respond to antibiotics, then a mammogram is performed. Often ultrasound is helpful in trying to distinguish between the two.
- Similarly, an **abscess** can be difficult to differentiate on imaging from **invasive carcinoma** as both present as masses. Typically, **breast cancer** is **not tender,** whereas an **abscess** is almost **always tender** (Fig. 30.22).

Breast Trauma

- Trauma to the breast can result in a **hematoma** and/or **fat necrosis.** Initial imaging findings of fat necrosis may be subtle, but often evolves into classical **oil cysts** (fibrous-walled collections from focal fat necrosis) with or without calcifications.
- A **seatbelt injury** creates a specific pattern of trauma to the inner breast along the site of the seatbelt, with the driver injuring the upper-inner left breast and lower-inner right breast (Fig. 30.23). On a mammogram a band-like asymmetry and/or hematoma may be seen and later there are often multiple **oil cysts** along the path of the seatbelt's impact (Fig. 30.24). **Oil cysts** are a manifestation of healing from **fat necrosis** in the breast, which may occur from trauma.

Fig. 30.23 Seatbelt Injury. These injuries occur from a three-point lap-shoulder seatbelt during a motor vehicle collision. They can produce painful chronic fat necrosis in the breast in a characteristic pattern across those areas the shoulder belt traverses, often the upper inner quadrant of one breast and lower inner quadrant of the opposite breast.

Fig. 30.22 Breast Abscess. Abscesses are almost always a complication of mastitis, usually nonlactational. They develop in those whose mastitis or cellulitis does not respond to antibiotic treatment. (A) Mediolateral oblique and (B) craniocaudal views demonstrate a mass (*solid white arrows*) with associated skin thickening (*dotted white arrows*).

Fig. 30.24 Seatbelt Injuries: Mammograms. (A) Craniocaudal and (B) mediolateral oblique views show typical pattern of multiple thin-walled oil cysts (*solid white arrows*) in a patient complaining of breast lumps after a motor vehicle accident. In another patient (C) craniocaudal and (D) mediolateral oblique views demonstrate similar pattern of calcified (*solid white arrows*) and noncalcified (*dotted white arrows*) oil cysts along the inner breast.

Dense Breasts

- **Dense breasts (heterogeneously dense or extremely dense)**, which occur in approximately 50% of the population, create challenges for breast cancer diagnosis. Although concern for the difficulties of imaging dense breast tissue has been cited as a reason not to screen young women, many young women **do not have** dense breasts. The use of **digital breast tomosynthesis** has been shown to be **helpful** for women with dense breasts and **can be performed as part of a routine screening** or **diagnostic mammogram**. Other studies, such as breast MRI and breast ultrasound can be useful, but are not routinely recommended for average-risk patients.

Postoperative Breast

- The postoperative breast includes the breast in patients with a history of reduction mammoplasty, breast augmentation, lumpectomy or breast-conserving therapy, and benign breast biopsies.
- **Reductions** often have typical findings on mammography related to surgery as well as signs of fat necrosis (Fig. 30.25).
- **Breast implants** are most commonly either **saline** or **silicone** and may be placed behind the pectoralis muscle (**subpectoral**) or in front of the pectoralis muscle (**subglandular**).
- **Saline implants** are either intact (normal) or deflated; **silicone implants** rupture by leaking silicone within the **fibrous capsule** that normally forms around the implant (**intracapsular rupture**) or by leaking silicone outside the capsule (**extracapsular rupture**).
- Mammographic signs of an **extracapsular rupture** will show silicone along the outside of the capsule, within the breast tissue (Fig. 30.26), and/or within axillary lymph nodes that will look denser than normal.

Fig. 30.25 Reduction Mammoplasty; Before and After. (A) and (B) show the prereduction fatty breast. (C) and (D) After reduction the breast has decreased in size and there are postsurgical changes (*solid white arrows*). Postsurgical distortion and fat necrosis may be seen in postoperative mammoplasties, especially in the inferior part of the breast.

Fig. 30.26 Extracapsular Silicone Implant Rupture. (A) Mediolateral oblique view with implant shows a silicone subglandular implant (*solid white arrows*). (B) A special implant-displaced view helps to reveal more breast tissue and, in this case, demonstrates dense white material (*dotted white arrows*), indicating free silicone. (C) Ultrasound image demonstrates what is called the **snowstorm** appearance, markedly echogenic areas with sharp anterior margins and indistinct posterior margins from the free silicone (*solid white arrows*).

- **Intracapsular rupture** findings can be subtle, such as a change in the implant contour. The **contents** of the implant can be contained by the fibrous capsule while the **shell** of the implant itself can collapse inward (Fig. 30.27).
- **MRI is the gold standard for evaluating the integrity of silicone breast implants.** Contrast is not used in these studies. The older an implant is, the more likely it is to rupture or leak.
- Patients with a history of a **surgical biopsy** or **lumpectomy** may have distortion, asymmetry, and calcifications. These findings tend to be more pronounced in breast cancer patients because of the addition of **radiation** to the treated breast. At times, patients may also have a seroma or hematoma at their surgical site.
- Careful follow-up of these patients is required to ensure that the postoperative findings stabilize by two years. Findings that worsen or change after two years in patients with a history of breast-conserving therapy should be thoroughly investigated.

Fig. 30.27 Intracapsular Breast Implant Rupture: MRI. A sagittal image of an implant (the breast tissue surrounding the implant is dark on this MRI image) shows a hypointense, wavy line within the implant (*black arrows*), which is a piece of the free-floating, collapsed implant envelope. This is called the **linguine sign.** It seems appropriate that the last image in the body of this textbook is named after a food, as you might want to celebrate your accomplishment of completing the text with a tasty treat.

🏠 TAKE HOME POINTS

- Breast imaging utilizes primarily mammography, ultrasound, and MRI for the evaluation of various breast symptoms and for the detection of breast cancer.
- Mammographic examinations are divided into two different categories: **screening**, done primarily on **asymptomatic women**, and **diagnostic mammography**, done in **women** with **breast symptoms**, patients **recalled** for a more extensive examination, and often in those with a **history of breast cancer** or with **breast implants.**
- Dense breasts produce challenges for imaging because they might mask a carcinoma. Digital breast tomosynthesis and breast MRI may be helpful.
- **Breast ultrasound** is the initial study that is used in average-risk symptomatic patients under 30 years of age. It is most commonly used in conjunction with diagnostic mammography and is helpful in distinguishing cystic from solid breast masses and as a problem-solving tool.
- **Breast MRI**, the most sensitive of all breast imaging modalities, is used with gadolinium-enhancement for screening certain high-risk patients, evaluating patients who have received breast implants, or adjuvant chemotherapy.
- **Screening mammograms** consist of two views of each breast: the **craniocaudal (CC) view** and the **mediolateral oblique (MLO) view.**
- The **American College of Radiology's** (ACR) recommendations for screening mammography are described.
- **Diagnostic mammograms** may involve a variety of additional mammographic views to those used in a standard screening protocol, such as compression or spot views, as well as the use of ultrasound.

- **Four basic signs** of breast disease on mammography are described and illustrated. They are masses, asymmetry, architectural distortion, and calcifications.
- Several characteristics of preinvasive and invasive breast cancers are described.
- **Ultrasound** plays a key role in the differentiation between cystic and solid breast masses.
- **Cyst aspiration** is used to relieve symptoms, such as pain, and to further study any presumed cyst that does not fulfill the strict criteria for a benign cyst.
- Lesions such as DCIS, and invasive carcinoma require **surgical excision** with needle localization of the lesion helping guide the surgeon to the abnormality.
- **Galactoceles** are one of the abnormalities that can occur during lactation (or pregnancy). They characteristically contain fat seen on mammography.
- Most **nipple discharges** are a consequence of a benign etiology. Solitary papillomas can cause a bloody nipple discharge.
- **Mastitis** is an inflammation of the breast most often caused by *Staphylococcus aureus.* **Breast abscesses** tend to form from mastitis. Both can appear clinically similar to inflammatory carcinoma of the breast.
- **Breast trauma** can lead to hematomas and fat necrosis. Seatbelt shoulder restraints can produce a characteristic pattern of injury from a motor vehicle collision.
- MRI is the gold-standard for evaluating **silicone breast implants**. Implant ruptures are divided into intracapsular or extracapsular.

🛜 More information on breast imaging is available to registered users online.

BIBLIOGRAPHY

Texts

Arnold W, DeLegge M, Schwaitzberg S. *Enteral Access: The Foundation of Feeding*. 1st ed. Dubuque, Iowa: Kendall Hunt Publishing; 2002.

Fraser RS, Pare P, Fraser R, Pare PD. *Synopsis of Diseases of the Chest*. 2nd ed. Philadelphia: W.B. Saunders; 1994.

Goodman LR. *Principles of Chest Roentgenology*. 3rd ed. Philadelphia: Saunders Elsevier; 2007.

Greenspan A. *Orthopedic Radiology: A Practical Approach*. 3rd ed. Philadelphia: Lippincott Williams and Wilkins; 2000.

Grossman RL, Yousem DM. *Neuroradiology: The Requisites*. St. Louis: Mosby; 1994.

Guyton AC, Hall J. *Textbook of Medical Physiology*. 11th ed. Philadelphia: W.B. Saunders; 2005.

Harris JH, Harris WH. *The Radiology of Emergency Medicine*. 4th ed. Philadelphia: Lippincott Williams and Wilkins; 2000.

Juhl JH, Crummy AB. *Essentials of Radiologic Imaging*. 6th ed. Philadelphia: Lippincott; 1993.

Love M. *An Introduction to Diagnostic Ultrasound*. 1st ed. Springfield: Charles C. Thomas; 1980.

Manaster BJ, Disler DG, May DA. *Musculoskeletal Imaging: The Requisites*. 2nd ed. St. Louis: Mosby; 2002.

McCloud T. *Thoracic Radiology: The Requisites*. 1st ed. St. Louis: Mosby; 1998.

Mettler F, Guiberteau M. *Essentials of Nuclear Medicine Imaging E-Book*. 6th ed. Saunders; 2012.

Meyers MA. *Dynamic Radiology of the Abdomen: Normal and Pathological Anatomy*. 2nd ed. New York: Springer-Verlag; 1982.

Nutritional Considerations in the Intensive Care Unit: Science, Rationale, and Practice. American Society for Parental and Enteral Nutrition. April, 2002.

Resnick D. *Diagnosis of Bone and Joint Disorders*. 2nd ed. Philadelphia: W.B. Saunders; 1981.

Resnick D. *Diagnosis of Bone and Joint Disorders*. 4th ed. Philadelphia: W.B. Saunders; 2002.

Rumack C, Wilson S, Charboneau WJ. *Diagnostic Ultrasound*. 2nd ed. St. Louis: Mosby; 1998.

Schultz RJ. *The Language of Fractures*. Huntington, NY: Robert E. Krieger; 1972.

Swischuk L. *Imaging of the Newborn, Infant, and Young Child*. 5th ed. Lippincott Williams & Wilkins; 2003.

Webb WR, Brant WE, Helms CA. *Fundamentals of Body CT*. Philadelphia: W.B. Saunders; 1991.

Weissleder R, Wittenberg J, Harisinghani MG. *Primer of Diagnostic Imaging*. 3rd ed. St. Louis: Mosby; 2003.

Journal Articles

Aberle DR, Wiener-Kronish JP, Webb WR, Matthay MA. Hydrostatic versus increased permeability pulmonary edema: diagnosis based on radiographic data in critically ill patients. *Radiology*. 1988;168: 73–79.

Almeida A, Roberts I. Bone involvement in sickle cell disease. *Br J Haematol*. 2005;129:482–490.

Amjadi K, Alvarez GG, Vanderhelst E, Velkeniers B, Lam M, Noppen M. The prevalence of blebs or bullae among young healthy adults: a thoracoscopic investigation. *Chest*. 2007;132(4): 1140–1145.

Baskin KM, Jimenez RM, Cahill AM, et al. Cavoatrial junction and central venous anatomy: implications for central venous access tip position. *J Vasc Interv Radiol*. 2008;19(3):359–365.

Bates D, Ruggieri P. Imaging modalities for evaluation of the spine. *Radiol Clin North Am*. 1991;29(4):675–690.

Boudiaf M, Soyer P, Terem C, Pelage J, Maissiat E, Rymer R. CT Evaluation of small bowel obstruction. *Radiographics*. 2001;21: 613–624.

Boyse TD, et al. US of soft-tissue foreign bodies and associated complications with surgical correlation. *Radiographics*. 2001;21: 1251–1256.

Burney K, Burchard F, Papouchado M, Wilde P. Cardiac pacing systems and implantable cardiac defibrillators (ICDs): a radiological perspective of equipment, anatomy, and complications. *Clin Radiol*. 2004;59(8):699–708.

Clinical translational oncology. *Springer*. 2008;10(12):777–785.

Cohen SM, Kurtz AB. Biliary sonography. *Clin Radiol*. 1991;29(6): 11-71-1198.

Connolly B, Mawson JB, MacDonald CE, Chait P, Mikailian H. Fluoroscopic landmark for SVC-RA junction for central venous catheter placement in children. *Pediatr Radiol*. 2000;(10):692–695.

Cury RC. Coronary CT angiography versus standard of care for assessment of chest pain in the emergency department. *J Cardiovasc Comput Tomogr*. 2013;7(2):79–82.

Dalinka MK, Reginato AJ, Golden DA. Calcium deposition disease. *Semin Roentgenol*. 1982;17(1):39–47.

de Jong EM, Felix JF, de Klein A, Tibboel D. Etiology of esophageal atresia and tracheoesophageal fistula: "Mind the gap". *Curr Gastroenterol Rep*. 2010;12(3):215–222.

Doubilet PM, Benson CB, Bourne T, Blaivas M. Diagnostic criteria for nonviable pregnancy early in the first trimester. *N Engl J Med*. 2013;369:15, for the Society of Radiologists in Ultrasound Multispecialty Panel on Early First Trimester Diagnosis of Miscarriage and Exclusion of a Viable Intrauterine Pregnancy.

Dyer DS, Moore EE, Mestek MF, et al. Can chest CT be used to exclude aortic injury? *Radiology*. 1999;213:195–202.

Edeiken J. Radiologic approach to arthritis. *Semin Roentgenol*. 1982;17(1):8–15.

Edwards MO, Kotecha SJ, Kotecha S. Respiratory distress of the term newborn infant. *Paediatr Respir Rev*. 2013;14(1):29–37.

Ellis K, Austin J, Jaretzki A. Radiologic detection of thymoma in patients with myasthenia gravis. *AJR Am J Roentgenol*. 1988;151: 873–881.

Epelman M, et al. Necrotizing enterocolitis: review of state-of-the-art imaging findings with pathologic correlation. *Radiographics*. 2007; 27:285–305.

Garcia MJ. Could cardiac CT revolutionize the practice of cardiology? *Cleve Clin J Med*. 2005;72(2):88–89.

Gaskill MF, Lukin R, Wiot JG. Lumbar disc disease and stenosis. *Radiol Clin North Am*. 1991;29(4):75–764.

Gluecker T, Patrizio C, Schnyder P, et al. Clinical and radiologic features of pulmonary edema. *Radiographics*. 1999;19:1507–1531.

Goodman A, Perera P, Mailhot T, Mandavia D. The role of bedside ultrasound in the diagnosis of pericardial effusion and cardiac tamponade. *J Emerg Trauma Shock*. 2012;5(1):72–75.

Gould MK, Tang T, Liu IL, et al. Recent trends in the identification of incidental pulmonary nodules. *Am J Respir Crit Care Med*. 2015;192(10):1208–1214.

Haus BM, Stark P, Shofer SL, Kuschner WG. Massive pulmonary pseudotumor. *Chest.* 2003;124(2):758–760.

Hendrix RW, Rogers LF. Diagnostic imaging of fracture complications. *Radiol Clin North Am.* 1989;27(5):1023–1033.

Henschke CI, Yankelevitz DF, Wand A, Davis SD, Shiau M. Accuracy and efficacy of chest radiography in the intensive care unit. *Radiol Clin North Am.* 1996;34(1):21–31.

Henry M, Arnold T, Harvey J. British Thoracic Society's guidelines for the management of spontaneous pneumothorax. *Thorax.* 2003;58(suppl 2):39–52.

Henry-Tillman RS, Klimberg VS. In situ breast cancer. *Curr Treat Options Oncol.* 2000;1:199–209.

Herold CJ. Management of solid and sub-solid lung nodules. *Cancer Imaging.* 2014;14(suppl 1).

Horrow MM. Ultrasound of the extrahepatic bile duct: issues of size. *Ultrasound Q.* 2010;26(2):67–74.

Husain LF, Hagopian L, Wayman D, Baker WE, Carmody KA. Sonographic diagnosis of pneumothorax. *J Emerg Trauma Shock.* 2012;5(1):76–81.

Indrajit IK, Shreeram MN, d'Souza JD, Multislice CT. A quantum leap in whole body imaging. *Indian J Radiol Imaging.* 2004;14(2):209–216.

Ingram MD, Watson SG, Skippage PL, Patel U. Urethral injuries after pelvic trauma: evaluation with urethrography. *Radiographics.* 2008;28:1631–1643.

Iqbal J, Narod SA. Choices for young women at intermediate risk of breast cancer. *Curr Oncol.* 2012;19(3):e112–e114.

Johnson JL. Pleural effusions in cardiovascular disease. *Postgrad Med.* 2000;107(4):95–101.

Karlo CA, Leschka S, Stolzmann P, Glaser-Gallion N, Wildermuth S, Alkadhi H. A systematic approach for analysis, interpretation, and reporting of coronary CTA studies. *Insights Imaging.* 2012;3(3):215–228.

Kim H, Min Park C, Koh JM, Lee SM, Goo JM. Pulmonary subsolid nodules: what radiologists need to know about the imaging features and management strategy. *Diagn Interv Radiol.* 2014;20(1):47–57.

King JB. Calcification of the costal cartilages. *Br J Radiol.* 1939;12(133):2–12.

Kundel HL, Wright DJ. The influence of prior knowledge on visual search strategies during the viewing of chest radiographs. *Radiology.* 1969;93:315–320.

Lingawi SS. The naked facet sign. *Radiology.* 2001;219:366–367.

Management of ingested foreign bodies and food impactions, position paper. American Society for Gastrointestinal Endoscopy. *Gastrointest Endosc.* 2011;73(6):1085–1091.

National Clinical Practice Guidelines in Oncology. National Comprehensive Cancer Network 4(9): 516–525. Sep 2007.

Neu J, Walker WA. Necrotizing enterocolitis. *N Engl J Med.* 2011;364:255–264.

Old JL, Calvert M. Vertebral compression fractures in the elderly. *Am Fam Physician.* 2004;69(1):111–116.

Pathria MN, Petersilge CA. Spinal trauma. *Radiol Clin North Am.* 1991;29(4):847–865.

Riddervold HO. Easily missed fractures. *Radiol Clin North Am.* 1992;30(2):475–494.

Shifrin RY, Choplin RH. Aspiration in patients in critical care units. *Radiol Clin North Am.* 1996;34(1):83–95.

Sik B, Kim M, Li BT, et al. Diagnosis of gastrointestinal bleeding: a practical guide for clinicians. *World J Gastrointest Pathophysiol.* 2014;5(4):467–478.

Smith-Bindman R, Miglioretti DL, Larson EB. Rising use of diagnostic medical imaging in a large integrated health system. *Health Aff (Millwood).* 2008;27(6):1491–1502.

Steenburg SD, Ravenel JG. Acute traumatic thoracic aortic injuries: experience with 64-MDCT. *AJR Am J Roentgenol.* 2008;191:1564–1569.

Thomas EL, Lansdown EL. Visual search patterns of radiologists in training. *Radiology.* 1963;81:288–292.

Tie MLH. Basic head CT for intensivists. *Crit Care Res.* 2001;3:35–44.

Tocino I, Westcott JL. Barotrauma. *Radiol Clin North Am.* 1996;34(1):59–81.

Veltman CE, de Graaf FR, Schuijf JD, et al. Prognostic value of coronary vessel dominance in relation to significant coronary artery disease determined with non-invasive computed tomography coronary angiography. *Eur Heart J.* 2012;33:1367–1377.

Yu S, Haughton VM, Rosenbaum AE. Magnetic resonance imaging and anatomy of the spine. *Radiol Clin North Am.* 1991;29(4):675–690.

Yuh W, Quets J, Lee H, et al. Anatomic distribution of metastases in the vertebral body and modes of hematogenous spread. *Spine.* 1996;21(19):2243–2250.

Chapter 1 Quiz Answers

These are the answers to the quiz cases that appear in Chapter 1. If you have turned right to the answers, you show remarkable curiosity and inquisitiveness. If you have waited until reading the whole text, you are someone who shows great self-discipline and a thirst for the core of knowledge. In either case, here are the answers.

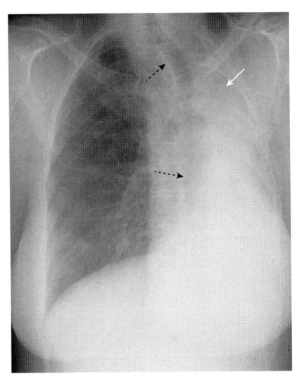

ANSWER FOR FIGURE 1.3 Case Quiz 2: The "Case of the Disappearing Heart." This patient had previously undergone a **left-sided pneumonectomy**, which is removal of the entire left lung for the tumor. The left 5th rib has been surgically excised (*white arrow*) as part of the procedure. In the absence of the air-filled left lung, a combination of fluid and fibrous tissue filled the "empty" hemithorax, but the overall loss of volume has produced a shift of the normal midline structures to the left (*dotted black arrow*). Normally, we see the heart on chest x-rays because of the difference in densities between it and the surrounding air-filled lung. Because the heart is surrounded by soft tissue in this patient, it becomes "invisible" on conventional radiography. This is an example of the **silhouette sign (see Chapter 5).**

ANSWER FOR FIGURE 1.2 Case Quiz 1. There is a large, left-sided, tension pneumothorax (*white arrows*). The left lung is partially collapsed as the pleural space fills with air. The heart is shifted from its normal position toward the right (*black arrow*), which means the pneumothorax is under tension. This is a medical emergency. A chest tube was rapidly inserted into the left hemithorax to release the pressure and reexpand the lung **(see Chapter 25).**

ANSWER FOR FIGURE 1.6. Case Quiz 3. There is a large area of low attenuation (outlined in black) in the distribution of flow of the right middle cerebral artery. There is a shift of the normal midline structures of the brain to the left (*white arrow*) from mass effect. This patient has had a **nonhemorrhagic infarct** of the brain **(see Chapter 27).**

ANSWER FOR FIGURE 1.8 Case Quiz 5. The most likely cause of this patient's pain is a large, **herniated disk** at the L4-L5 level (*dotted white arrow*). The disk extends posteriorly into the spinal canal and compresses the nerves of the cauda equina (*dotted black arrows*). Normal disks contain more water and are brighter (*solid white arrows*) than abnormal ones (*solid black arrow*) **(see Chapter 21).**

ANSWER FOR FIGURE 1.7 Case Quiz 4. This patient has **gallstones** (*solid white arrow*) that lie along the dependent (posterior) surface of the gallbladder (GB). The gallbladder is echo-free because it contains fluid (bile), but the stones are hyperechoic. They absorb most of the ultrasound, producing a paucity of shadows beyond the stones called **acoustical shadowing** (*dotted arrows*). F, Foot; H, head. **(see Chapter 19).**

ANSWER FOR FIGURE 1.10 Case Quiz 6: The "Case of the Upside-Down Stomach." This patient has an unusual condition in which the stomach has rotated upward and toward the patient's right side along an axis between the fundus (F) and the antrum (A) as shown by the arrow, most likely into a large hiatal hernia in the chest. The greater curve of the stomach comes to lie superiorly, rather than in its normal inferior position. This is called an **organoaxial volvulus of the stomach.** It produces this "upside-down" appearance to normal anatomy. Patients with this abnormality may present with pain or vomiting.

Page numbers followed by *f* indicate figures; *t*, tables; *b*, boxes.